Pharmacology Condensed

Commissioning Editor: Laurence Hunter
Project Development Manager: Barbara Simmons
Project Manager: Frances Affleck
Designer: Erik Bigland
Illustrator: Peter Lamb

Pharmacology Condensed

M. M. Dale MB BCh PhD
Senior Teaching Fellow
Department of Pharmacology
University of Oxford;
Honorary Lecturer
Department of Pharmacology
University College
London
UK

D. G. Haylett BSc PhD
Senior Lecturer
Department of Pharmacology
University College
London
UK

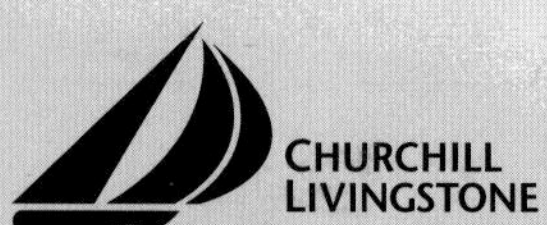

EDINBURGH LONDON NEW YORK OXFORD PHILADELPHIA ST LOUIS SYDNEY TORONTO 2004

CHURCHILL LIVINGSTONE
An imprint of Elsevier Limited

First published 2004
Reprinted 2005 (twice)

ISBN 0 443 07049 0

British Library Cataloguing in Publication Data
A catalogue record for this book is available from the British Library

Library of Congress Cataloging in Publication Data
A catalog record for this book is available from the Library of Congress

Notice

Medical knowledge is constantly changing. Standard safety precautions must be followed, but as new research and clinical experience broaden our knowledge, changes in treatment and drug therapy may become necessary as appropriate. Readers are advised to check the most current product information provided by the manufacturer of each drug to be administered to verify the recommended dose, the method and duration of administration, and contraindications. It is the responsibility of the practitioner, relying on experience and knowledge of the patient, to determine dosages and the best treatment for each individual patient. Neither the Publisher nor the authors assumes any liability for any injury and/or damage to persons or property arising from this publication.

The Publisher

The Publisher's policy is to use **paper manufactured from sustainable forests**

Typeset by IMH(Cartrif), Loanhead, Scotland
Printed in China

Preface

Pharmacology Condensed is, in essence, a companion volume to Rang, Dale, Ritter and Moore's *Pharmacology*, having condensed each chapter of that book to a few pages in this one. Consequently this book is best used with Rang et al. but could also be used on its own or in conjunction with another pharmacology textbook.

Pharmacology is not a conceptually difficult science – it does not have the abstruse concepts that characterise theoretical physics or higher mathematics. The problem in studying pharmacology is that there are a great many disparate facts and ideas that have to be mastered, along with a multitude of hard-to-remember drug names. To get to grips with the facts and concepts in pharmacology it is essential to appreciate fully how drugs work; and to do this it is necessary to understand the underlying patho-physiological processes on which drugs act. Having accomplished this by study of a textbook of pharmacology (such as Rang et al.) which covers the material in detail, the next problem is that of making sure the information stays securely and accessibly in your memory for when you need it later in your professional life. A useful way to do this is to decide, for any particular topic, what the essential points are. These should be easier to remember and when brought to mind could call up, by association, fuller details of the topic concerned. In this book we have set out to delineate, in text and summary diagrams, these essential points.

Our chapters follow fairly closely the sequence of chapters in Rang et al., and within each chapter we have used a similar approach in dealing with the material. We have included short summaries of the two chapters in Rang et al. which describe the cellular mechanisms that are affected by many important drugs described in later chapters of both books. Some figures are derived from, or based on those in Rang et al., but many are new and have been specially designed to summarise textual material. And in order to help with the dauntingly large number of drug names, we have selected one or two important drugs from each group and set them out in bold type, putting other examples in non-bold type.

The main object of this book then is to make available the essential aspects of pharmacology so that the reader can lodge them securely in his/her mind as pointers to the more detailed material buried 'deeper in'. But it might also be of value in preparing for examinations, which is after all a not unacceptable aim.

2004 MMD
DGH

Acknowledgements

We would like to thank the following for their help and advice in the preparation of this book: Professor J. Mandelstam, Professor R J P Williams, Professor J R Ritter. We are grateful to Frank Kennedy for dealing efficiently with the often refractory main computer; his technological expertise was invaluable. We wish to record our appreciation of the team at Elsevier who worked on the book; the team included among others: Laurence Hunter (commissioning editor and éminence grise), Barbara Simmons (project development manager), Frances Affleck (project manager), Erik Bigland (designer), Jane Ward (freelance copy editor), Ian Hunter (freelance typesetter), and Merrall-Ross International Ltd (freelance indexers). Barbara Simmons in particular dealt with problems raised by the authors with gentle, cheerful competence and we owe her a special vote of thanks. We are also indebted to Ian Hunter, who was a tower of strength in coping with necessary last-minute corrections to the figures and the text.

Contents

1 General principles of drug action

Pharmacology concerns the study of how drugs affect the function of host tissues or combat infectious organisms. In most cases, drugs bind selectively to target molecules within the body, usually proteins but also other macromolecules. The main drug targets are receptors, enzymes, ion channels, transporters (carriers) and DNA. There are few instances (e.g. osmotic purgatives and antacids) of drugs acting without binding to a specific target.

It is generally desirable that a drug should have a higher affinity for its target than for other binding sites. First, it ensures that the drug's free concentration (and hence action) is not reduced by non-productive binding to the much greater number of non-target molecules in the body. Secondly, lower doses can be used, which automatically reduces the risks of unwanted actions at other sites. Chapter 2 deals specifically with the consequences of drug binding to these targets. The rest of this chapter will deal predominantly with the principles of receptor pharmacology.

Receptors as drug targets

Receptors are protein macromolecules—on or in cells—that act as recognition sites for endogenous ligands such as neurotransmitters, hormones, inflammatory/immunological mediators, etc. Many drugs used in medicine make use of these endogenous receptors. The effect of a drug may be to produce the same response as the endogenous ligand or to prevent the action of an endogenous (or exogenous) ligand. A drug (or endogenous chemical) that binds to a receptor and activates the cell's response is termed an *agonist.* A drug that reduces or inhibits the action of an agonist is termed an *antagonist.*

Consider what happens when an agonist drug acts on a receptor. Essentially several drug molecules will be present in the vicinity of the receptor, moving at random, and occasionally some drug molecules will make contact with receptors. The action of an inflammatory mediator, histamine, on bronchiolar smooth muscle can be taken as an example. There are two aspects to this action:

- the agonist-receptor (drug-receptor) interaction
- the agonist-induced (drug-induced) response.

With the drug-receptor interaction, we will be dealing with the concepts of affinity and *occupancy*. With the drug-induced response, we will meet the concept of *efficacy*.

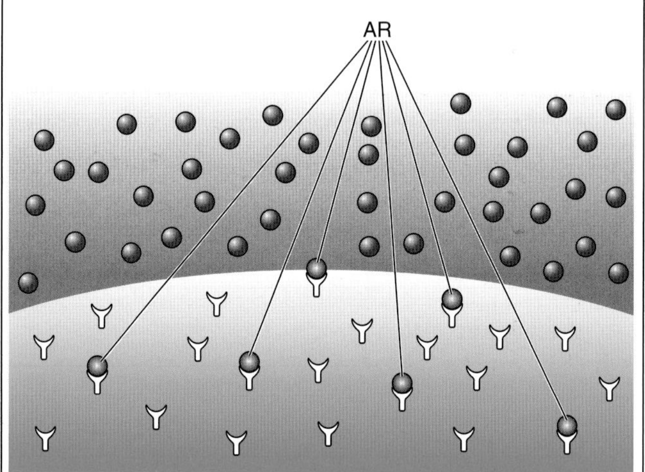

Fig. 1.1 Schematic diagram illustrating receptors (R) occupied by drug A (e.g. histamine) on the surface of smooth muscle.

The agonist–receptor (drug–receptor) interaction

In Figure 1.1 the smooth muscle surface is represented by the blue curved segment. The receptors (shown as cups) are representative of the total number of receptors on the muscle (R_{tot}). The histamine molecules are represented by the grey circles. When the muscle is exposed to a concentration of histamine [A] and allowed to come to equilibrium, the drug will occupy a number of receptors (AR). We now need to consider the relationship between [A] and the occupancy of the receptors $[AR]/[R_{tot}]$.

Drug–receptor interaction is usually freely reversible and can be represented by the following equation:

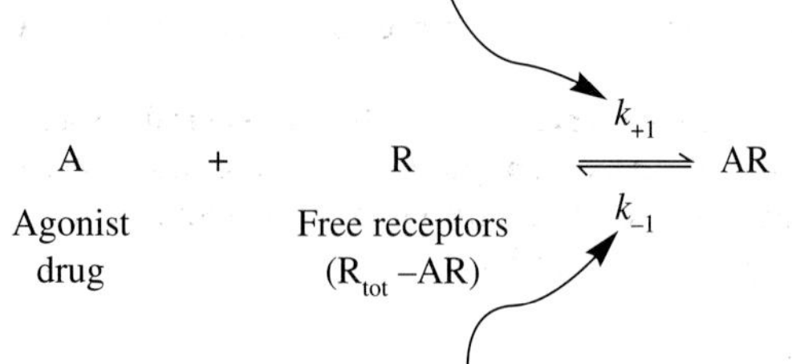

The Law of Mass Action (the rate of the reaction is proportional to the product of the concentrations of the reactants) can be applied to the reaction. At equilibrium the forward and reverse rates are equal, i.e.

$$k_{+1}\,[A][R] = k_{-1}[AR]$$

so that

$$\frac{[A][R]}{[AR]} = \frac{k_{-1}}{k_{+1}} = K_A$$

... and as we are dealing only with equilibrium conditions, and not with kinetics, we can form a new constant K_A from $\frac{k_{-1}}{k_{+1}}$

K_a is the dissociation equilibrium constant for the binding of drug to receptor; it has the dimensions of concentration. (It is the reciprocal of the affinity constant, i.e the higher the affinity of the drug for the receptors, the lower the value of K_A). A high K_A specifies a low affinity, which means that there are fewer drug-receptor complexes overall.

The relationship between K_A, the concentration of agonist drug, and the proportion of receptors occupied (i.e. the occupancy p_A is given by

$$p_A = \frac{[AR]}{[R_{tot}]} = \frac{[A]}{K_A + [A]}$$

This is self-evident (i.e. the concentration of receptors occupied over the total receptor concentration)

But this may not be obvious to every student; it is the Hill–Langmuir equation

The value of K_A is equal to the concentration of the agonist drug that at equilibrium results in occupancy of 50% of the receptors.

For example if the concentration of the drug is 10 µmol/l and the K_A is 10 µmol/l, then:

$$p_A = \frac{10}{10 + 10} = 0.5$$

The relationship between occupancy and drug concentration specified in the Hill–Langmuir equation (identified above) can be represented graphically as shown in Figure 1.2

The theoretical curves given are for occupancy. Now let us consider the agonist-induced response.

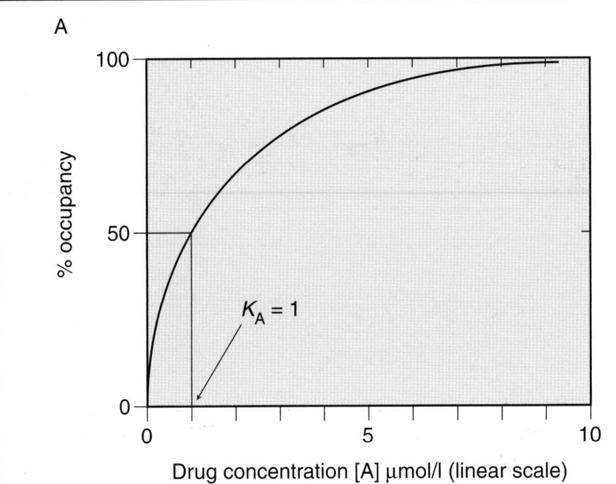

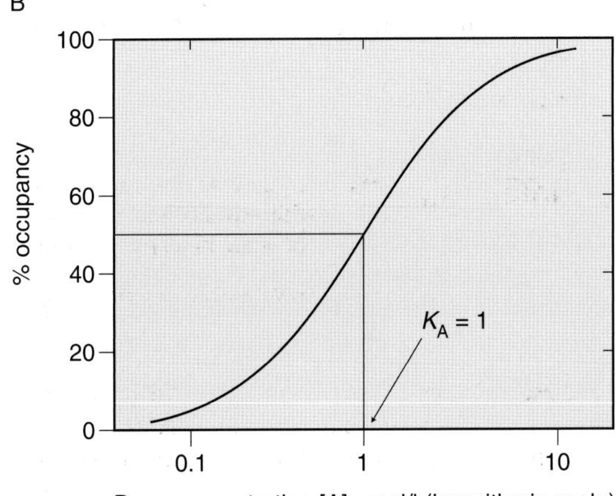

Fig. 1.2 Occupancy, according to the Hill–Langmuir equation, plotted against drug concentration. The graph shows that when concentration of agonist drug and K_A both equal 1 µmol/l, the occupancy of receptors is 50%.

The agonist-induced (drug-induced) response

An agonist-induced response—if it is *a graded response*—can be plotted as a concentration–effect or dose–response curve (Fig. 1.3). The concentration producing a response 50% of the maximum is termed the EC_{50} (EC, effective concentration).

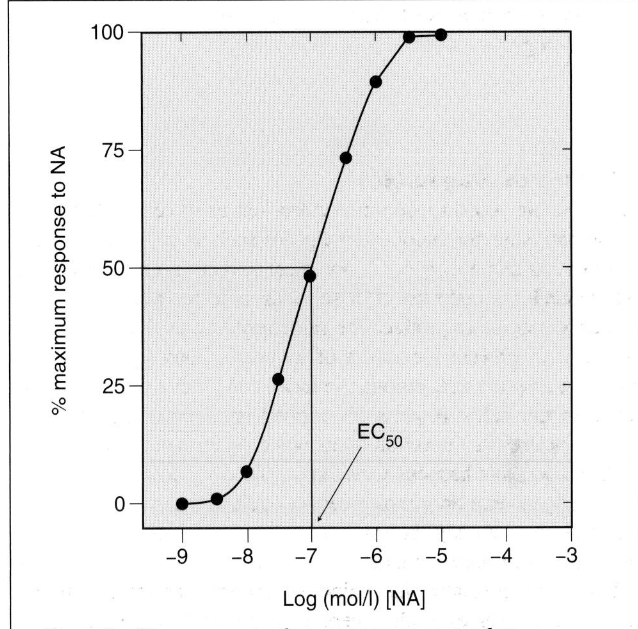

Fig. 1.3 The concentration–response curve for noradrenaline (NA)-mediated contraction of smooth muscle in vitro.

Can one make the assumption that responses such as these are directly proportional to occupancy at the relevant receptors?

Certainly the log concentration–response curve in Figure 1.3 looks very like the theoretical log concentration–occupancy curve in Figure 1.2. However, even with the simple in vitro response of smooth muscle to noradrenaline, it is not possible to know, with certainty, the concentration of drug at the receptors. Factors such as enzymic degradation, binding to tissue components, problems related to diffusion of drug to the site of action, and so on, complicate the picture.

The relationship between occupancy and response is generally unknown and, almost certainly, not linearly related to occupancy. Consequently, although concentration–response (or dose–response) curves look very similar to concentration–occupancy curves, they cannot be used to determine the agonist affinity for the respective receptors.

This applies even more to those pharmacological responses that are 'all-or-none' rather than graded. (An 'all-or-none' response is one in which the drug either does or does not produce an effect.) An example is given in Figure 1.4.

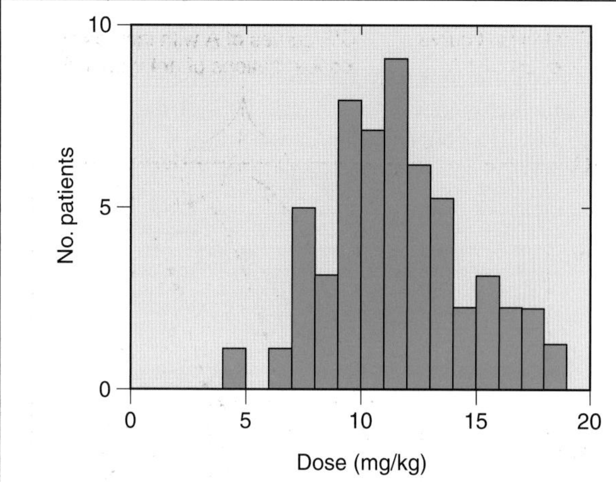

Fig. 1.4 The responses of individual patients to increasing doses of a hypnotic. The drug was infused until the patient felt drowsy. The most sensitive person felt drowsy when 4 mg/kg had been infused, the least sensitive when 18 mg/kg had been infused.

The data in Figure 1.4 can be plotted as a cumulative frequency distribution curve in which the response is the percentage of patients who felt drowsy with increasing doses of hypnotic drug (Fig. 1.5). The dose that produced a response in 50% of the individuals is termed the ED_{50} (ED, effective dose).

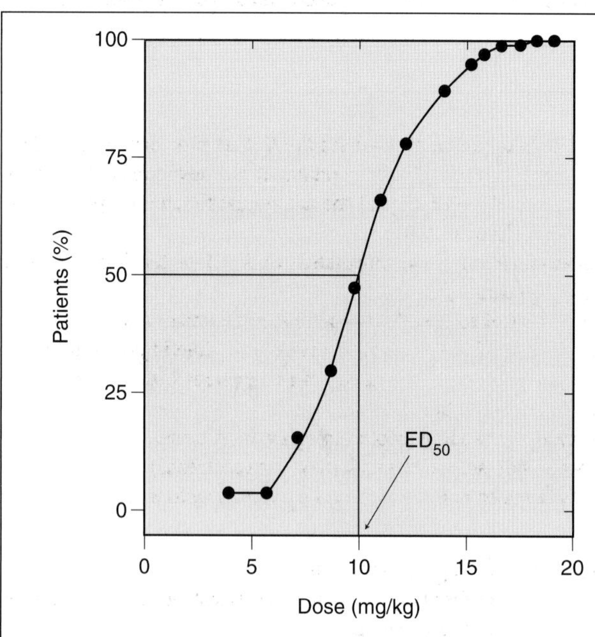

Fig. 1.5 The cumulative dose–response curve for patients who felt drowsy with increasing doses of hypnotic. (Note that here the distribution is approximately normal with respect to dose whereas it is usually normal with respect to log dose.)

With some drugs, the maximum response produced corresponds to the maximum response that the tissue can give. These are termed *full agonists*. The action depicted in Figure 1.3 is that of a full agonist. Other drugs—that are believed to act on the same receptors—do not give the maximum tissue response in any concentration. These are termed *partial agonists.*

Partial agonists

The concentration–response curves of some full and partial agonists on the muscarinic receptors of smooth muscle of the gastrointestinal tract are shown in Figure 1.6. It can be seen that both acetylcholine and propionylcholine are full agonists but propionylcholine requires a larger concentation to produce a maximum response. Butyrylcholine even in very high concentration never produces as great a response as acetylcholine—it is a partial agonist.

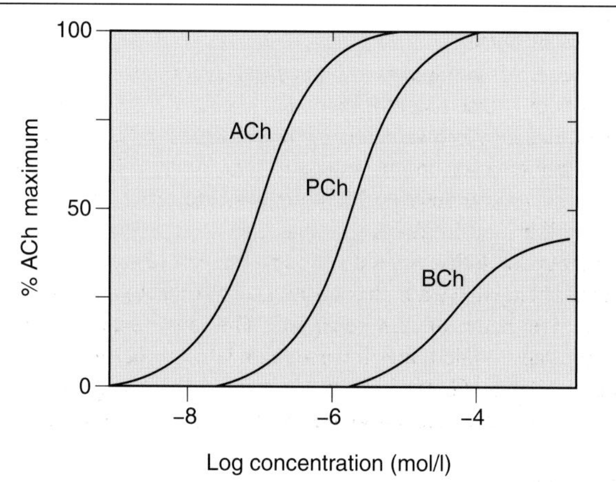

Fig. 1.6 Log dose–response curves for full and partial agonists on gastrointestinal smooth muscle. ACh, acetylcholine; PCh, propionylcholine; BCh, butyrylcholine.

What is the explanation for the different responses of partial and full agonists? Experiments have shown that this is not because the partial agonists bind to fewer receptors, but that they are less able to elicit a response from the receptors to which they do bind. They are, in fact, less potent. They are said to have less *intrinsic activity* (or *lower efficacy*).

Efficacy

Efficacy is a complex concept that, in simple terms, describes the ability of the drug, after binding to the receptor, to activate transduction mechanisms that lead to a response.

Partial agonist action can be best interpreted in terms of a two-state model of the molecular events at a single receptor on interaction with agonist A. The model envisages that an occupied receptor can exist in two states: a 'resting' state (R) and an 'activated' state (R*).

$$A + R \underset{}{\overset{K_{A1}}{\rightleftharpoons}} AR \underset{}{\overset{K_{A2}}{\rightleftharpoons}} AR^*$$

The equilibrium between AR and AR* will determine the magnitude of the maximum response. Normally, if there is no drug present, the equilibrium favours R. A full agonist would bind preferentially to, and shift the equilibrium to, R*:

$$A + R \underset{}{\overset{K_{A1}}{\rightleftharpoons}} AR \underset{}{\overset{K_{A2}}{\rightleftharpoons}} \mathbf{AR^*}$$

An equilibrium that favours AR, with few receptors in the activated state, would make the drug A a partial agonist (i.e. a drug with low efficacy):

$$A + R \underset{}{\overset{K_{A1}}{\rightleftharpoons}} \mathbf{AR} \underset{}{\overset{K_{A2}}{\rightleftharpoons}} AR^*$$

Note that because partial agonists occupy receptors, they competitively antagonise the action of a full agonist while producing a small effect of their own. A clinical example is oxprenolol, a β-blocker (a partial agonist on β_1-adrenoceptors in the heart, causing tachycardia and increased force in its own right) that antagonises the action of endogenous noradrenaline.

Inverse agonists

The model of drug–receptor interaction, specified in this chapter so far, assumes that receptors are inactive in the absence of bound ligand. It is now known that some receptors can adopt the active, R*, conformation even in the absence of an agonist. They are said to show *constitutive* activity. It is then possible that a drug might shift the equilibrium in favour of the non-active form, so reducing background activity. Such drugs exist and are referred to as *inverse agonists*. They have a higher affinity for the inactive compared with the active state of the receptor. The best examples are the β-carbolines, which are inverse agonists at the benzodiazepine binding sites on $GABA_A$ receptors. Rather than being anxiolytic, as most benzodiazepines, these agents are anxiogenic (see Ch. 37).

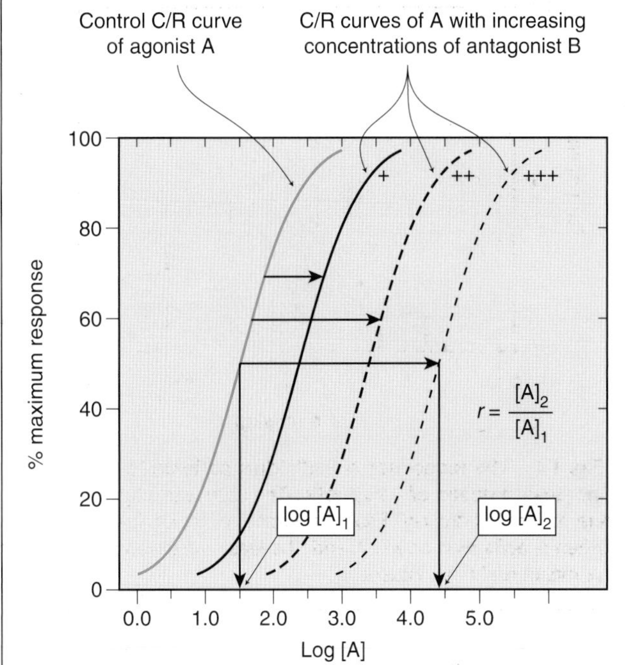

Fig. 1.7 Reversible competitive antagonism. Increasing concentrations of a competitive antagonist prazosin (indicated by +, ++, +++) produce increasing shifts of the control log concentration–response curve of agonist A (noradrenaline) to the right. The response is expressed as a percentage of maximum contraction of the rat vas deferens. The shift can be expressed as a ratio *r*. C/R, concentration versus response.

Antagonists

In simple terms, an antagonist can be defined as a drug that reduces the action of an agonist: which may be an endogenous ligand or a drug. Many of the clinically most useful drugs are antagonists. Drug antagonism can be produced by a variety of mechanisms, the most important being competitive antagonism.

Competitive antagonism

Numerous drugs (e.g. propranolol, naloxone) exert their clinical action by competitive antagonism at receptors. A competitive antagonist binds to the receptor and prevents the binding of an agonist. If the antagonist binds reversibly, then the effect of the antagonist can be overcome by raising the concentration of the agonist so that it competes more effectively for the binding sites. For a given concentration of reversible competitive antagonist, the log concentration–response curve of the agonist drug (A) will be displaced to the right in a parallel fashion (Fig. 1.7). The shift is expressed as a ratio *r* (termed 'dose ratio' or 'concentration ratio'), which is defined as the factor by which the agonist concentration must be increased in the presence of the antagonist to restore the response to that given by agonist alone. The magnitude of the shift is given by the Schild equation:

$$r - 1 = \frac{[B]}{K_B}$$

where [B] is the concentration of antagonist producing the shift and K_B is the dissociation equilibrium constant for the binding of the antagonist.

The Schild equation underlies the Schild plot, which is widely used to estimate K_B for the binding of the antagonist. It is thus possible to find the *affinity* of the antagonist for the receptors since this is the reciprocal of K_B.

An explanation of the calculation of K_B from the Schild plot is given in Appendix 1.

Examples of reversible competitive antagonism are:

- the block by H_2 receptor antagonists (e.g. cimetidine, used to treat peptic ulcer) of the action of endogenous histamine on gastric acid secretion.
- the block by β-adrenoceptor antagonists (e.g. atenolol, used for hypertension and other cardiovascular conditions) of the action of endogenous noradrenaline on β_1-adrenoceptors in the heart.

Other forms of drug antagonism

There are some other ways in which the effect of one drug can be reduced by the action of another.

Irreversible competitive antagonism

In irreversible competitive antagonism, the antagonist binds irreversibly, usually because of the formation of covalent bonds, effectively reducing the number of receptors available for binding. There may then be insufficient receptors available for the agonist to regain its maximum response as its concentration is increased (Fig. 1.8). Note: In some tissues there are spare receptors, that is more

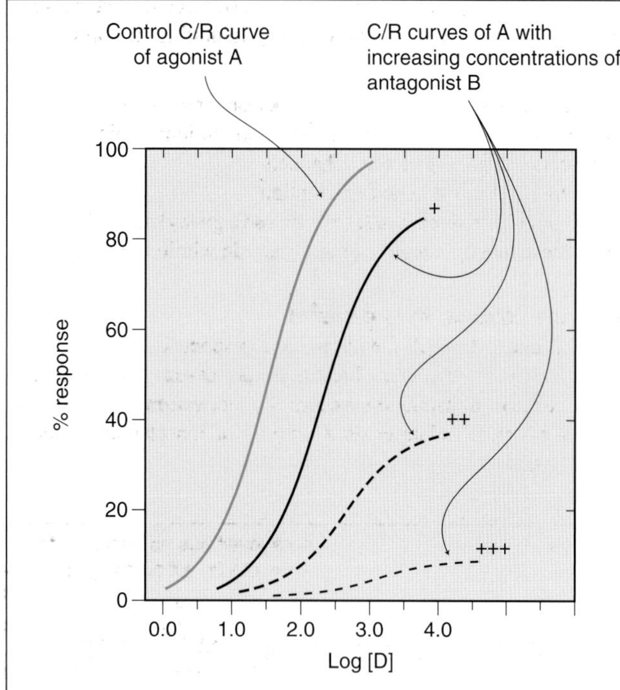

Fig. 1.8 Irreversible competitive antagonism. Increasing concentrations of an irreversible antagonist, B, causes progressively greater depressions of the maximum response of agonist A. C/R, concentration versus response.

receptors are present than must be occupied to give a full response; under these conditions a limited exposure to an irreversible antagonist might produce a parallel shift—hinted at in Figure 1.8.

An example is the block of α_1-adrenoceptors by phenoxybenzamine (used to treat pheochromocytoma), which forms a covalent bond with the receptor.

Physiological (functional) antagonism

In physiological antagonism, the 'antagonist' has the opposite biological action of the agonist, reducing the agonist effect by action on a different receptor (on which it is itself an agonist). An example of physiological antagonism is salbutamol (used to treat the acute asthmatic attack; albuterol in USA), which, by acting as an agonist (a smooth muscle relaxant) on β_2-adrenoceptors in bronchiolar smooth muscle, antagonises the bronchoconstrictor action of endogenous leukotrienes acting on leukotriene C_4 receptors.

Non-competitive antagonism

In non-competitive antagonism, the antagonist does not block the receptor itself but blocks the signal transduction process initiated by receptor activation, e.g. Ca^{2+} channel blockers will prevent smooth muscle contraction elicited by various agonists.

Pharmacokinetic antagonism

The antagonist reduces the free concentration of drug at its target either by reducing drug absorption or by accelerating renal or hepatic elimination. For example, induction of the cytochrome P450 drug-oxidising system by phenobarbital can reduce the effectiveness of many drugs.

Chemical antagonism

A chemical antagonist combines with the drug (in plasma or gut lumen) to produce an insoluble and inactive complex, e.g. protamine sulfate neutralises the action of heparin.

Desensitisation and tolerance

There are many examples of the failure of drug action to be maintained despite continued administration. Receptors can be converted to an inactive, desensitised form either by a simple isomerisation (e.g. the very rapid desensitisation of nicotinic receptors) or by a slower phosphorylation e.g. of G-protein-coupled receptors (GPCRs). There are indeed specific enzymes that mediate the phosphorylation and hence inactivation of GPCRs. Receptors can also be removed from the cell surface by internalisation subsequent to agonist binding. This process of receptor downregulation may take several days to reverse.

Homeostatic mechanisms may also come into play to reduce drug action. For example, the antihypertensive effect of thiazide diuretics is blunted by a slow activation of the renin–angiotensin system.

2 Molecular aspects of drug action

Drugs produce effects in the body mainly in the following ways: (i) by acting on *receptors*, (ii) by inhibiting *carriers* (molecules that transport one or more ions or molecules across the plasma membrane), (iii) by modulating or blocking *ion channels*, (iv) by inhibiting *enzymes*.

RECEPTORS AS TARGETS FOR DRUG ACTION

Receptors are protein molecules in or on cells whose function is to interact with the body's endogenous chemical messengers (hormones, neurotransmitters, the chemical mediators of the immune system, etc.) and thus initiate cellular responses. They enable the responses of the body's cells to be coordinated. Drugs used in medicine make use of these chemical 'sensors'—either stimulating them (drugs that do this are termed agonists) or preventing endogenous mediators or agonists from stimulating them (drugs that do this are termed antagonists).

There are four types of receptor:

- receptors coupled to G-proteins (GPCR: guanine nucleotide-binding proteins); also termed metabotropic receptors
- receptors linked to ion channels; also termed ionotropic receptors or ligand-gated ion channels
- receptors that affect gene transcription
- receptors linked to enzymes (e.g. kinases, guanylate cyclase, etc); these mostly initiate a kinase cascade within the cell.

Receptors coupled to G proteins

GPCRs occur in the cell membrane and respond in seconds. They have a single polypeptide chain that has seven transmembrane helices. Signal transduction occurs by activation of particular G-proteins that modulate enzyme activity or ion channel function (Figs 2.1–2.3).

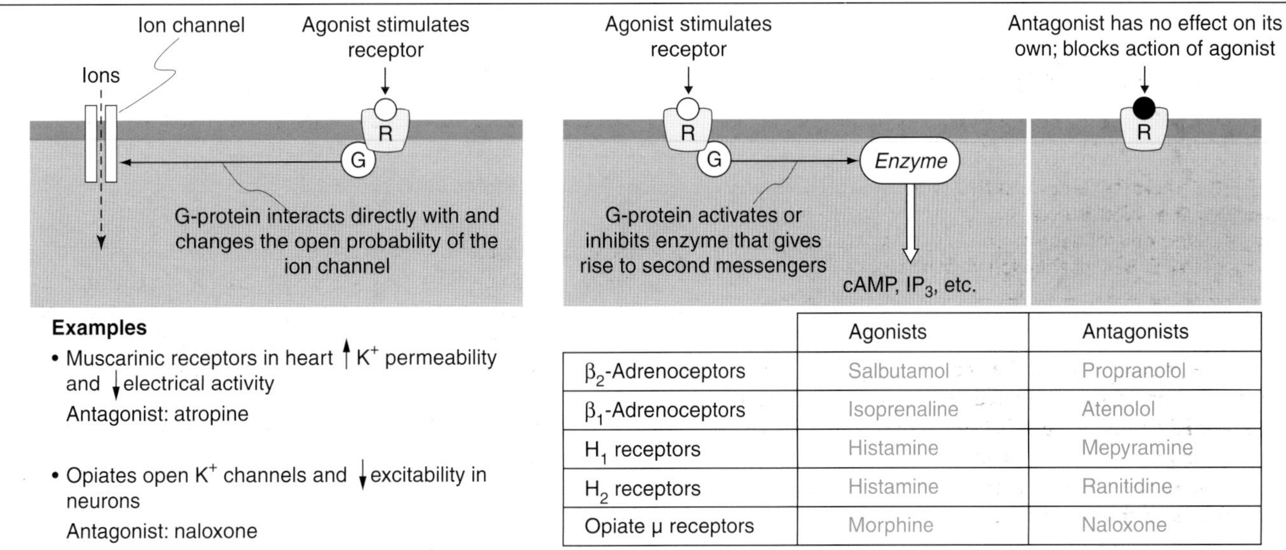

	Agonists	Antagonists
β_2-Adrenoceptors	Salbutamol	Propranolol
β_1-Adrenoceptors	Isoprenaline	Atenolol
H_1 receptors	Histamine	Mepyramine
H_2 receptors	Histamine	Ranitidine
Opiate μ receptors	Morphine	Naloxone

Fig. 2.1 Receptors coupled to G-proteins with examples of drugs acting on them. Each receptor couples to several G-proteins (not shown), resulting in amplification of the response.

G-proteins	Targets activated	Example of receptor involved	Typical effect	Produced by agonists	Antagonist
G_q (+)	Phospholipase C → PIP_2; → IP_3 — Releases Ca^{2+} from intracellular stores; → DAG — Activates protein kinase C	H_1-histamine	Smooth muscle contraction (↑IP_3); A variety of effects due to protein phosphorylation	Histamine Ch. 15	Mepyramine
G_s (+)	Adenylate cyclase: ATP → cAMP — Activates protein kinase A	β_2-Adrenoceptor →	Smooth muscle relaxation (↑cAMP)	Adrenaline Ch. 11, salbutamol Ch. 24	Propranolol
G_i (−)	Adenylate cyclase	M_2-muscarinic →	Decreased force of contraction of the heart (↓cAMP)	Acetylcholine	Atropine
G_i (+)	K^+ channels in cell membrane — Increased opening of the channels resulting in hyperpolarisation	M_2-muscarinic →	Cardiac slowing	Acetylcholine Ch. 10	Atropine

Fig. 2.2 Examples of G-protein-coupled actions. The pathways are shown for three different G-proteins. IP_3, inositol trisphosphate, PIP_2, phosphatidylinositol 4,5-bisphosphate.

G-proteins are attached to the membrane and consist of 3 subunits α, β and γ, the last two being closely associated:

In the free G protein, GDP occupies the binding site on the α-subunit. The α subunit and the β/γ complex can each activate intracellular targets. **Subtypes of all 3 subunits exist; the particular subunit determines which targets are activated**

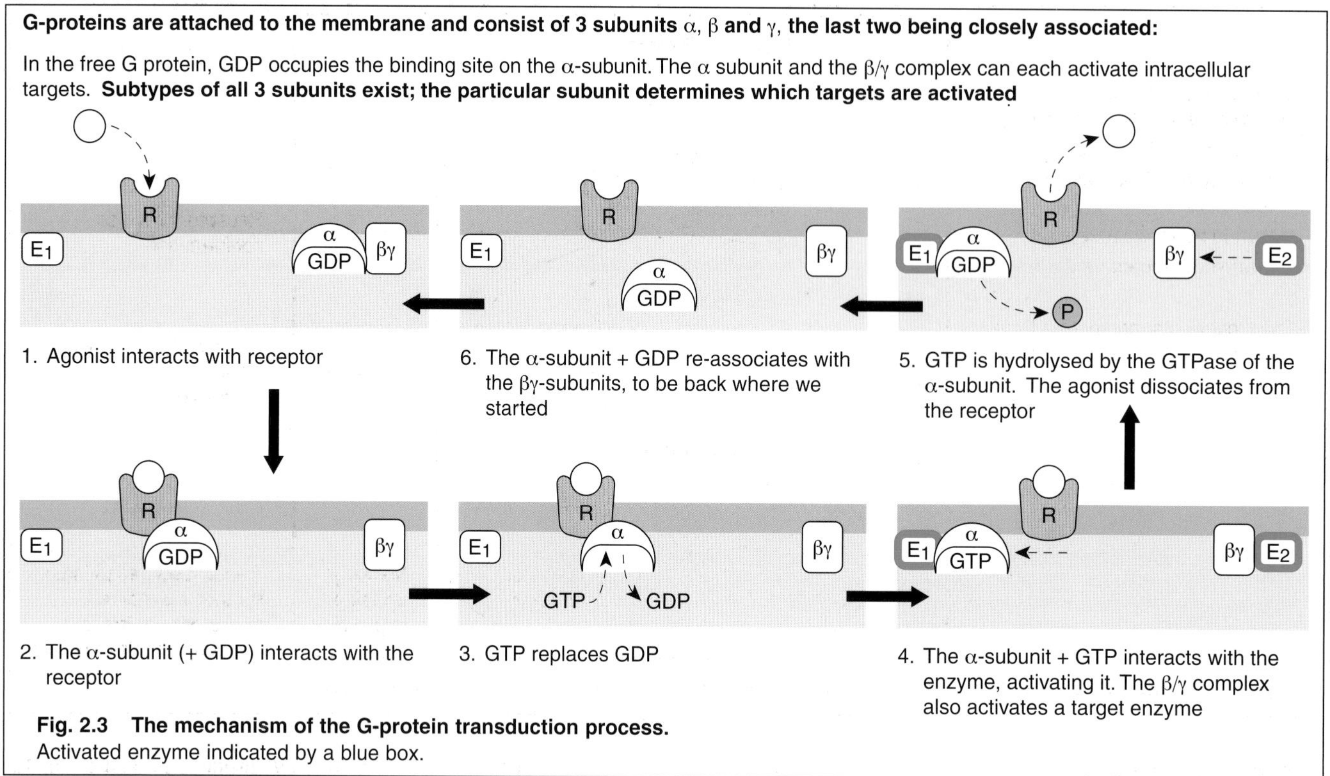

Fig. 2.3 The mechanism of the G-protein transduction process. Activated enzyme indicated by a blue box.

Receptors linked to ion channels (i.e. ionotropic receptors)

Receptors linked to ion channels are located in the cell membrane and respond in milliseconds. The channel forms part of the receptor. The nicotinic receptor for acetylcholine (see Ch. 10) is an example (Fig. 2.4).

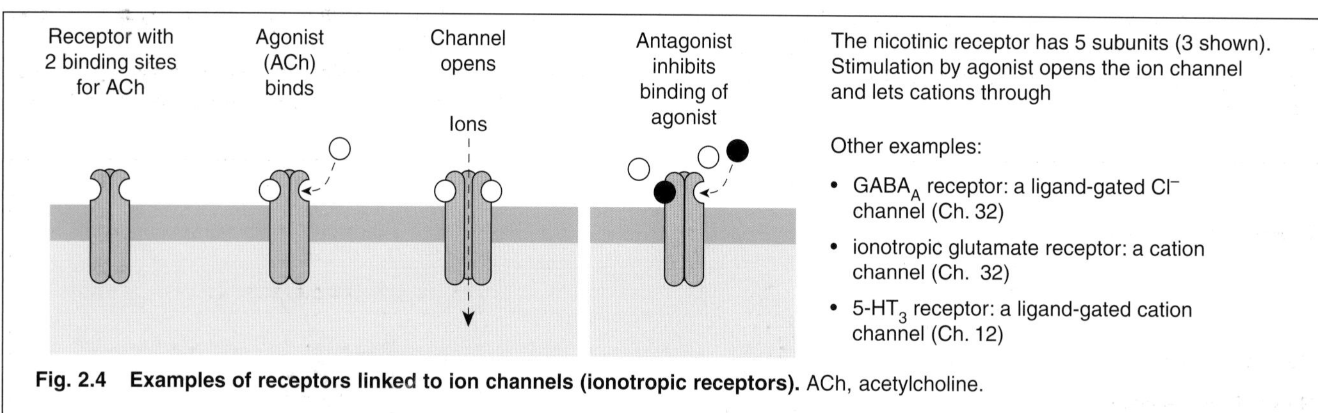

Fig. 2.4 Examples of receptors linked to ion channels (ionotropic receptors). ACh, acetylcholine.

Receptors linked to gene transcription

The receptors that regulate gene transcription are called nuclear receptors although some are located in the cytosol (e.g. glucocorticoid receptors) and migrate to the nucleus after binding a ligand (Fig. 2.5).

Receptors linked to enzymes

These receptors are transmembrane proteins with a large extracellular portion that contains the binding sites for ligands (e.g. growth factors, cytokines) and an intracellular portion that has integral enzyme activity—usually tyrosine kinase activity (Fig. 2.6). Activation initiates an intracellular pathway involving cytosolic and nuclear transducers and eventually gene transcription. Cytokine receptors activate Jak kinases, which, in turn, activate Stat transcription factors and these activate gene transcription (Fig. 2.6).

CARRIERS AS TARGETS FOR DRUG ACTION

The classification of membrane transport proteins varies between authorities, but in essence there are two main types:

- ATP-powered ion pumps
- transporters (Table 3.1)

Both are transmembrane proteins. In Rang et al. *Pharmacology*, these are termed 'carriers'.

ION CHANNELS AS TARGETS FOR DRUG ACTION

Some drugs produce their actions by directly interacting with ion channels. Three examples are given in Figure 2.9. Note that these ion channels transport ions across the plasma membrane. They are not receptors and should be distinguished from ion channels that function as ionotropic receptors (see above).

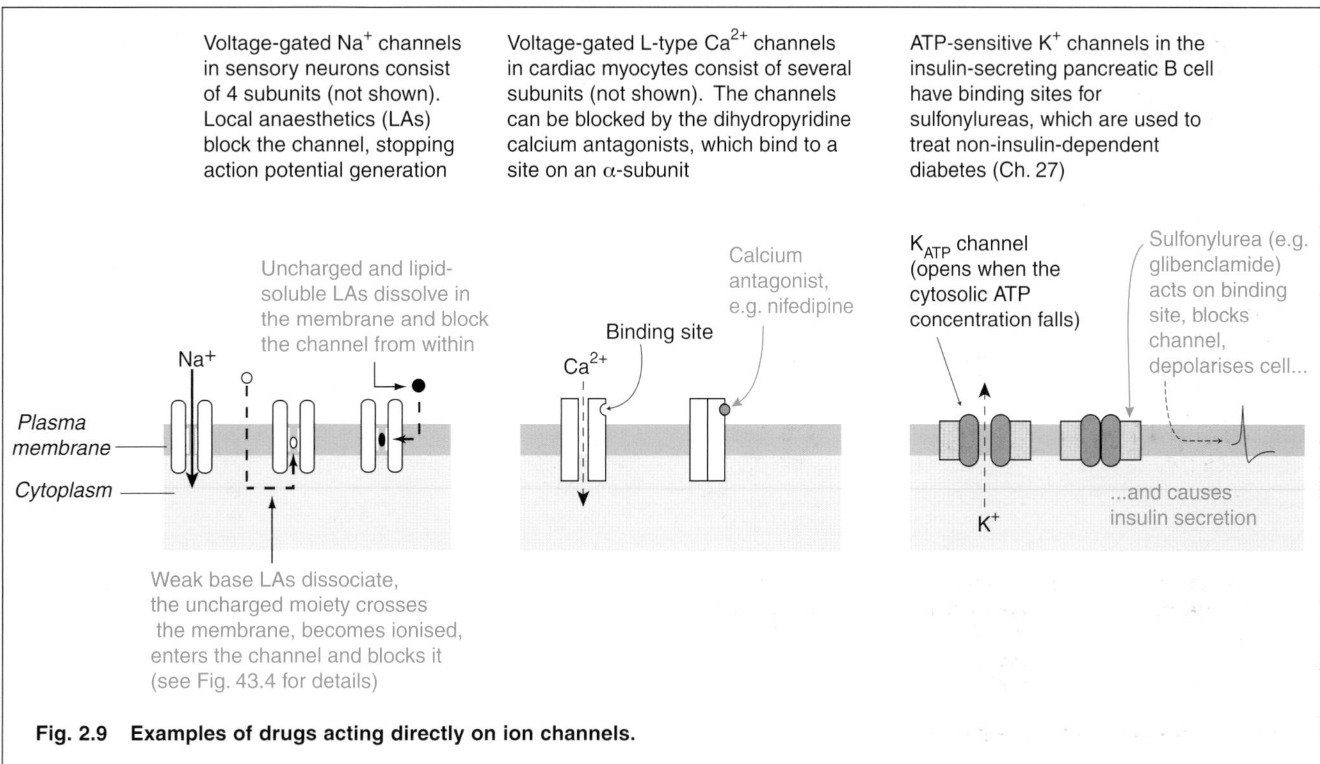

Fig. 2.9 Examples of drugs acting directly on ion channels.

ENZYMES AS TARGETS FOR DRUG ACTION

Drugs can produce effects on enzyme reactions by substrate competition or by reversibly or irreversibly modifying the enzyme. Some examples are given in Table 2.1.

Table 2.1 Drugs acting through alteration of enzyme reactions

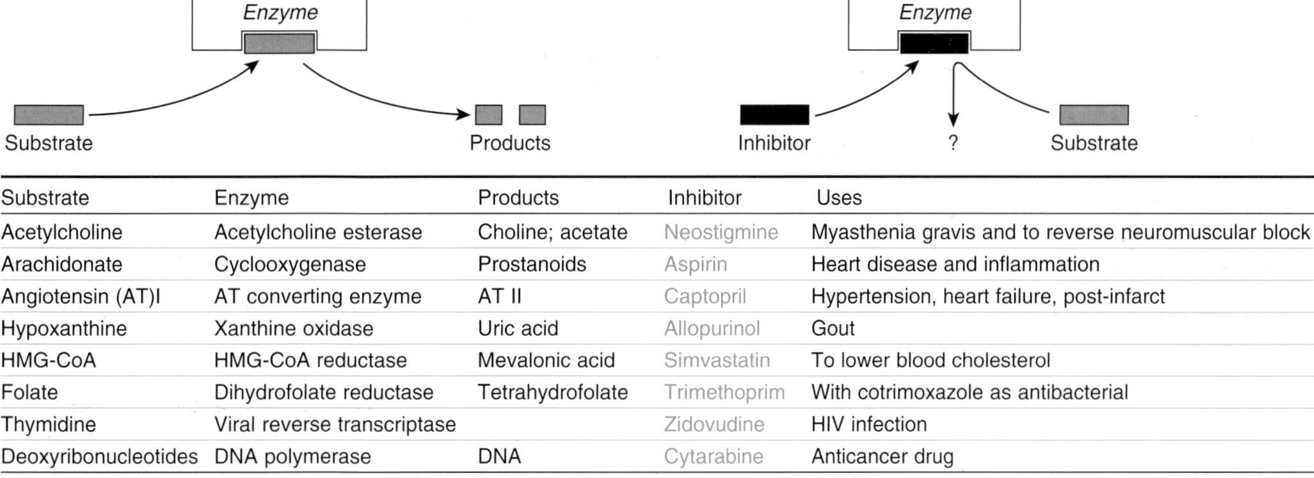

Substrate	Enzyme	Products	Inhibitor	Uses
Acetylcholine	Acetylcholine esterase	Choline; acetate	Neostigmine	Myasthenia gravis and to reverse neuromuscular block
Arachidonate	Cyclooxygenase	Prostanoids	Aspirin	Heart disease and inflammation
Angiotensin (AT)I	AT converting enzyme	AT II	Captopril	Hypertension, heart failure, post-infarct
Hypoxanthine	Xanthine oxidase	Uric acid	Allopurinol	Gout
HMG-CoA	HMG-CoA reductase	Mevalonic acid	Simvastatin	To lower blood cholesterol
Folate	Dihydrofolate reductase	Tetrahydrofolate	Trimethoprim	With cotrimoxazole as antibacterial
Thymidine	Viral reverse transcriptase		Zidovudine	HIV infection
Deoxyribonucleotides	DNA polymerase	DNA	Cytarabine	Anticancer drug

3 Excitable tissues and secretory mechanisms

In this chapter we examine some of the key cellular processes that operate over a brief time scale to control tissue responses; we also consider their potential as targets for drug action.

THE IMPORTANT REGULATORY ROLE OF CALCIUM

The short-term control of processes such as *excitation*, *contraction* and *secretion* commonly depends on Ca^{2+}-dependent regulation of enzymes, channels, contractile proteins, vesicle proteins, etc. Many drugs act by changing the concentration of Ca^{2+} in the cytosol, $[Ca^{2+}]_i$. $[Ca^{2+}]_i$ is affected by:

- the flux of Ca^{2+} through Ca^{2+} channels and transporters in the plasma membrane
- the storage and release of Ca^{2+} by intracellular organelles.

Many of the actions of $[Ca^{2+}]_i$ are mediated by the calcium-binding protein calmodulin.

Regulation of $[Ca^{2+}]_i$

Nearly all of the Ca^{2+} in cells is sequestered in the endoplasmic or sarcoplasmic reticulum (ER or SR) and the mitochondria; the free $[Ca^{2+}]_i$ is only about 10^{-7} mol/l. Extracellularly, $[Ca^{2+}]_o$ is about 1.5 mol/l; consequently, there is a large concentration gradient for Ca^{2+} entry. $[Ca^{2+}]_i$ is kept low by (a) active transport of Ca^{2+} across the plasma membrane and into intracellular compartments, and (b) the normally low Ca^{2+} permeability of the cell membranes. Changes in $[Ca^{2+}]_i$ result from net movements of Ca^{2+} between the cytosol, storage compartments and cell exterior (Fig. 3.1).

Processes lowering $[Ca^{2+}]_i$

Calcium is actively transported into organelles and from cells by Ca^{2+}-dependent ATPases (Ca^{2+} pumps). It is also extruded from cells by *Na^+/Ca^{2+} exchange*, the energy for extrusion coming from the electrochemical gradient for Na^+.

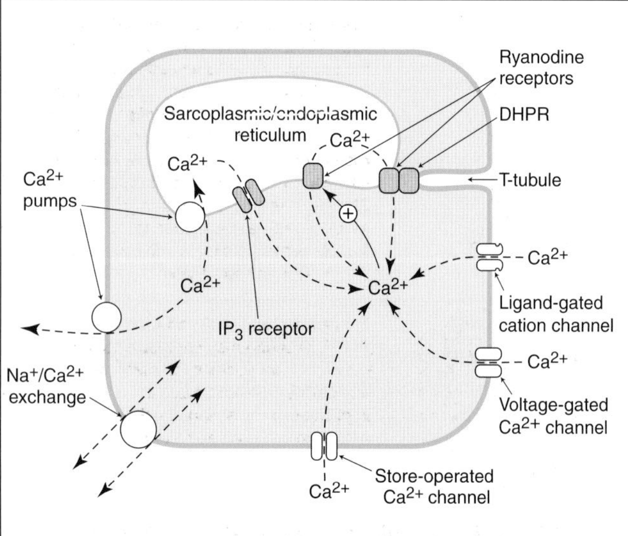

Fig. 3.1 A stylised cell showing the processes influencing $[Ca^{2+}]_i$. DHPR, dihydropyridine receptor; IP_3, inositol trisphosphate.

Processes raising $[Ca^{2+}]_i$

$[Ca^{2+}]_i$ is raised by Ca^{2+} entry across the cell membrane and Ca^{2+} release from the ER or SR. These movements are controlled by the following process.

Calcium entry across the cell membrane

Voltage-gated Ca^{2+} channels These channels open when the cell is depolarised, for example, by a conducted action potential. L, T, N, P/Q and R subtypes of voltage-gated Ca^{2+} channel are found. A pore-forming α_1-subunit is associated with other subunits (α_2, β, γ, δ) that modify channel properties. L channels are important in the contraction of cardiac and smooth muscle; N and P/Q channels are involved in neurotransmitter and hormone release, while T channels are found in neurons and in cardiac pacemaker cells. 'Calcium antagonists' (e.g. **nifedipine** and **verapamil**) that block L-type channels are therapeutically useful (Chs 17–19). The opening of Ca^{2+} channels can be modified indirectly by the action of G-protein-coupled receptors.

Ligand-gated channels Many ligand-gated cation channels are relatively non-selective and conduct Ca^{2+} as well as Na^+ and K^+. NMDA glutamate receptors (Ch. 33) have a high permeability to Ca^{2+}, and their excessive activation causes substantial Ca^{2+} uptake by neurons, which can lead to cell death (*excitotoxicity*, Ch. 35) The P_{2X} receptor (Ch. 12), activated by ATP, is an important route of entry for Ca^{2+} into some smooth muscle.

Na^+/Ca^{2+} exchange If $[Na^+]_i$ rises excessively, the exchanger, mentioned above, can operate in reverse to transport Ca^{2+} into the cell.

'Store-operated' Ca^{2+} channels (SOCs) SOCs in the plasma membrane open when the ER stores are depleted. How the ER communicates with the SOC is not known. They amplify the rise in $[Ca^{2+}]_i$ that follows release from the ER.

Calcium release from the ER or SR

The inositol trisphosphate (IP_3) receptor This ligand-gated ion channel occurs in the ER membrane and is activated by IP_3. It is responsible for the increase in $[Ca^{2+}]_i$ caused by the activation of G_q-coupled receptors (Ch. 2).

Ryanodine receptors (RyRs) These receptors get their name from being blocked by the alkaloid ryanodine. They are particularly important in cardiac and skeletal muscle, where they are responsible for Ca^{2+} release from the SR.

ELECTRICAL EXCITABILITY OF CELLS

All cells maintain a high $[K^+]_i$ and a low $[Na^+]_i$ (compared with the external concentrations). The *equilibrium potential** for Na^+, E_{Na}, is thus positive and that for K^+, E_K, negative (Table 3.1).

Since the cell membrane has a much greater permeability to K^+ than to Na^+, the resting membrane potential lies closer to E_K than to

*The *equilibrium potential* for an ion is the membrane potential at which ion movement due to the concentration gradient is balanced by movement due to the electrical gradient and no net current flows.

Table 3.1 Intracellular and extracellular ion concentrations and equilibrium potentials for skeletal muscle

Ion	Concentration		Equilibrium potential (mV)
	Extracellular	Cytosolic	
Na^+	145 mmol/l	12 mmol/l	+67
K^+	4 mmol/l	150 mmol/l	−97
Cl^-	125 mmol/l	4.25 mmol/l	−90
Ca^{2+}	1.5 mmol/l	0.1 μmol/l	+129

Notes: $[Cl^-]_i$ has been calculated assuming Cl^- is passively distributed at a resting membrane potential of −90 mV; not all external Ca^{2+} is ionised, $[Ca^{2+}]_o$ being only about half total extracellular [Ca].

E_{Na}, yielding an internal potential between −30 and −90 mV. An increase in Na^+ permeability causes an inward current of Na^+ and membrane depolarisation, whereas an increase in K^+ permeability causes an outward current and hyperpolarisation.

The *action potential* usually involves:

- a rapid, regenerative activation of voltage-gated Na^+ channels when the membrane is depolarised beyond approximately −50 mV (for example by transmitter action); in many cells (e.g. cardiac and smooth muscle cells), voltage-gated Ca^{2+} channels contribute to action potential generation.
- a slower, more prolonged increase in K^+ permeability.

The action potential peak approaches E_{Na}, following which the cell repolarises rapidly as the Na^+ channels inactivate. In most cells, repolarisation, and action potential termination, is aided by the opening of voltage-gated K^+ channels. Drugs that enhance the opening of Na^+ or Ca^{2+} channels increase excitability, whereas increasing K^+ conductance reduces it. Channel blockers have the opposite effects.

Use-dependent and voltage-dependent channel block

Voltage-gated channels can exist in three states: *resting* (closed), *activated* (open, induced by depolarisation) and *inactivated* (self-blocked). The slow recovery of the voltage sensitivity of Na^+ channels after an action potential renders the membrane temporarily *refractory*.

Sodium channel blockers (e.g. **antidysrhythmics**, **local anaesthetics**) often bind more strongly to one or other of these states (Chs 17 and 43). Those binding most strongly to the inactivated state may produce *use-dependent block,* since the drug effect increases with the rate of action potential discharge, as the proportion of inactivated channels increases.

Most Na^+ channel blockers are positively charged at physiological pH and their action is influenced by the voltage gradient across the cell membrane; their blocking action (from the inside of the membrane) is increased by depolarisation as the ion responds to the increased driving force. *Voltage-dependent block* can enhance the action of **antidysrhythmic** and **antiepileptic** drugs since the dysrhythmias and seizure activity may arise in depolarised cells of damaged tissue.

Sodium channels

The complex structure of Na^+ channels is shown in Figure 43.1 (p. 98).

Potassium channels

Potassium channels have important actions on *excitability*, the *duration* of the action potential and action potential *frequency*. They fall into three main classes (Fig. 3.2). Mutations of K^+ channels contribute to a number of inherited diseases, for example the long-QT syndrome, associated with mutations in cardiac voltage-gated K^+ channels.

Muscle contraction

Skeletal, cardiac and smooth muscle differ in the linkage between membrane events and increase in $[Ca^{2+}]_i$, and in the mechanism by which $[Ca^{2+}]_i$ mediates contraction.

Skeletal muscle

In skeletal muscle, the propagated action potential in the cell membrane is conducted passively down the T-tubules. Here *dihydropyridine receptors*, closely related to the L-type Ca^{2+} channel, respond to the depolarisation by activating *ryanodine receptors* in the adjacent SR membrane, causing Ca^{2+} release from the SR into the sarcoplasm (see Fig. 3.1). The rise in $[Ca^{2+}]_i$ is transient and results in a 'twitch' response.

Cardiac muscle

Details of the cardiac action potential and the effects of drugs on the rate and rhythm of the heart are described in Ch. 17. In cardiac muscle, contraction is triggered by the entry of Ca^{2+} through voltage-gated Ca^{2+} channels (L-type), in the cell membrane or T-tubule, during the action potential plateau. The amount of Ca^{2+} entering the myocyte is not sufficient by itself to activate the contractile machinery. However, the rise in $[Ca^{2+}]_i$ activates ryanodine receptors (different from those of skeletal muscle) to release Ca^{2+}

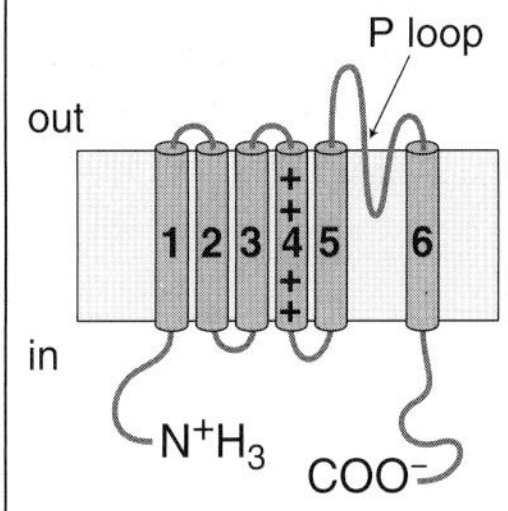

Voltage-gated channels (K_V)

Ca^{2+}-activated K^+ channels (K_{Ca}) are included in this group though not all are voltage gated. Many of these channels are blocked by tetraethylammonium and 4-aminopyridine

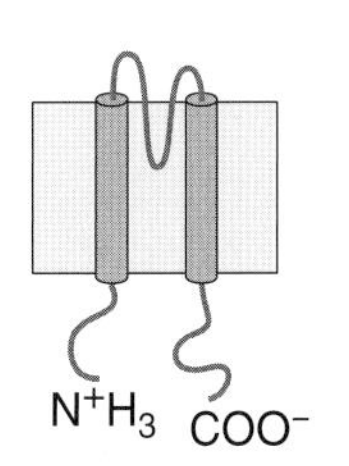

Inwardly rectifying K^+ channels (K_{ir}) allow K^+ to pass much more readily into the cell than out. Some of these channels are activated by G-protein subunits and thus mediate the inhibitory effects of many agonists acting on G-protein-coupled receptors. The K_{ATP} channels, which are inhibited by antidiabetic sulfonylureas (Ch. 27), are members of this family. Similar sulfonylurea-sensitive channels in smooth muscle are targets for K^+ channel-opening drugs, such as cromakalim

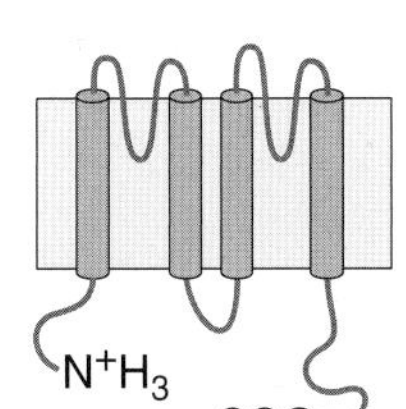

Two-pore domain K^+ channels (e.g. TWIK, TRAAK) may contribute to the resting K^+ conductance in many cells, and certain subtypes have been implicated in the action of volatile anaesthetics, such as halothane

Fig. 3.2 Alpha-subunits of K^+ channels. Four K_v or K_{ir} subunits combine to form a functional channel, whereas only two 2-pore subunits are required. Additional β-subunits (e.g. the SUR subunit, Ch. 27) modulate channel properties.

from the SR. The rise in $[Ca^{2+}]_i$ produces a regenerative activation of ryanodine receptors, which raises $[Ca^{2+}]_i$ sufficiently to cause contraction. L-type Ca^{2+} channel blockers have useful cardiac effects (see Chs 17–19).

Smooth muscle

The regulation of smooth muscle contraction is less well understood. The action potential of smooth muscle propagates more slowly than that of cardiac and skeletal muscle and is, in most cases, generated by L- (or T-) type Ca^{2+} channels rather than Na^+ channels. This provides one important route of Ca^{2+} entry. Calcium may also enter via ligand-gated cation channels (e.g. the P_{2X} ATP receptor). Calcium ions are also released from the SR either by IP_3 receptor activation or by ryanodine receptor activation (Ca^{2+}-induced Ca^{2+} release). Contraction of smooth muscle occurs when the *myosin light chain* is phosphorylated. This phosphorylation is catalysed by *myosin light chain kinase* (MLCK), which is activated when it binds to Ca^{2+}-calmodulin. A second enzyme, *myosin phosphatase*, reverses the phosphorylation, and causes relaxation. The activity of MLCK and myosin phosphatase is regulated by cAMP and cGMP, and many drugs that contract or relax smooth muscle modify the concentration of these second messengers. Figure 3.3 summarises the main mechanisms involved in the control of smooth muscle contraction and the action of drugs thereon.

RELEASE OF CHEMICAL MEDIATORS

Calcium plays a central role in the release of neurotransmitters, hormones and inflammatory mediators.

Mediators are conveniently divided into:

- preformed mediators packaged in storage vesicles from which they are released by exocytosis, e.g. neurotransmitters, hormones
- those produced on demand (e.g. nitric oxide (Ch. 14) and prostanoids (Ch. 15)) and released by diffusion or by membrane carriers.

A rise in $[Ca^{2+}]_i$ is important in both cases. It initiates exocytosis and is often the main activator of the enzymes responsible for the synthesis of diffusible mediators.

Exocytosis

Exocytosis is the main mechanism for release of transmitter from nerves, hormone from endocrine cells and histamine from mast cells. Exocytosis requires the fusion of storage vesicles with the inner surface of the plasma membrane. In fast synaptic transmission, Ca^{2+} enters the nerve ending through voltage-gated Ca^{2+} channels, mainly of the N and P type, and promotes the docking and exocytosis of synaptic vesicles at *active* zones. These are situated close to the Ca^{2+} channels and opposite receptor-rich areas of the postsynaptic

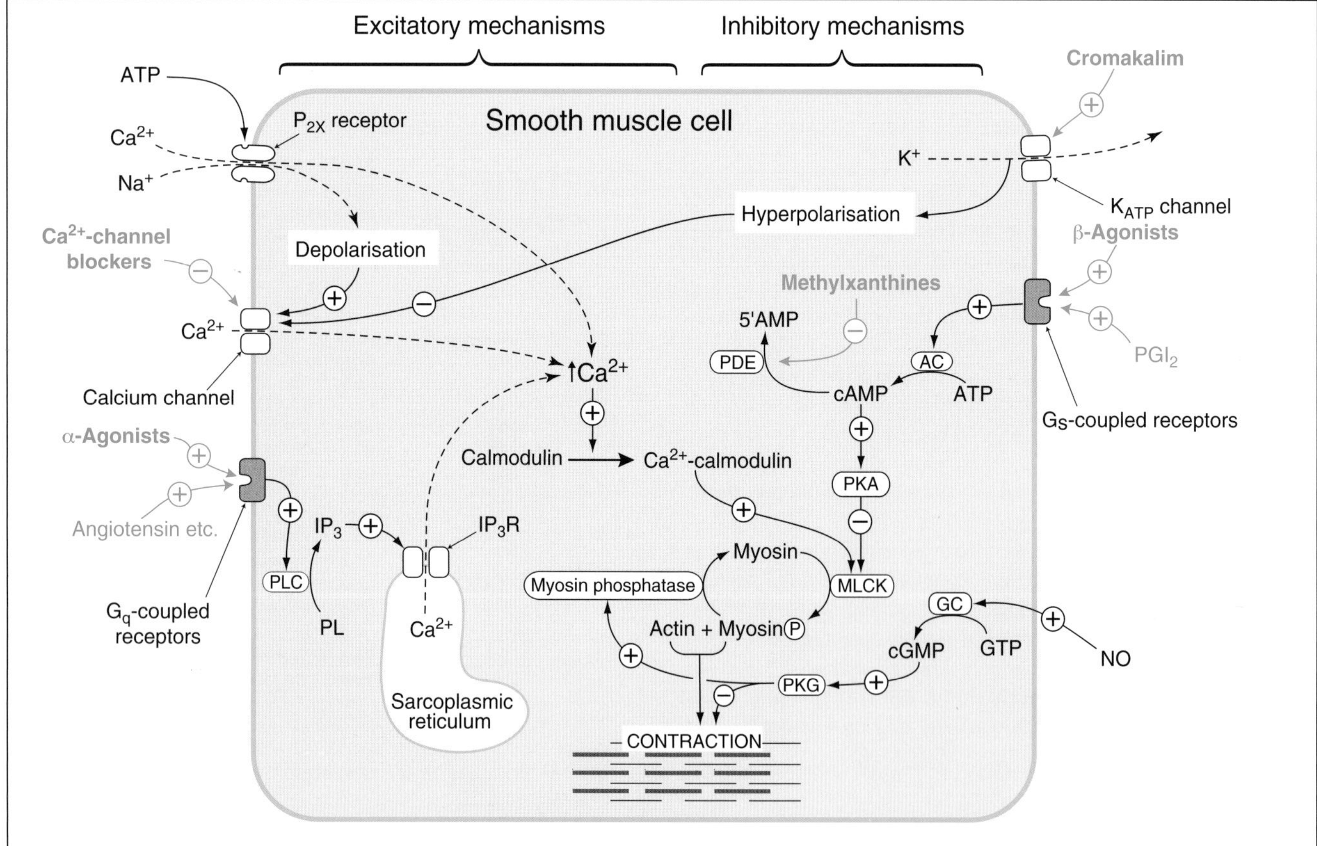

Fig. 3.3 The role of ion channels and receptors in the regulation of $[Ca^{2+}]_i$ and contraction as typified by smooth muscle. AC, adenylate cyclase; GC, guanylate cyclase; IP_3, inositol trisphosphate; MLCK, myosin light chain kinase; NO, nitric oxide; PDE, phosphodiesterase; PGI_2, prostaglandin I_2; PKA, protein kinase A; PKG, protein kinase G; PL, phospholipid; PLC, phospholipase C.

membrane. Recent evidence suggests that Ca^{2+} binds to a protein, *synaptotagmin*, on the vesicle surface and that this promotes the binding of a second vesicle-bound protein, *synaptobrevin*, to *syntaxin* on the inner surface of the plasma membrane. This binding promotes membrane fusion. After releasing its content, the vesicle is recaptured by endocytosis, and its membrane is recycled into new vesicles.

Non-vesicular release mechanisms

In addition to exocytosis, transmitters can move out of nerve endings via carriers in the cell membrane or by diffusion. For example, the release of monoamines from nerve terminals by amphetamines (see Ch. 11) utilises the monoamine transporter (acting in reverse). Non-vesicular release though slower than exocytosis is nevertheless fast enough for nitric oxide to function as a true transmitter (Ch.14).

Epithelial ion transport

In fluid-secreting epithelia (e.g. those of the renal tubule and gastrointestinal tract), fluid secretion generally involves both Na^+ and Cl^- transport. The epithelial cells form sheets separating one compartment (e.g. the plasma-perfused compartment) from the luminal compartment. Secretion occurs because Na^+ is pumped out of one side of the cell by the Na^+/K^+ ATPase, taking water with it while drawing Na^+ in passively from the other side through specific epithelial Na^+ channels (ENaCs). ENaCs are regulated mainly by *aldosterone*, which enhances Na^+ reabsorption by the kidney. Aldosterone, like other steroid hormones, exerts its effects by regulating gene expression (see Ch. 2). An increase in the number of ENaCs increases the rate of Na^+ and fluid transport. ENaCs are selectively blocked by the diuretic drug *amiloride* (Ch. 25).

Chloride transport has an important role in the airways and gastrointestinal tract. In the airways, it is essential for fluid secretion, whereas in the colon, it mediates fluid reabsorption; the difference results from the different arrangement of various transporters and channels with respect to the polarity of the cells. In epithelia the main Cl^- channel is the *cystic fibrosis transmembrane conductance regulator* (*CFTR*). This is defective in the inherited disorder cystic fibrosis and the resulting impairment of secretion, particularly in the airways, causes the severe symptoms. Efforts are being made to find drugs that restore CFTR function. Both Na^+ and Cl^- transport are regulated by intracellular messengers, notably by Ca^{2+} and cAMP. Activation of the CFTR by cAMP in the gastrointestinal tract causes a large increase in the rate of fluid secretion. This underlies the diarrhoea produced by cholera infection.

4 Cell proliferation and apoptosis

Cell proliferation—an event that takes place over a longer time scale than the events depicted in Ch. 3— occurs continuously in the human body, billions of new cells being generated daily from existing cells, with equivalent numbers of cells being removed by apoptosis (programmed cell death; cell suicide).

Pathophysiology

Cell proliferation is involved in:

- the growth of tissues and organs
- the replenishment of cells, e.g. of the gastrointestinal epithelium, of red and white blood cells
- the repair and healing after injury
- acute and chronic inflammation
- hypertrophy/hyperplasia, e.g. of blood vessels and/or cardiac muscle in cardiovascular disease, of bronchial epithelium in respiratory disease.

Angiogenesis (the development of new blood vessels) necessarily accompanies many of these processes.

Apoptosis is involved in:

- embryogenesis, during which it eliminates redundant cells, thus helping to sculpt organs and tissues
- the development of self-tolerance in the immune system
- the regression of mammary gland cells after lactation
- the shedding of the intestinal lining
- the death of neutrophils once these have played their part in inflammation
- the pathophysiology of autoimmune, neurodegenerative and cardiovascular diseases and the acquired immune deficiency syndrome (AIDS)
- the pathophysiology of cancer: it acts as a defence against mutations, eliminating cells with abnormal DNA that could become malignant.

New drug development

New drugs affecting cell proliferation, angiogenesis and apoptosis are being actively sought for many of the conditions specified above, particularly cancer. Some new agents are already in the pipeline.

Cell proliferation and the cell cycle

Dividing cells go through a *cell cycle* during which all the cell constituents are duplicated giving rise to two *daughter cells*. The phases of the cycle are shown in Figure 4.1.

Growth factor action and/or interaction between the cell and the matrix are the main triggers for starting off the cell cycle. Subsequent progress is controlled by special kinases (cyclin-dependent kinases, cdks) whose activity is activated by binding to proteins termed *cyclins*. The cyclin/cdk complexes act sequentially to drive the cell cycle: when bound to the relevant cyclin, cdks phosphorylate and thus activate some enzymes and inhibit others, the cyclin being degraded after the cdk has acted.

Several factors (shown in Fig. 4.1) modulate cycle progress:

- cdk inhibitors
- the Rb protein, a protein coded for by the Rb gene (**r**etino**b**lastoma gene, so-called because mutations of this gene are associated with retinblastoma tumours)
- the p53 protein, coded for by gene *p53*.

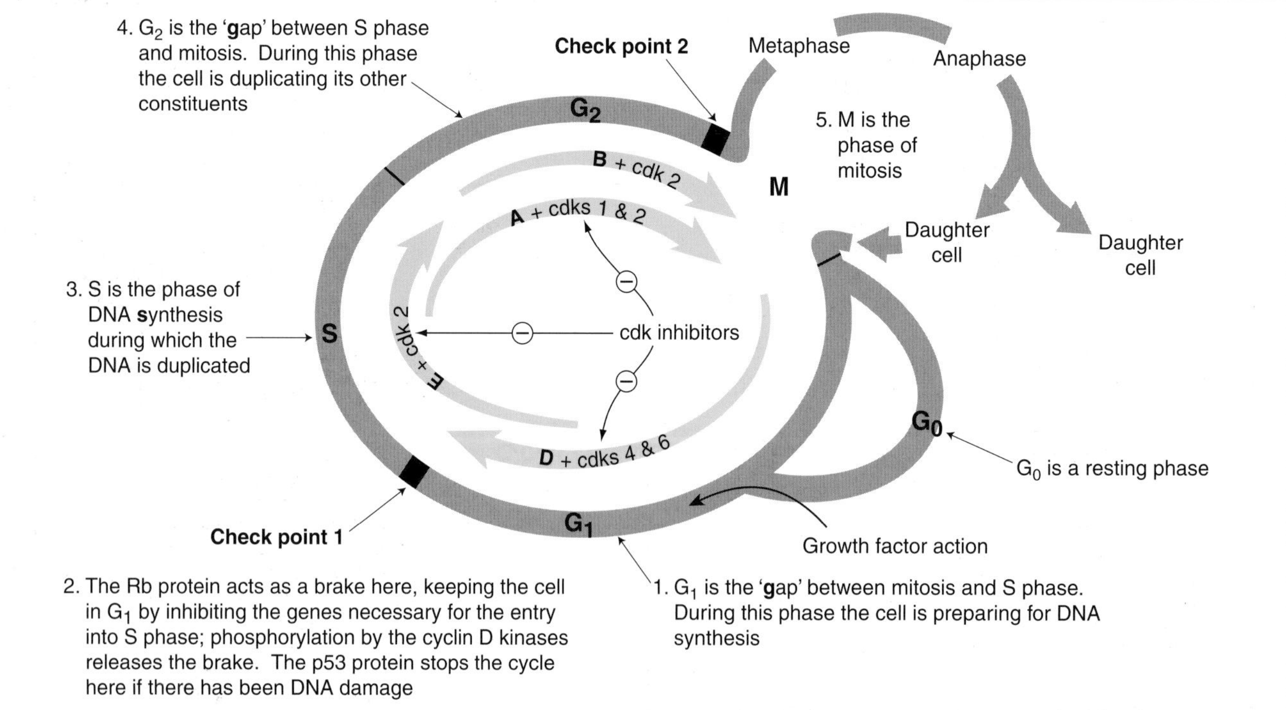

Fig. 4.1 The cell cycle of dividing cells. Cells in G_0 are not in the cell cycle but enter the cycle when stimulated by the action of growth factors or integrins. The cyclins (D, E, A and B) are shown as blue arrows, each with their respective cyclin-dependent kinases (cdks). The thickness of the arrows indicates the intensity of action of the cdks. Various cdk inhibitors control the activity of the cdks.

The action of growth factors and integrins

Growth factors (GFs)—such as fibroblast, epidermal, platelet-dependent, vascular endothelial—act through receptor tyrosine kinases or receptor-coupled kinases to stimulate the production of the positive and negative regulators of the cell cycle (Fig. 4.2).

Integrins are transmembrane receptors that interact with components of the extracellular matrix to cooperate with GFs in the production of the cell cycle transducers.

GFs can stimulate cells to release *metalloproteinases*; these degrade the local matrix making space for the increased cell numbers. The metalloproteinases, in turn, release and activate GFs sequestered on matrix components.

Apoptosis

Apoptosis is a programmed sequence of biochemical processes; it is thus quite unlike *necrosis*, which is disorganised disintegration of damaged cells, resulting in products that trigger the inflammatory response.

Apoptosis is a default response in that continuous stimulation of the cell by *survival factors* (e.g. cytokines, integrins, hormones, adhesion factors) is necessary for the cell to survive. If this essential signalling by the *anti-apoptotic pathway* ceases, the cell's self-destruct machinery is activated; this may be termed 'death by neglect'.

The apoptotic pathways The mechanism of programmed cell death involves the *apoptotic pathways,* which can be activated by the cell's death receptors (this is 'death by design') and also by DNA damage through the mitochondrial pathway. The enzymes that bring about cell death are a family of *caspases*, which act selectively on specific enzymes or structural elements inhibiting some and stimulating others. There are two main apoptotic pathways (Fig. 4.3).

The death receptor pathway This is activated when death ligands (e.g. tumour necrosis factor; TNF) stimulate the death receptors (such as members of the TNF receptor family, e.g. Fas), triggering *initiator* caspase 8; this, in turn, activates *effector* caspases (e.g. caspase 3).

The mitochondrial pathway This can be brought into play by DNA damage or by withdrawal of survival factor action. DNA damage stimulates pro-apoptotic members of the Bcl-2 family to promote the release from the mitochondria of cytochrome *c,* which complexes with a protein termed Apaf-1 (**a**poptotic **p**rotease-**a**ctivating **f**actor-1). The complex activates the initiator caspase 9, which, in turn, activates the *effector* caspases (e.g. caspase 3). If the survival pathway ceases to function, anti-apoptotic members of the Bcl-2 family compete with their pro-apoptotic siblings and prevent the activation of the mitochondrial pathway.

Caspase actions

The effector caspases *degrade* various cell constituents: proteins, structural components, enzymes, etc. They *activate* other cell constituents, e.g. a DNAase that cuts up the DNA into fragments. The cell is eventually reduced to a cluster of membrane-bound bodies each containing a variety of organelles. The dying cell displays 'eat-me' signals that are recognised by macrophages, which obligingly comply. The caspases are under the control of IAPs.

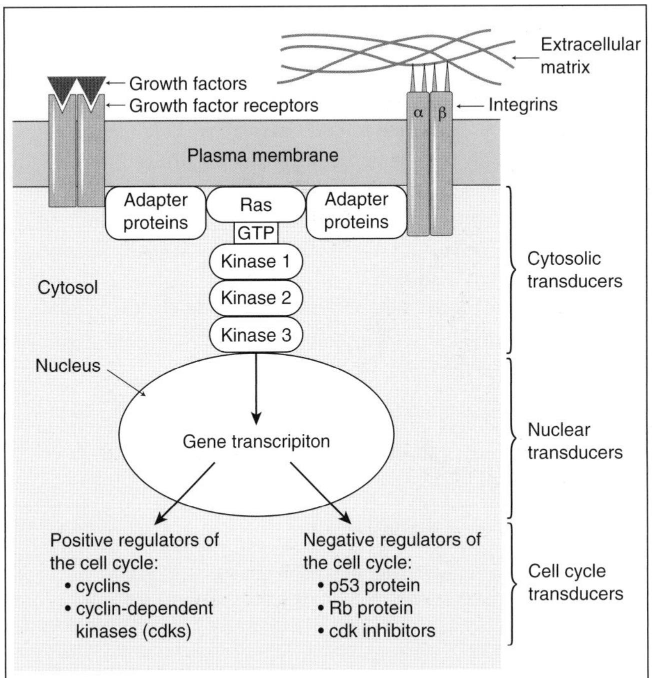

Fig. 4.2 Schematic diagram showing how activation of growth factor receptors and integrins gives rise to the cell cycle transducers. RAS is a GTP-binding protein involved in signal transduction.

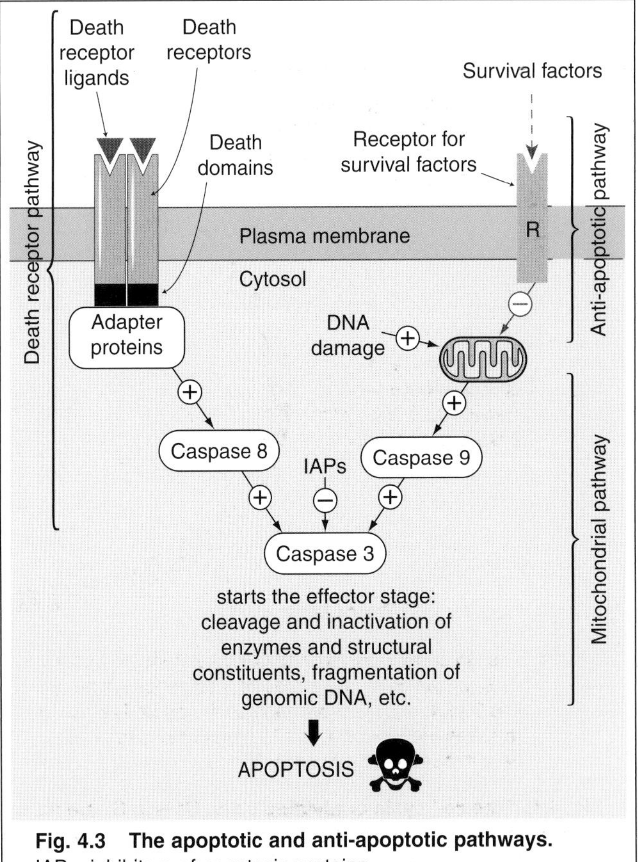

Fig. 4.3 The apoptotic and anti-apoptotic pathways. IAPs, inhibitors of apoptosis proteins.

5 Measurement of drug action

The action of drugs is usually measured by bioassay, which is the measurement of potency or activity of a drug using a biological response. It is used when it is necessary (a) to measure the activity of new/chemically unknown substances in research work or in new drug development, (b) to investigate endogenous mediators/transmitters, and (c) to measure unwanted actions of drugs. A clinical trial in which, for example, a new drug is compared with one already in use is a special form of comparative bioassay.

Principles of bioassay

Most bioassays involve measurements of the responses of isolated tissue or groups of animals. In the usual type of bioassay, the response of the unknown (or test) drug is compared with that of a standard (or control) drug. The response to a drug may be:

- graded, e.g. the contraction of a smooth muscle, the change in heart rate.
- all or none ('quantal'), e.g. the absence or presence of a pinch reflex, the sucess of maze-running in a stipulated time.

For accurate estimation, a parallel line assay is required (though in many cases this may not be feasible).

Graded responses

Taking the contraction of an isolated tissue such as a strip of smooth muscle as an example, the log of the dose is plotted against the response expressed as the percentage of the maximal response (Fig. 5.1). When two agents act on the same receptor and have the same intrinsic activity (see Ch. 1), the log dose–response curves will be parallel and their relative potency can be obtained from the separation of the two curves (Log M in Fig. 5.1).

All-or-none responses

In all or none situations (usually an in vivo response), the response is expressed as the percentage of individuals giving the all-or-none response. If a parallel log dose–response curve can be obtained, the potency ratio of unknown (or test) drug to control (standard) can be obtained as for a graded response. However, the two drugs may not have identical mechanisms of action and thus will not necessarily have parallel curves. This is the case with comparative bioassays, which seek to compare the biological activity of different drugs: for example to assess whether a new local anaesthetic is more potent than procaine, or whether a new antihypertensive vasodilator acting by a novel mechanism is more or less potent than the calcium antagonist nifedipine.

In comparative assays, a comparison of the ED_{50} (the dose which produces the particular outcome in 50% of the population) of each drug can be used to get a rough estimation of their relative potencies. Note in this case the shape of the curve is determined by the statistical distribution of sensitivities of the individuals. A small standard deviation will produce a steep log dose–response curve and vice versa. Comparative assays are often used during the development of new drugs and in clinical trials (Fig. 5.2).

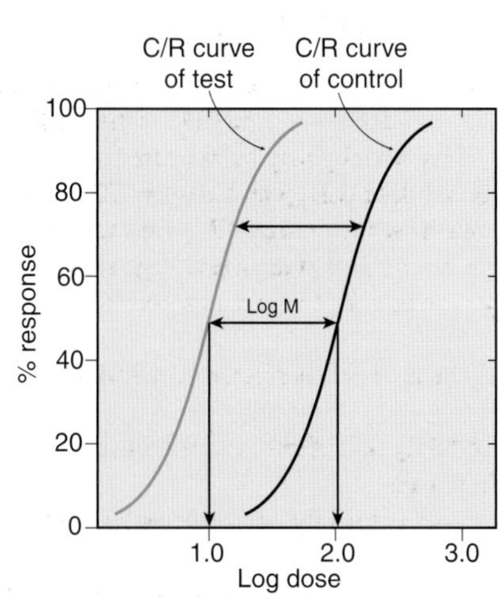

Fig. 5.1 Comparison by bioassay of the potency of the unknown (test) drug with standard (control). Since the concentration–response (C/R) curves are parallel, log M (the potency ratio) is the same at all points of the curve.

New drug developmnent

Before a new drug can receive a product licence it must be tested for effectiveness and toxicity. Preclinical tests on isolated tissues and in intact animals* should ensure that the drug has the required mechanism of action (e.g. β-adrenoceptor block) and at least in animals will produce appropriate 'system' responses (e.g. analgesia). At this stage the new drug will be tested against standard drugs in comparative assays. Toxicity tests in animals should in most cases allow some prediction of toxic/adverse effects in humans.

Clinical testing

In comparisons of drugs used clinically, potency does not necessarily relate directly to therapeutic usefulness; it is important to consider also the maximum achievable response and the incidence of unwanted effects.

Clinical testing in humans involves four phases:

Phase I Measurement of pharmacological activity, pharmacokinetics and side effects in healthy volunteers (unless exposure of healthy individuals is unethical, e.g. trials of potentially toxic anticancer drugs can only be done in cancer patients).

Phase II Pilot studies in small groups of patients to confirm that the drug works in the target condition and to establish the dosage regimen to be used in phase III.

Phase III Formal clinical trials in a large number of patients to determine the drug's efficacy compared with existing treatment and to determine the incidence of unwanted effects.

Phase IV Post-marketing surveillance to establish efficacy and toxicity in general use. The detection of rare, adverse effects is most likely to occur in this phase.

*__Animal models.__ Initial tests of the potency of a drug such as a new vasodilator drug have necessarily to be done on animals. But there can be hazards in extrapolating such data to the use of the new agent as an antihypertensive drug in humans. Animal 'models' can, however, be devised that attempt to mimic closely human conditions (such as anxiety, pain or hypertension) and which might provide valuable information on a drug's potential before exposure of human subjects. For example, animal models of hypertension have been established in which high blood pressure is induced by compromising renal function or by the selective breeding of strains that develop hypertension spontaneously.

CLINICAL TRIALS

The object of a clinical trial is to obtain an objective assessment of two or more methods of treatment. This frequently involves comparing a new drug with a standard drug—as is necessary in Phase III of clinical testing (see above).

Principles of clinical trials

Ideally the log dose–response curve of the new 'test' drug is compared with the log dose–response curve of the standard 'control' drug. This is rarely feasible. In practice, two points on the dose–response curves of each may be used, chosen in a preliminary trial (Fig. 5.2). More commonly still, single doses of each are compared. In essence, most clinical trials give information on the *comparative efficacy* not the *comparative potency* of the two drugs.

Two important principles in the conduct of a clinical trial are:

- random allocation of patients to test and control groups
- a 'double-blind' design.

Random allocation of patients to test and control groups

There is a real possibility that bias could affect the allocation of patients to 'test' or 'control' treatment. To minimise such bias, it is essential to allocate patients to new or old treatments on a random basis. For a large group of patients, randomisation should ensure that each group has an equivalent spectrum of ages, males or females, severity of disease, etc. In some trials, with smaller numbers of participants, and where the patients' condition is stable, a *cross-over design* allows each patient to receive both treatments.

Double-blind design

If either the patient or doctor knows which treatment is being administered, the assessment may be subject to bias according to the expectations of either or both. This is normally countered by a 'double-blind' design, i.e. neither the patient nor the investigator knows which treatment is being given. The importance of a patient's belief is emphasised by the *placebo* effect. This means that an inert preparation can have a demonstrable effect if the patient believes it to be pharmacologically effective.

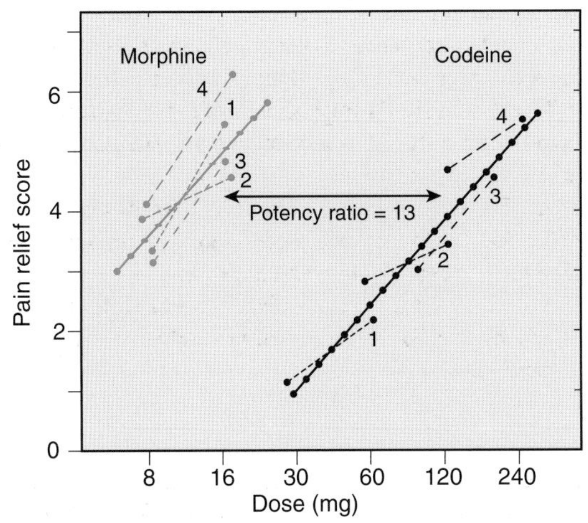

Fig. 5.2 Comparative assay of morphine versus codeine in humans. Each of four patients was given by intramuscular injection, on successive occasions, in random order, four different treatments (high and low doses of morphine and high and low doses of codeine). The subjective pain relief score was calculated for each treatment. The calculated regression line (solid line with dots) gave a potency ratio estimate of 13. (After Houde RW et al. 1965 In: Analgetics. Academic Press NY.)

Number of subjects required

The number of patients needed for a trial depends on the significance level sought and the power of the trial. These are influenced by consideration, respectively, of type I errors (proposing a difference when none exists) and type II errors (failure to detect a real difference). If it is thought to be worthwhile to detect a small improvement (such as a 1 or 2% decrease in death rate) then a large number of patients will be required. Statisticians determine the detailed design of a trial, including the number of patients required to meet the declared aim.

A more recent and instructive means of expressing the benefits (or risks) of a treatment is based on an assessment of the absolute risk reduction (ARR) and the number needed to treat (NNT). The NNT is the number of patients who must be treated to produce one individual who has the given response, either desired or harmful. For example, if a treatment reduces the mortality of a disease from 5% to 2.5%, the ARR is 0.025 and, on average, the NNT (given by 1/ARR) is 40. For every 40 treated, one life would be saved.

Meta-analysis

For some conditions, it may be difficult to recruit many subjects, and the ensuing small trials may produce inconclusive results. Meta-analysis is a procedure for combining the results of several independent trials with the hope of achieving a significant result. (The constituent trials must of course have been properly designed.)

Ethical principles

Ethical principles are clearly a major issue in clinical trials. Independent ethics committees should always approve the design and conduct of clinical trials.

The therapeutic index, TD_{50} and LD_{50}

A proper measure of a drug's value depends on a benefit–risk assessment. Very few drugs have no untoward effects; the amount of risk that is tolerated depends on the seriousness of the condition being treated. Greater risks will be accepted in the treatment of a life-threatening condition than for a trivial ailment (headache). A simple measure of benefit versus risk is the therapeutic index, (TI), where:

$$TI = \frac{TD_{50}}{ED_{50}} \text{ or } \frac{LD_{50}}{ED_{50}}$$

The TD_{50} is the dose required to produce a toxic effect in 50% of the subjects (the median toxic dose) and the ED_{50} is the median effective dose. In animal studies, toxicity may be measured by death, in which case the median lethal dose (LD_{50}) replaces the TD_{50}. Clearly if the TD_{50}, or LD_{50}, is much greater than the ED_{50} then the TI will be large and the drug might be considered to have a large safety margin. The LD_{50}, necessarily measured in animals, is a poor measure of human toxicity since:

- it measures only death, not other potentially serious sublethal effects
- it will almost certainly be different in experimental animals compared with humans
- it is a measure of acute toxicity and neglects long-term adverse effects
- it takes no account of idiosyncratic responses, i.e. it will not allow for the rare individuals who are much more sensitive to the drug (often genetically determined).

Although it is almost impossible to quantify the TI in a satisfactory way, the concept is a valuable one.

6 Absorption and distribution of drugs

It is clinically important to know how drug concentrations in the tissues change with time, i.e. to understand the pharmacokinetic aspects of drug action. The time course of drug action usually follows that of the concentration at the target site. Important exceptions are drugs that bind irreversibly (e.g. organophosphorous anticholinesterases), where the effect can outlive the concentration. Following absorption, drugs are carried to their targets in the body and their sites of elimination by the blood circulation. Well-perfused tissues, such as the lungs and kidney, can equilibrate with the plasma concentration quickly, whereas, poorly perfused tissues, such as fat, will only take up and release drugs slowly. Once a drug arrives at a tissue, it must pass out of the blood capillaries and possibly cross cell membrane barriers, either to reach its target or to pass into the urine or bile. Accordingly, a drug's ability to cross cell membranes is of major concern in pharmacokinetics.

Membrane permeation by drugs

The plasma membrane of cells constitutes a hydrophobic lipid barrier and drug permeation can occur by:

- direct diffusion through the lipid
- carrier-mediated transport
- diffusion through aqueous pores
- pinocytosis.

The first two mechanisms are most important; aqueous pores are too small to allow the passage of most drugs (which typically have molecular weights in the range 200–1000) and pinocytosis is thought to be important for only a few large molecules (e.g. insulin penetration of the blood–brain barrier).

Diffusion through membrane lipid

Diffusion of a drug depends on its concentration gradient and its diffusion coefficient. The concentration gradient established within the cell membrane depends on the drug's lipid/water partition coefficient. This is conveniently estimated by the drug's distribution between water and a simple organic solvent, such as heptane. (There is a good correlation between such partition coefficients and drug absorption.)

Ionisation

Most drugs, being weak acids or weak bases, ionise to some extent in aqueous solution. The ionised form is *lipophobic*, so that ionisation impedes passive membrane permeation.

The fractional ionisation can be determined from the *Henderson–Hasselbalch* equation:

$$\text{for a weak acid: } \log_{10} c_i/c_u = \text{pH} - \text{p}K_a$$

$$\text{for a weak base: } \log_{10} c_i/c_u = \text{p}K_a - \text{pH}$$

Where c_i is the concentration of drug in ionised form, c_u is that in unionised form, pK_a is $-\log_{10}$ of the acid dissociation constant for the drug and pH is $-\log_{10}$ of the hydrogen ion concentration.

Ionisation thus depends on the pH of the aqueous environment and the drug's acid dissociation constant (a strong acid has a low pK_a and a strong base has a high pK_a; Fig. 6.1).

Ion trapping

Where a lipid membrane separates solutions of different pH, the difference in ionisation on the two sides can lead to an uneven distribution. The ionised molecules do not readily cross the membrane and there is an effective trapping of them on the side promoting ionisation. A weak base such as morphine, even when given intravenously, will achieve a high concentration in the acidic gastric lumen (Fig. 6.2).

Active transport

Carriers are important for membrane transport of essential nutrients that have low lipid solubility. Most drugs are exogenous substances of no nutritional value and are not substrates for the carriers involved in nutrient absorption or delivery to cells (exceptions include the anticancer agent 5-fluorouracil, an analogue of uracil, which can utilise the transporter for pyrimidines in the gut). Active transport systems in the kidney and liver are, by comparison very important in the elimination of drugs from the body. (Such carriers have probably evolved for the clearance of toxic substances that might have been ingested and whose rapid elimination would have survival value.) Active transport (via the P-glycoprotein transporter) is also an important mechanism for resistance to anticancer drugs.

Features of active drug transport are:

- uphill transport (allowing high renal clearances)
- a finite number of transporter molecules leading to:
  —Saturation.
  —Competition between drugs for transport. Exacerbated by the low substrate specificity of many carriers.

Drug absorption

Drugs can be administered via the gut (enteral) or by other routes (parenteral).

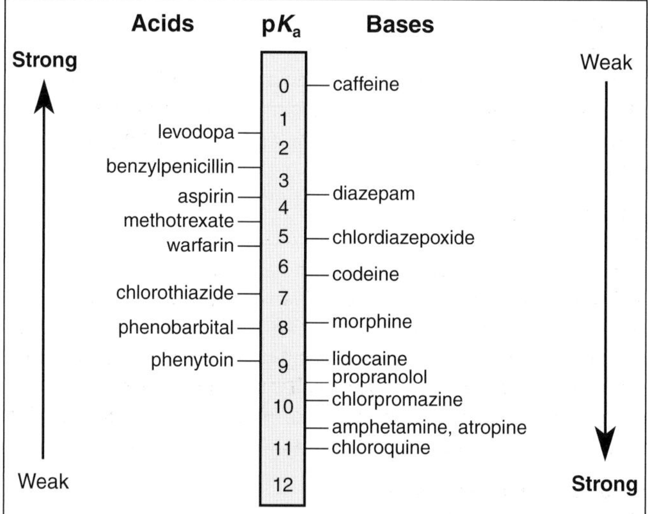

Fig. 6.1 Examples of some pK_a values of selected drugs.

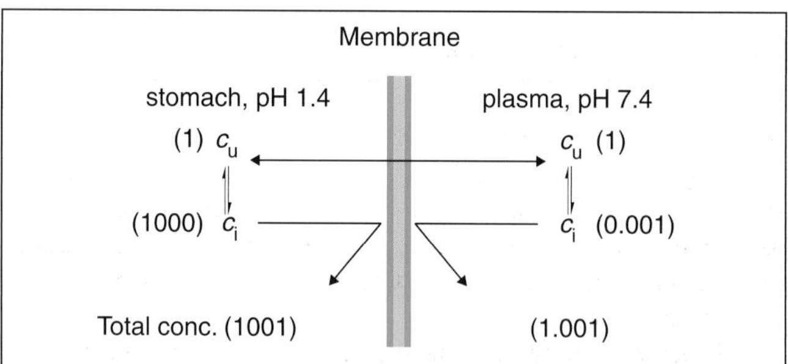

Fig. 6.2 Ion trapping. In this theoretical example, a weak base with a pK_a of 4.4 is shown concentrating in the stomach.

Enteral administration

Oral absorption from the stomach or intestines, after the drug is swallowed, is the most convenient and acceptable route. An important consideration is that oral absorption will deliver the drug directly to the liver, the major site of drug metabolism, via the portal circulation; this may result in substantial *first-pass elimination*. Drug absorbed from the mouth (*sublingual* or buccal) and the lower rectum does not enter the hepatic portal vein and so avoids first-pass metabolism. Sublingual glyceryl trinitrate is rapidly absorbed to provide quick relief of anginal pain (it is ineffective if swallowed). Rectal administration is suitable for some irritants and if vomiting prevents oral medication.

Factors controlling oral absorption

Lipid solubility and ionisation This is discussed above. Note that the intestine with its villi and microvilli is the main absorptive area, so that weak acids, which will be less ionised in the stomach, will, nevertheless, be mostly absorbed in the more alkaline intestine. Rapid passage of drug from the stomach to intestine is likely to speed up drug absorption.

Drug formulation Drugs must dissolve to establish a concentration gradient for absorption, the rate and extent of absorption depending on the pharmaceutical formulation. Rapid absorption of a tablet requires its disintegration into small particles that readily dissolve. Note that while a drug is more water soluble in its ionised form, it is the unionised form that is membrane permeable. *Sustained release* formulations release the drug slowly to prolong drug action and reduce the frequency of administration.

Gastrointestinal motility Stasis can slow oral absorption while diarrhoea, predictably, may allow insufficient time for complete absorption.

Interactions with other substances in the gut Food in general will slow absorption by simply reducing the drug's concentration. More specific interactions can also occur; for example tetracyclines will interact with Ca^{2+} in food to form an incompletely absorbed, insoluble complex.

Bioavailability

Bioavailability is a term applied particularly to oral preparations and expresses the extent to which a dose is absorbed. The most useful definition is *the proportion of the administered dose that reaches the systemic circulation*. Incomplete release from the dosage form, destruction within the gut, poor absorption and first-pass elimination are important causes of low bioavailability. For drugs with a low therapeutic index, it is important that repeat prescriptions provide medicines of equivalent bioavailability (*bioequivalence*).

Parenteral administration

These routes are useful for

- rapid effects (e.g. in status asthmaticus)
- drugs that are poorly absorbed from the gut (e.g. pancuronium, insulin)
- irritants (some anticancer agents)
- localisation of action (e.g. inhaled bronchodilators, mydriatics).

Intravenous (i.v.) injection is the most rapid route, i.v. infusions allowing tight control of drug concentration in the plasma. *Intramuscular* (i.m.) and *subcutaneous* (s.c.) injection have found particular utility in providing long-term therapy from *depot* preparations (e.g. contraceptive steroid implants or slowly released antipsychotic agents).

Inhalation is used for anaesthetic gases and in treatment of bronchial asthma with bronchodilators and anti-inflammatory steroids.

Topical application of drugs to the skin is used mainly for local actions, but systemic absorption of very lipid-soluble substances is possible (e.g. hyoscine patches to prevent motion sickness).

Drug distribution

Most drugs entering the body do not spread rapidly throughout the whole of body water to achieve a uniform concentration. Large molecules (heparin, insulin) cannot easily enter interstitial and intracellular spaces whereas smaller and lipid-soluble molecules can.

A drug's penetration into these compartments is indicated by its *apparent volume of distribution* (V_d): the volume of fluid that would be required to hold the amount of drug in the body at the measured plasma concentration. It can be estimated by the equation:

$$V_d = \text{Dose}/c_p$$

where c_p is the concentration of drug in the plasma after it has equilibrated in its distribution volume but before a significant fraction has been eliminated. Examples of V_d values (l/kg) are:

- heparin 0.05–0.1
- tubocurarine 0.2–0.4
- ethanol 1.0
- propranolol 2–5
- nortriptyline >20.

Binding to protein and other tissue components

Tetracyclines bind to calcium in bones and teeth (which can produce abnormalities in tooth development in children). Many drugs bind to plasma proteins of which albumin is generally the most important, although α-acid glycoprotein is of greater importance for some basic drugs (e.g. propranolol). For some drugs, more than 95% of drug in plasma may be bound to protein. Binding to plasma proteins is of finite capacity and of low specificity and has several consequences:

- Bound drug is usually inactive.
- The reduction in free drug concentration may reduce elimination (by reducing glomerular filtration) or, conversely, protein binding may serve to deliver drug to the kidney and liver, and so enhance elimination.
- One drug may prevent the binding of another, and so enhance pharmacological activity. (This is of significance only for highly bound drugs, such as warfarin, whose displacement and resulting increased activity can cause bleeding)

Accumulation in lipid

Lipid-soluble drugs may concentrate in adipose tissue. For example, halothane can concentrate in fat during long operations and its slow release can lead to prolonged CNS depression postoperatively.

Penetration of drugs into the brain

The endothelial cells lining brain capillaries are joined to each other by tight junctions to produce an unbroken cell membrane lining, which is the main element of the blood–brain barrier. This prevents passive entry into the brain of lipophobic/ionised molecules. An additional feature is the turnover of cerebrospinal fluid. This is produced by the choroid plexuses, flows through the ventricles and after reaching the outer surface of the brain drains into the blood at the arachnoid villi. Drugs that penetrate slowly will be removed by 'washout' in this way and achieve a steady-state concentration much below the plasma concentration.

7 Drug metabolism and excretion

The effects of a drug depend not only on its pharmacological actions but also on how it is handled in the body. When a drug enters the body, it is subjected, in essence, to the processes that have been developed for dealing with toxic foreign molecules—it is metabolised and/or excreted. The liver is the main site of drug metabolism and the kidney the main site of excretion. Metabolism involves two main processes: first, the molecule is made more lipophobic so as to reduce the possibility of reabsorption in the renal tubules; secondly, it is conjugated so as to reduce its effects and aid excretion. With some drugs, the metabolites share the actions of the parent drug (e.g. diazepam and its metabolite nordazepam). With other drugs the metabolite may be responsible for toxicity (e.g. paracetamol). Some drugs are prodrugs–inactive themselves but converted into an active drug within the body; for example, enalapril is hydrolysed to the active compound enalaprilat and minoxidil is activated by conjugation. Some drugs can modify their own metabolism and that of other drugs by induction of the hepatic enzymes. For many drugs there are two phases of metabolism.

The phases of drug metabolism

Phase I comprises the following reactions:
- oxidation (Fig. 7.1), e.g. propranolol, paracetamol
- reduction, e.g. prednisone
- hydrolysis, e.g. procaine, suxamethonium.

Phase II comprises the following conjugation reactions:
- glucuronidation, e.g. morphine
- glycosidation
- sulfation, e.g. paracetamol
- methylation
- acetylation, e.g. sulfonamides, isoniazid
- amino acid (esp. glycine) conjugation
- glutathione conjugation, e.g. paracetamol.

The phase I oxidation reactions by the hepatic P450 monooxygenase system are perhaps the most important.

The P450 monooxygenase system

The oxidation of a drug by the monooxygenase system requires:
- the cytochrome P450 haem protein: a membrane protein in the smooth endoplasmic reticulum
- molecular oxygen
- cytochrome P450 reductase (which is closely associated with cytochrome P450)
- NADPH.

The cytochrome P450 reductase catalyses the following reaction (cyto, cytochrome):

$$\text{NADPH} + \text{Oxidised cyto} + \text{H}^+ \rightarrow \text{Reduced cyto} + \text{NADP}^+$$

During the reaction, two electrons—required for the subsequent oxidation reaction—are generated. During the oxidation of a drug molecule by the P450 system, the cytochrome P450 undergoes cyclic oxidation/reduction as shown in Figure 7.1. Table 7.1 gives examples of drugs metabolised by oxidation.

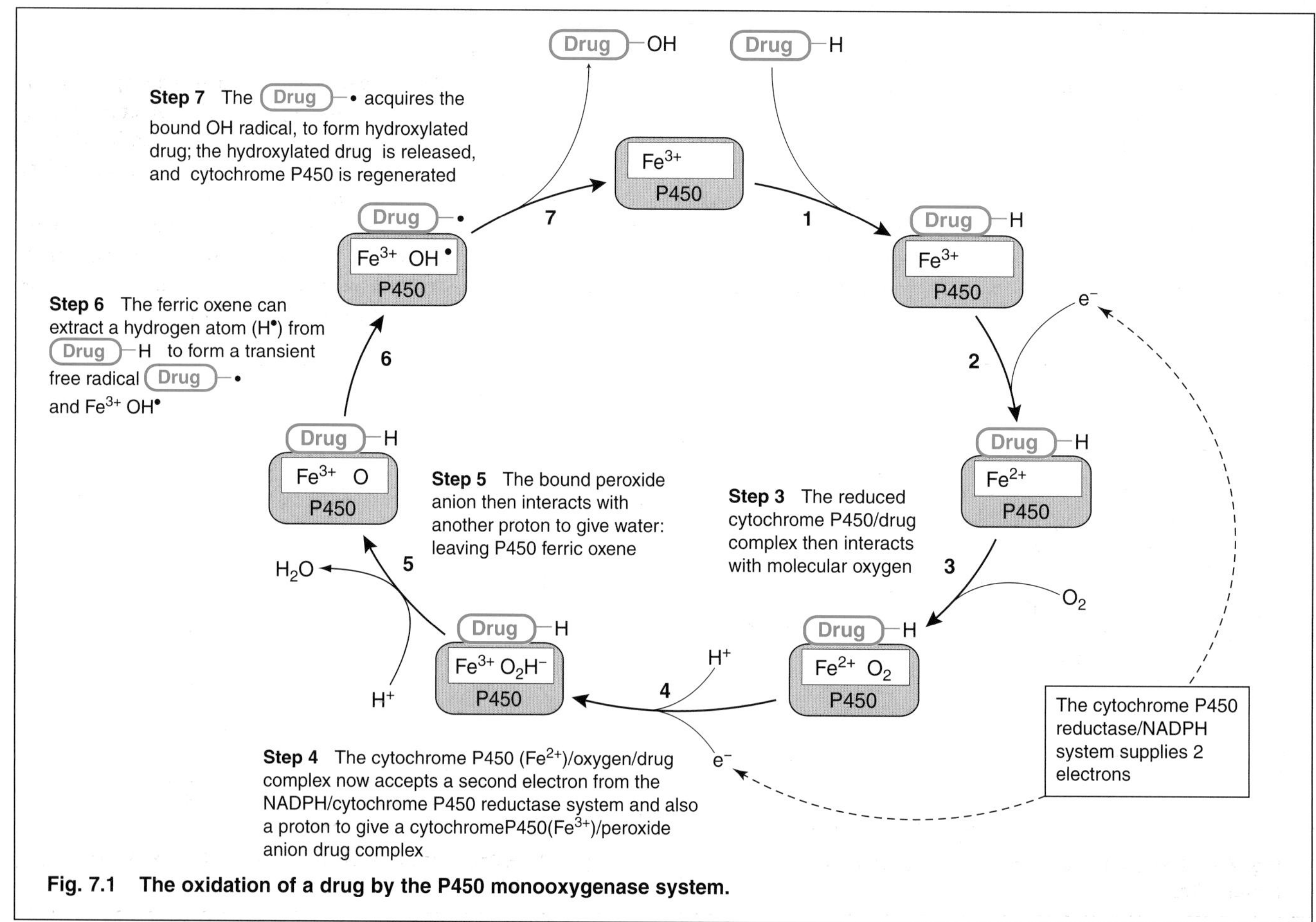

Fig. 7.1 The oxidation of a drug by the P450 monooxygenase system.

Table 7.1 Examples of drugs metabolised by P450 monooxygenase oxidation reactions

Reactions	Drugs
O-dealkylation	Codeine, dextromethorphan (Ch. 41), indometacin (Ch. 15)
Aliphatic hydroxylation	Ibuprofen (Ch. 15), ciclosporin (Ch. 16)
Deamination	Amphetamines (Chs 11 and 42)
N-dealkylation	Morphine (Ch. 40), diazepam (Ch. 36), tamoxifen (Ch. 49)
N-oxidation	Chlorphenamine (Ch. 15), dapsone (Ch. 49)
S-oxidation	Cimetidine (Ch. 26), thioridazine (Ch. 38)
Aromatic hydroxylation	Propranolol (Ch. 11), phenytoin (Ch. 40)

The activity of the cytochrome P450 system can be markedly increased by exposure to other drugs or dietary factors; such enzyme induction can reduce the effect of a drug. Other drugs may potentiate drug action by inhibiting the P450 system.

The excretion of drugs and their metabolites

The kidney is the principal organ of excretion of drugs and their metabolites but some compounds are excreted in the bile and some by other routes such as the lungs.

Renal excretion

Renal excretion involves the following processes.

Filtration in the glomerulus Arterial blood pressure forces an ultrafiltrate from the glomerular capillaries into Bowman's capsule (Fig. 7.2). Small drug molecules (M_r < 5000) in both charged and uncharged states cross the glomerular membranes readily, achieving a concentration in the filtrate identical to their free concentration in the plasma. (Negatively charged sialoproteins in the capillary wall can impede the filtration of larger, negatively charged molecules.) Drug molecules bound to plasma proteins are not filtered.

Active tubular secretion This occurs in the proximal convoluted tubule. About 80% of drugs or metabolites pass from the glomerulus via the efferent arterioles to the peritubular capillaries that surround the proximal convoluted tubule; here the agents become available for active transport into the tubule. In the basolateral area of the tubule, there are low-specificity carriers for organic anions and organic cations, which transport endogenous substances and drugs from the plasma into the tubular cell from where they pass into the filtrate by facilitated diffusion (Fig. 7.2).

Drugs actively secreted Some organic acids that are secreted are the **penicillins**, **probenecid**, some diuretics (**furosemide**, **thiazides**) and various conjugates (glycine, glucuronic acid, sulfate). Some organic cations that are secreted are morphine, amiloride (a K^+-sparing diuretic) and quaternary ammonium compounds such as the cholinoceptor agonists and antagonists. The carriers may have sufficient activity to clear the drug completely from the blood passing through the kidney. Tubular secretion of one drug may be competitively inhibited by another; in this way the half-life of penicillin is markedly increased by probenecid.

Reabsorption from the tubules

Drugs within the tubules in the unionised form and lipid-soluble will be reabsorbed. A weak acid, such as aspirin, will thus be more readily excreted in alkaline rather than acidic urine. The ratio of ionised to unionised acid is given by 10^{pH-pK_a}.

Taking the pK_a of aspirin as 3.4, the ratio of ionised to unionised drug in the urine at a pH value of 6.4 will be $10^{6.4-3.4} = 10^3$ = 1000:1. At pH 8.4, it will be $10^{8.4-3.4} = 10^5$ = 100000:1.

At both pH values, very little of the drug will be in the unionised, membrane permeant form. Nevertheless, the proportion at the lower pH will be 100 times that at the higher pH. This allows much more reabsorption at the lower pH and has a dramatic effect on the clearance of aspirin as shown in Figure 7.3. This is effectively an example of ion trapping as described in Ch. 6. The enhanced elimination of weakly acidic drugs at high urinary pH is made use of in the process of forced alkaline diuresis.

Hepatic excretion

Bile is produced at a daily rate of 0.5–1 litre and is a major route of excretion for a few drugs (e.g. cromoglycate) and rather more drug metabolites (e.g. morphine glucuronide). Drug excreted in bile may be reabsorbed from the intestine to undergo further cycles of biliary excretion: so-called *enterohepatic circulation*. A significant proportion of drug in the body may be held in this *enteric pool*, which may act to increase the drug's half-life. Drugs pass from blood to bile by active transport and competition may occur. The transporters differ from those found in the kidney.

Fig. 7.2 Renal sites of excretion of drugs and metabolites.

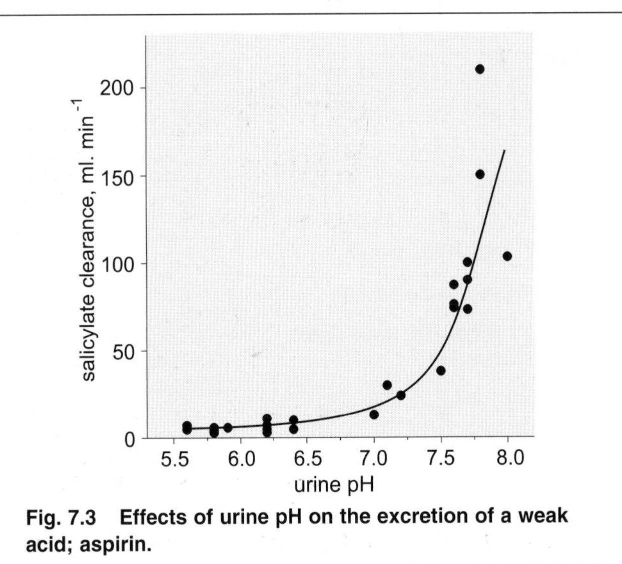

Fig. 7.3 Effects of urine pH on the excretion of a weak acid; aspirin.

8 Pharmacokinetics

Pharmacokinetics explores the changes in drug concentrations throughout the body with time. An appreciation of this is important for understanding drug effects. Let us start with the concept of compartments.

Compartments

Whole body autoradiographs and chemical analysis of tissues show that drugs do not penetrate uniformly throughout the body. Particular tissues may well show higher or lower concentrations of drug than the plasma. Some tissues, however, may behave similarly (i.e. have similar drug concentration versus time profiles); it is then convenient to consider them as belonging to a common *compartment*. It is usual to adopt the minimum number of compartments (usually one or two) that can adequately describe the time course of drug disposition and predict the changes in concentrations that occur following administration. For many drugs, the volume of distribution (V_d, see Ch. 6) appears to be a single entity and the situation is consistent with the *one-compartment model*. For other drugs, it is found that different tissues equilibrate with the drug at different rates. Where the tissues fall easily into two groups (e.g. well perfused and poorly perfused) a *two-compartment model* is sometimes applicable. Compartment 1 comprises the plasma and rapidly equilibrating tissues (e.g. lung and kidney). Compartment 2 represents the remaining more slowly equilbrating tissues (Fig. 8.1).

One-compartment distribution kinetics

Where passive diffusion is responsible for absorption or excretion, drug transport is often *first order*, i.e. the rate is proportional to the concentration gradient. First-order kinetics is exemplified by the exponentially declining plasma concentration of drug, c_p, which follows first-order elimination after i.v administration (Fig. 8.2A):

$$c_p = c_p(0)e^{-k_{el}t}$$

where c_p is the drug concentration in plasma, $c_p(0)$ is initial plasma concentration at time $t = 0$ and k_{el} is the elimination rate constant.

The relationship may be linearized by taking logarithms (Fig. 8.2B). For natural logarithms (ln):

$$\ln c_p = \ln c_p(0) - k_{el}t$$

A plot of ln c_p against t gives a straight line of slope $-k_{el}$.

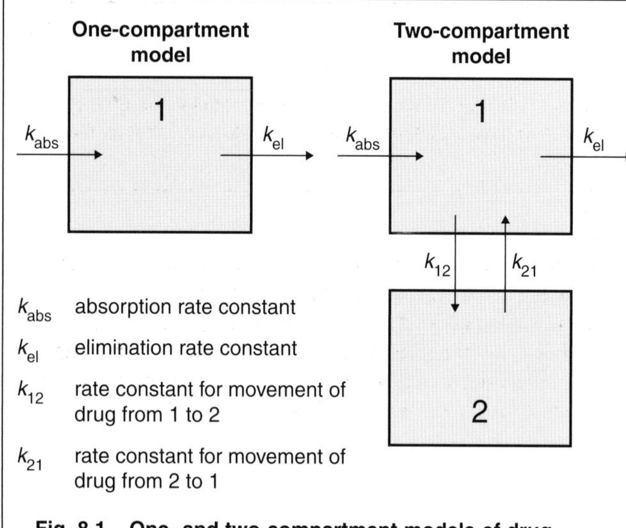

Fig. 8.1 One- and two-compartment models of drug distribution. In the 2-compartment model, absorption and elimination are to and from compartment 1, respectively.

The *plasma half-life*, ($t_{1/2}$ or $t_{0.5}$) applicable to drugs subject to first-order elimination is the time taken for any given plasma concentration to decrease by 50% ($t_{1/2}$ is inversely related to k_{el}: $t_{1/2} = 0.693/k_{el}$).

Zero-order kinetics refers to the situation where the rate of the process (e.g. drug metabolism) is independent of the drug's concentration.

Carrier-mediated transport of drugs and enzymic biotransformations are saturable phenomena that, in the steady state, follow *Michaelis–Menten* kinetics. Where such a process lowers c_p:

$$-\frac{dc_p}{dt} = \frac{V_{max}c_p}{c_p + K_M}$$

where V_{max} is the maximum rate of transport or biotransformation and K_M is the Michaelis constant. When the drug concentration is high (relative to K_m), this reduces to:

$$-\frac{dc_p}{dt} \approx V_{max}$$

At this point the elimination process is saturated and, being independent of concentration, obeys zero-order kinetics (c_p declines at a fixed rate, Fig. 8.2C). Zero-order kinetics applies to many drugs at high concentrations and to some at 'low' concentrations (e.g. ethanol).

Two-compartment kinetics

The kinetics of the two-compartment model will obviously be more complicated and the plot of ln c_p versus time after i.v. administration will not yield a straight line. Figure 8.3 shows drug concentrations in compartments 1 and 2 following i.v. injection. For first-order distribution and elimination, the decay of the plasma concentration of the drug will follow a biexponential curve.

Drug clearance

Drug clearance (*Cl*) is defined as the volume of plasma cleared of drug per unit time. (Usual units are ml/min.) Thus (assuming first-order, one-compartment behaviour):

$$\text{Clearance} = \frac{\text{Elimination rate}}{\text{Plasma concentration}}$$

The elimination rate is also given by the amount of drug in body (c_pV_d) multiplied by k_{el}. Therefore,

$$Cl = \frac{k_{el}c_pV_d}{c_p} = k_{el}V_d$$

As $k_{el} = 0.693/t_{½}$. clearance = $0.693V_d/t_{½}$.

Total body clearance is the sum of the clearances occurring by whatever routes are applicable to the drug in question; often only renal and hepatic clearances are important.

Repeated drug administration

Drugs are commonly given as repeated doses using a fixed *dosing interval*. Since most drugs are eliminated exponentially, whenever a second dose is administered some of the preceding dose will still be in the body and the new peak concentration achieved will exceed that after the first dose i.e. *cumulation* occurs (Fig. 8.4). With repeated doses c_p, and hence elimination, increases until a plateau is reached where the whole of the dose is eliminated during the dosing

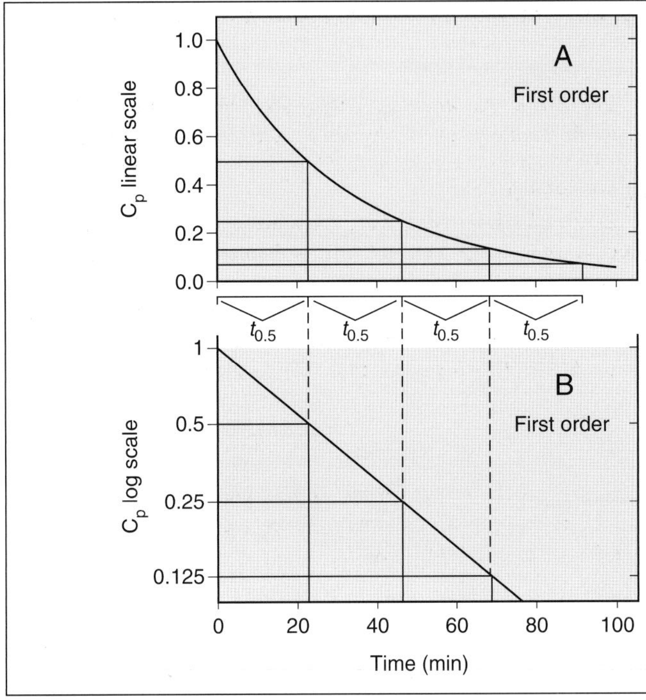

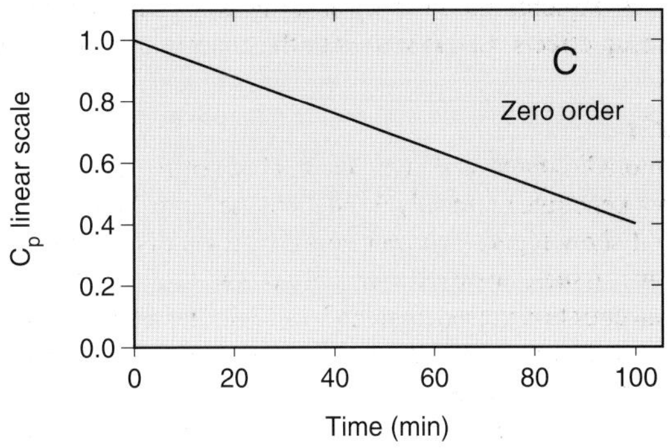

Fig. 8.2 Elimination of drugs. (A) First-order linear concentration scale; (B) first-order logarithmic scale. In first order, C_p decreases by half in successive half-lives (half-life here is 23 min) (C) shows the constant rate of elimination according to zero-order kinetics (here 0.006 units/min).

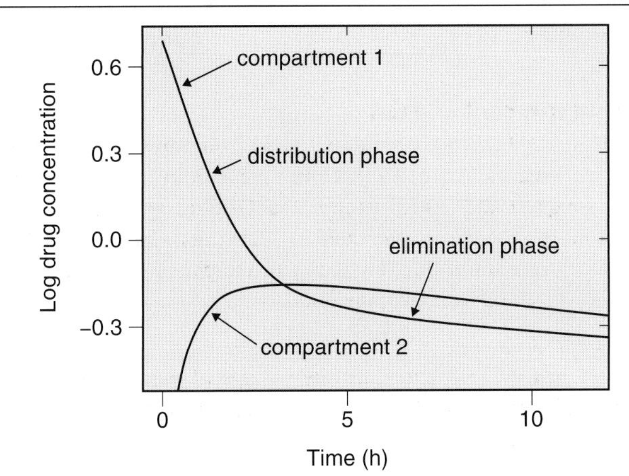

Fig. 8.3 Changes in drug concentrations in a two-compartment model of drug distribution following i.v. administration. Concentration falls quickly in compartment 1 as drug distributes into compartment 2. Note logarithmic concentration scale.

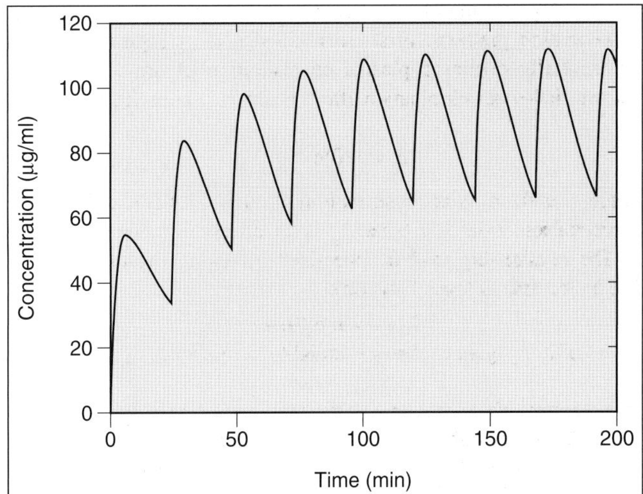

Fig. 8.4 Drug cumulation. Incomplete elimination of drug during the dosing interval results in a build up of drug in the plasma.

interval. Paradoxically, the rate of approach to the plateau is determined by the elimination rate constant rather than the absorption rate constant. A drug with a long half-life (e.g. digoxin) will thus approach the plateau concentration slowly. If this is undesirable, initial *loading doses* can be employed.

The clearance concept can be usefully employed to determine the expected steady-state concentration of drug in the plasma, c_{ss}, during an infusion or regular intermittent dosing. In the steady state, the rate of drug administration (e.g. 500 mg per day) will equal the rate of loss (elimination rate, i.e. $Cl \times c_{ss}$). Therefore, c_{ss} is given by the dose rate divided by the clearance. Alternatively, by knowing the clearance of a drug and the desired target plasma concentration it is possible to calculate the required dose rate ($c_{ss} \times Cl$).

9 The autonomic nervous system

The autonomic nervous system (ANS) regulates smooth muscle tone and cardiac function. It also has actions on exocrine and some endocrine secretions and on intermediate metabolism. An autonomic pathway consists of two neurons, pre- and postganglionic, with the synapse (junction between the axon of one nerve and the cell body of another) in the autonomic ganglion.

There are two major divisions of the ANS, the **parasympathetic** and **sympathetic** (see Fig. 9.1). The **enteric nervous system** of the gut, a third division, is under the influence of the former two. Sympathetic and parasympathetic actions are often in opposite directions (e.g. the control of heart rate and force and contraction of the smooth muscle of the iris or of the gastrointestinal (GI) tract) but in some tissues the action of one branch is unopposed (e.g. contraction of ciliary muscle by parasympathetic action).

The sympathetic nervous system

The cell bodies of sympathetic preganglionic neurons are found in the lumbar and thoracic spinal cord. The preganglionic nerve fibres synapse with postganglionic neurons either just outside the spinal cord, in the **paravertebral chains**, or in the **midline (prevertebral) ganglia**. The preganglionic fibres branch and synapse with postganglionic neurons in several segments above and below their

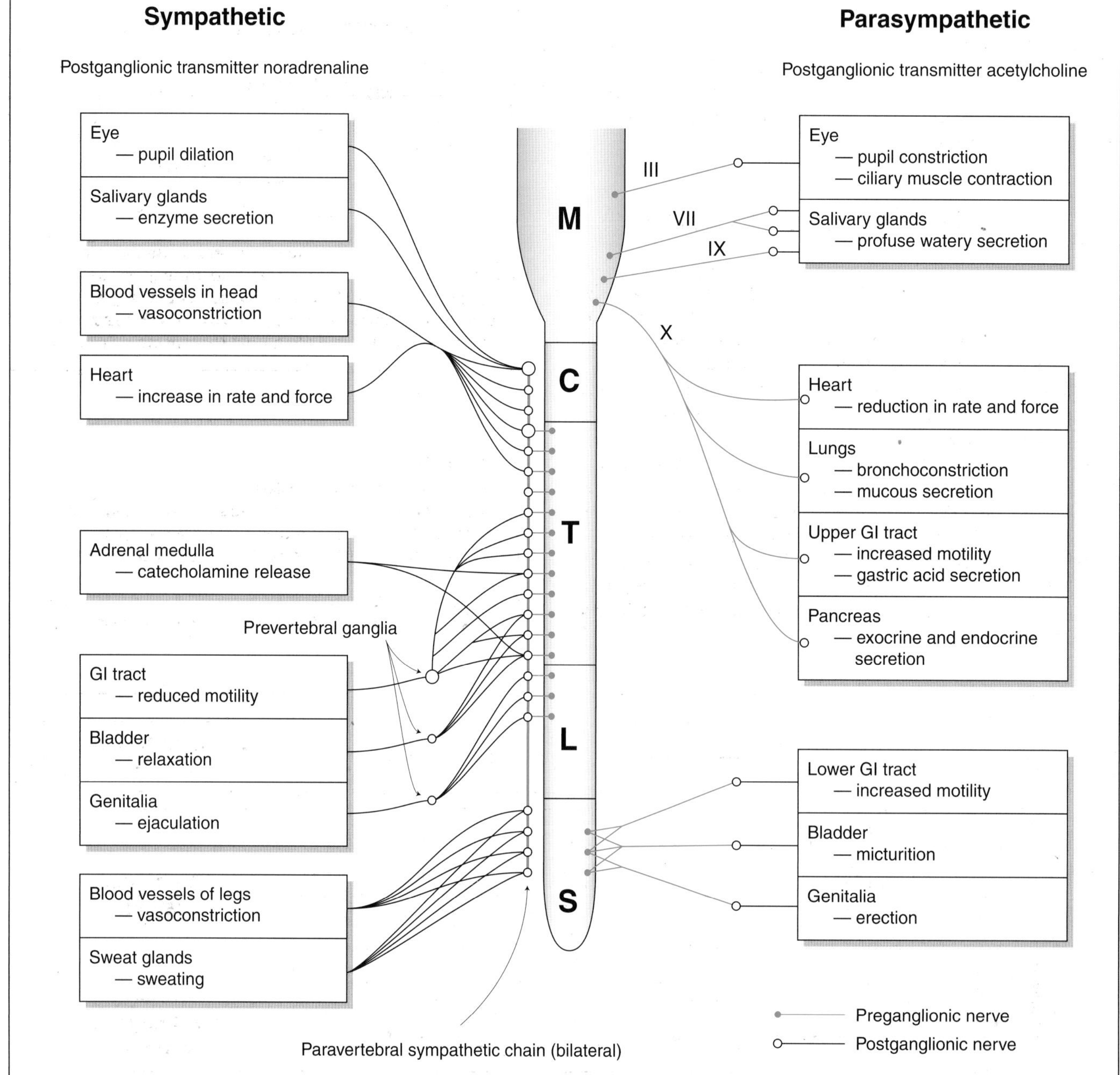

Fig. 9.1 The basic layout of the autonomic nervous system with illustrative actions. (M, medullary; C, cervical; T, thoracic; L, lumbar; S, sacral; III, VII, IX and X, cranial nerves.)

origin in the spinal cord — an anatomical basis for a diffuse response. Many of the postganglionic fibres from the sympathetic chain join the spinal nerves.

Widespread sympathetic effects also result from the release of catecholamines from the adrenal medulla.

The parasympathetic nervous system

Parasympathetic preganglionic fibres leave the CNS in the cranial nerves (III, VII, IX and X) and in spinal roots from the sacral region of the spinal cord. In contrast to their sympathetic counterparts, parasympathetic ganglia lie close to the target sites and the postganglionic fibres are often entirely within the tissue of the target organ. Most parasympathetic preganglionic fibres connect with only a few postganglionic fibres — an anatomical basis for discrete, localised responses.

The enteric nervous system

The enteric nervous system consists of neurons with cell bodies in the plexuses in the intestinal wall. Autonomic nerves terminate on these cells but the system can operate autonomously in the control of peristalsis and secretion.

NEUROTRANSMITTERS AND CO-TRANSMITTERS

Neurotransmitters are chemicals released by the terminus of an axon in order to transmit an impulse across the synaptic junction. The two main neurotransmitters in the ANS are **acetylcholine** (ACh) and **noradrenaline** (NA, or norepinephrine), released from postganglionic parasympathetic and sympathetic neurons, respectively (Fig. 9.2). An important exception is the autonomic innervation of sweat glands: although these are anatomically part of the sympathetic system the nerves utilise ACh.

All preganglionic neurons and somatic motor nerves release ACh. NANC (non-adrenergic, non-cholinergic) transmitters occur as primary transmitters in enteric neurons and sensory neurons and as co-transmitters with NA and ACh in autonomic nerves; examples include **ATP, GABA** (gamma-aminobutyric acid), **5HT** (5-hydroxytryptamine), **dopamine, NO** (nitric oxide) and **peptides** (e.g. enkephalins, somatostatin, vasoactive intestinal peptide and neuropeptide Y).

Co-transmitters are released together with neurotransmitters and commonly have a response speed that differs from that of NA or ACh (Fig. 9.3). The terminus of a presynaptic nerve carries several different kinds of presynaptic receptor that will modulate the release of the neurotransmitter (e.g. NA acting on α_2-adrenoceptors inhibits ACh release from parasympathetic nerves in the GI tract and stimulation of opioid receptors will inhibit NA release in various tissues).

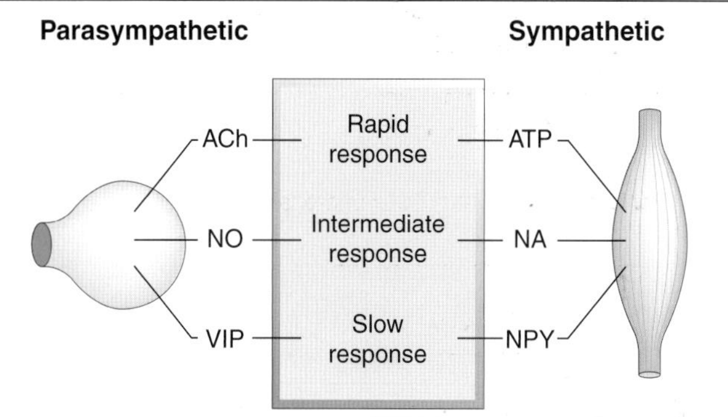

Fig. 9.3 The main co-transmitters at postganglionic parasympathetic and sympathetic neurons give rise to fast, intermediate and slow responses of the target tissue. (ACh, acetylcholine; NO, nitric oxide; VIP, vasoactive intestinal peptide; NA, noradrenaline; NPY, neuropeptide Y.)

Clinical uses

Drugs can be targeted to modulate
- release of ACh and NA directly through nerve stimulation
- release of ACh and NA through presynaptic receptors
- release of NANC (non-adrenergic, non-cholinergic) transmitters
- breakdown of ACh or NA
- postsynaptic reception of neurotransmitters/co-transmitters.

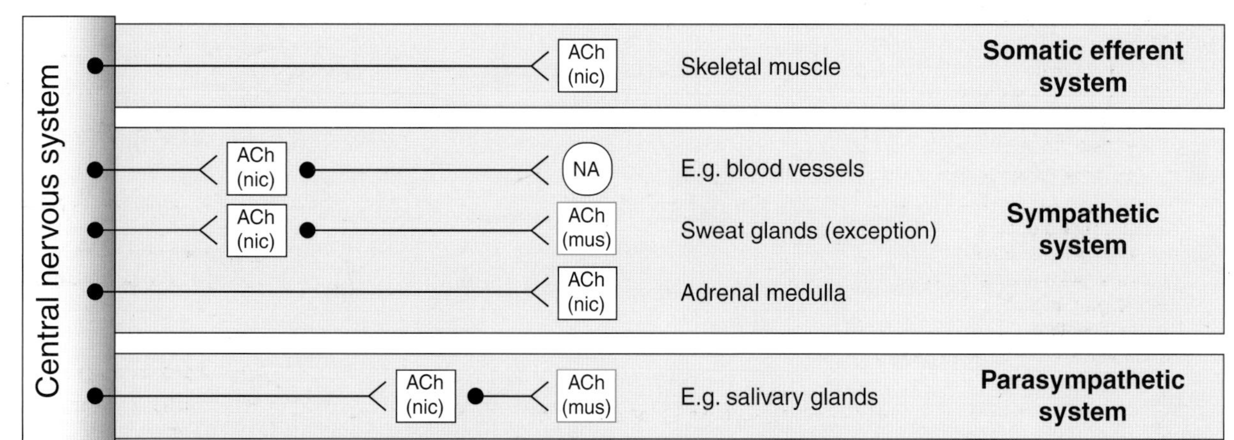

Fig. 9.2 Acetylcholine (ACh) and noradrenaline (NA) as transmitters in the peripheral nervous system. The location of nicotinic (nic) and muscarinic (mus) receptors are indicated

10 Cholinergic transmission

Acetylcholine (ACh) is the transmitter at the neuromuscular junction (NMJ), autonomic ganglia, postganglionic parasympathetic nerve endings and at various synapses in the CNS. It is produced in nerves and broken down by acetylcholinesterase (AChE). There are nicotinic and muscarinic receptors for ACh.

SYNTHESIS, STORAGE AND RELEASE OF ACETYLCHOLINE AND SUMMARY OF DRUG ACTION

ACh is an ester synthesised from choline and acetic acid (as acetyl-CoA) by choline acetyltransferase (CAT). It is stored in vesicles and released by Ca^{2+}-mediated exocytosis triggered by a nerve action potential. Uptake of choline into the nerve endings, and the storage and release of ACh, can each be inhibited though not in a clinically useful way. Modulation of ACh release by presynaptic receptors is likely to be an important physiological mechanism and may, for example, contribute to the effects of opioids on gut motility.

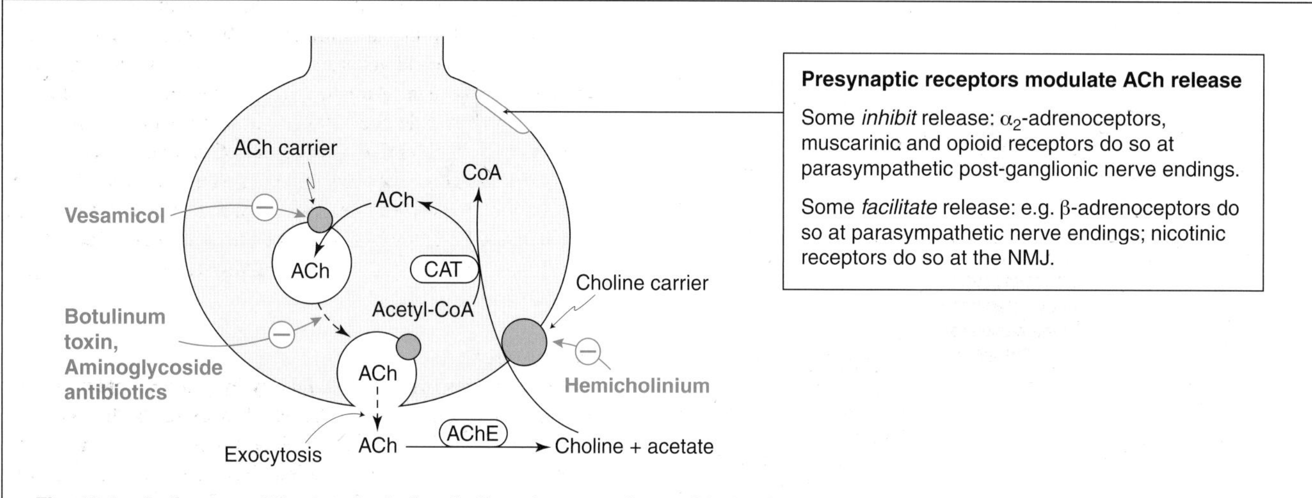

Fig. 10.1 A diagram of the terminal of a cholinergic nerve along with the drugs that can modify acetylcholine uptake into and release from the terminal acetylcholinesterase. AChE, acetylcholinesterase.

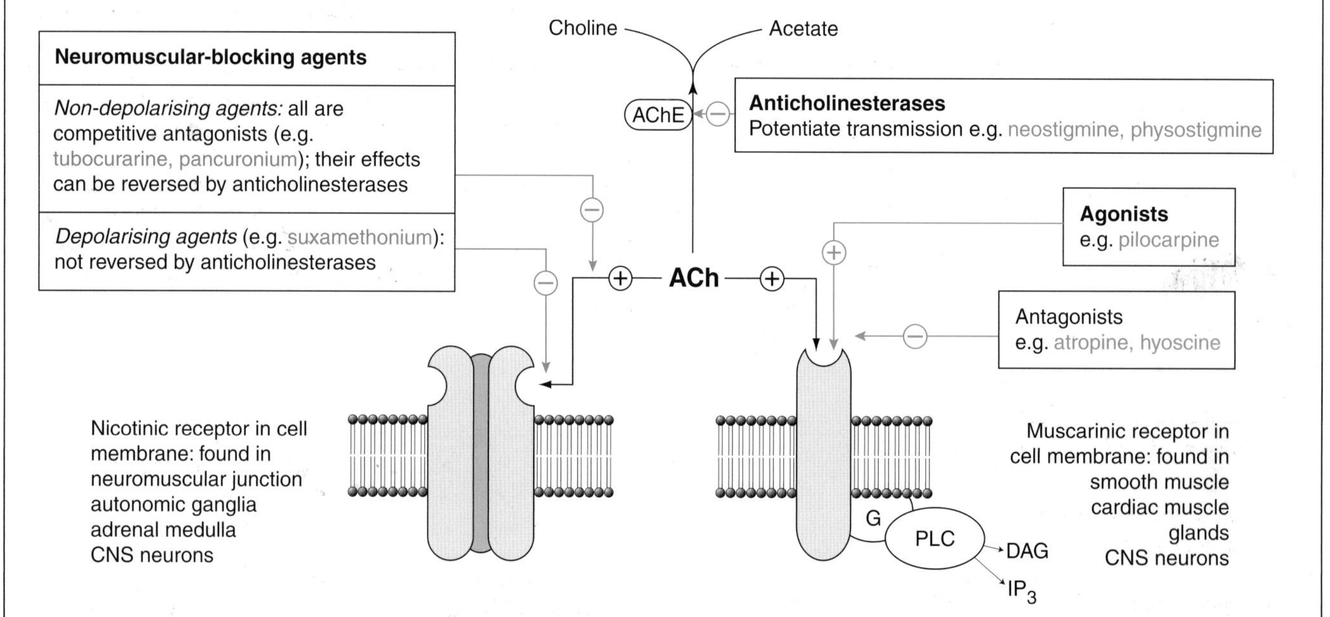

Fig. 10.2 Summary of the effects of released acetylcholine and the drugs that affect its actions. (PLC, phospholipase C; DAG, diacylglycerol; G, G-protein; IP_3, inositol trisphosphate; note that this PLC system is only one of several transduction systems that can be activated by muscarinic receptor stimulation in various cell types.)

NICOTINIC RECEPTORS

Drugs acting on nicotinic receptors

The main peripheral sites at which ACh acts on nicotinic receptors are:

- the NMJ at skeletal muscle
- autonomic (ANS) ganglia.

At both sites the receptors are mainly postsynaptic.

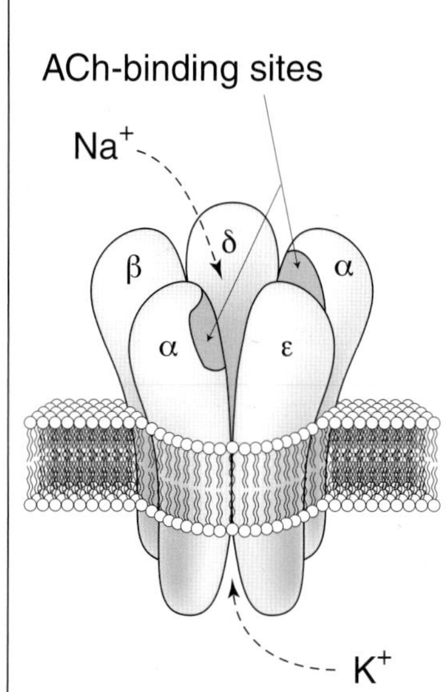

A nicotinic receptor is shown embedded in the cell membrane. It is a cation channel-forming protein comprising five subunits:

- NMJ: 2α, β, δ and ε
- neurons: 2α and 3β

To date, nine different α- and four different β-subunits have been cloned. Some drugs have selective actions on either neuronal or muscle type receptors. Channel opening allows Na^+ influx leading to membrane depolarization and action potential initiation.

Fig. 10.3 The structure of the nicotinic receptor.

Table 10.1 Examples of drugs acting on nicotinic receptors

	NMJ	ANS ganglia
Agonists	ACh*	ACh*
	Nicotine*	Nicotine*
	Suxamethonium	
	Decamethonium	
Antagonists	Tubocurarine	**Trimetaphan**
	Pancuronium	Mecamylamine
	Vecuronium	Hexamethonium*
	Atracurium	
	α-Bungarotoxin*	

*No clinical use, of historical or experimental interest.

Neuromuscular-blocking agents

Both agonists and antagonists can produce neuromuscular block (see table).

- ***Non-depolarising blocking agents.*** All those used clinically are competitive antagonists. Agents such as **pancuronium** reduce the size of the end-plate potential and so block transmission. Their effect can be reversed by anticholinesterases (see below), which increase the concentration of ACh at the receptor.
- ***Depolarising blocking agents.*** These activate the receptor and so, at least initially, cause some contraction of muscle fibres (e.g. **suxamethonium**). However, the maintained depolarisation which they produce causes the Na^+ channels in the muscle membrane adjacent to the end-plate to enter the inactivated state and thus prevents the end-plate potential from producing a propagated action potential. Anticholinesterases will not reverse depolarisation block since any increase in ACh concentration only serves to enhance the depolarisation.

Pharmacokinetic aspects

All the neuromuscular blockers are quaternary ammonium compounds, which penetrate cell membranes poorly. They are given intravenously. Durations of action are pancuronium, 1–2 h; vecuronium, 30–40 min; atracurium, <30 min; suxamethonium, 10 min. Pancuronium and vecuronium undergo both renal excretion and hepatic metabolism. Atracurium was designed to be largely broken down by a simple chemical reaction in the blood stream, so its duration of action, unlike that of the other antagonists, is not dependent on renal or hepatic function. The short half-life of suxamethonium, a choline ester, results from its rapid hydrolysis in the plasma. (A genetic variant — occurring in 1 in 2000 people — which reduces the activity of plasma cholinesterase can result in a duration of up to 2 h.)

Unwanted effects

Tubocurarine causes hypotension, mainly by ganglion block. It also releases histamine from mast cells, which adds to the hypotension and may cause bronchoconstriction. Pancuronium, vecuronium and atracurium are less prone to inducing these effects. Pancuronium has some antimuscarinic activity, which may cause tachycardia. Suxamethonium produces bradycardia (agonist action at muscarinic receptors) and a rise in intraocular pressure (contraction of extraocular muscles). In patients with severe trauma or burns, the K^+ efflux from skeletal muscle mediated by suxamethonium may increase plasma K^+ levels sufficiently to cause cardiac dysrhythmias.

Ganglion-blocking agents

Ganglion blockers have widespread and predictable actions consequent on blocking both sympathetic and parasympathetic transmission (e.g. hypotension from blocking sympathetic vasoconstriction, a dry mouth from blocking parasympathetic salivation, tachycardia by vagal block). Ganglion block is caused either by receptor antagonism (**trimetaphan**) or by direct channel block (**hexamethonium**). An excess of nicotine also causes ganglion block.

Clinical uses of drugs acting on nicotinic receptors

The main uses are in surgical procedures in anaesthetised patients.

- Neuromuscular-blocking drugs such as **suxamethonium**, **atracurium**, pancuronium, vecuronium, are used to produce muscle relaxation.
- A ganglion-blocking drug (**trimetaphan**) is used to produce controlled hypotension.

MUSCARINIC RECEPTORS

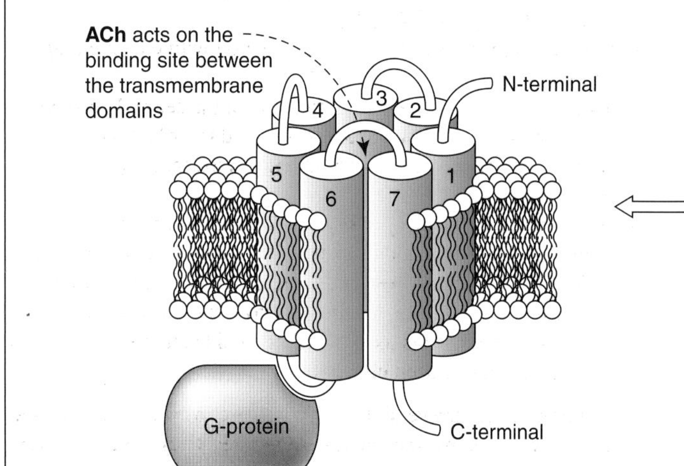

A muscarinic receptor is shown embedded in the cell membrane. Muscarinic receptors are members of the G-protein-coupled receptor family, having 7 transmembrane segments in their amino acid sequence. Five muscarinic receptor subtypes (M_1–M_5) have been cloned, though only 3 (M_1–M_3) are well characterised.

M_1 (neural) and M_3 (glandular) couple to G_q and increase cellular inositol trisphosphate and diacylglycerol concentrations. M_2 (cardiac) couple to G_i and inhibit adenylate cyclase and open K^+ channels. M_1 receptors can also inhibit K^+ channel opening. The cellular events triggered by G-protein activation are discussed in detail in Chapter 2

Fig. 10.4 The structure of the muscarinic receptor.

Table 10.2 Examples of drugs acting on muscarinic receptors

Agonists	Antagonists
ACh	**Atropine**
Carbachol	**Hyoscine**
Pilocarpine	Pirenzepine (M_1 selective)
	Benzatropine
	Ipratropium
	Tropicamide
	Cyclopentolate

Pharmacological actions

Muscarinic agonists cause

- smooth muscle contraction (e.g. gut, bladder) (M_3)
- pupillary constriction, ciliary muscle contraction
- decreased rate and force of heart beat (M_2)
- glandular secretion (salivary, sweat, exocrine pancreas) (M_3)
- gastric acid secretion (M_1)
- vasodilatation via nitric oxide (M_3)
- inhibition of neurotransmitter release (M_2; M_1 may *facilitate* release)
- slow excitation of ganglia (M_1)

Muscarinic antagonists all act in a reversible competitive fashion. Most show no selectivity between the receptor subtypes. They cause:

- inhibition of secretions (e.g. dry mouth)
- tachycardia
- pupillary dilatation and paralysis of accommodation
- relaxation of smooth muscle
- inhibition of gastric acid secretion
- CNS excitation (atropine) or depression (hyoscine)
- anti-emetic action
- antiparkinsonian action.

Pharmacokinetics

Atropine and **hyoscine** are well absorbed from the GI tract despite their quaternary ammonium structure and have half-lives of ~3 h. **Tropicamide** and cyclopentolate (tertiary amines) are used topically for effects on the eye and have a shorter duration of action than atropine.

Ipratropium (quaternary ammonium) is administered by inhalation and, given this way, has no systemic actions. Its effects on the airways last for ~4 h. **Benzatropine** is given orally but can be given i.v. or i.m.; it penetrates the brain well. **Pilocarpine** (tertiary amine) given as eyedrops can cross the conjunctival membrane to produce effects which last for a day.

Unwanted effects

Muscarinic antagonists can cause a wide range of unwanted effects. Some occur through parasympathetic block: constipation, urinary retention, blurred vision and raised intraocular pressure (problem in narrow-angle glaucoma). Some result from CNS actions, e.g. sedation (hyoscine) or excitement (atropine), and mental confusion.

Clinical uses of drugs acting on muscarinic receptors

- **Antagonists** affect a number of systems
  - —cardiovascular: to treat sinus bradycardia (**atropine**)
  - —ophthalmic: to dilate the pupils (**tropicamide,** cyclopentolate)
  - —respiratory: to reduce cholinergic bronchospasm (as adjunct to bronchodilators) in asthma (**ipratropium**; see Ch. 24), for anaesthetic premedication to reduce airway secretions during anaesthesia for surgery (**atropine, hyoscine**)
  - —gastrointestinal: as an antispasmodic (**dicyclomine**), to reduce acid secretion as part of the treatment of peptic ulcer (**pirenzepine**; M_1 selective)
  - —neurological: to prevent motion sickness (**hyoscine**), for Parkinson's disease (**benzatropine**).
- **Agonists**
  - —ophthalmic: to lower intraocular pressure in glaucoma (**pilocarpine**)
  - —gastrointestinal: to increase motility (bethanechol).

CHOLINESTERASE AND THE ANTICHOLINESTERASES

Cholinesterase

There are two forms of cholinesterase: acetylcholinesterase (AChE) and plasma or butyrylcholinesterase (BuChE). Both hydrolyse ACh and other esters but have differing locations and specificities (Table 10.3). AChE is the enzyme that terminates the action of ACh released from nerves. (In terms of the mechanism of termination of action, ACh thus differs from noradrenaline, which is taken back up into the nerve.)

Enzyme action

Hydrolysis of ACh occurs in three steps (Fig. 10.5):

1. ACh binds to the enzyme
2. The acetyl group binds to serine OH on the enzyme and is transferred, resulting in a transiently acetylated enzyme plus free choline
3. Hydrolytic cleavage of serine acetyl bond releases acetyl group.

Table 10.3 Differences between AChE and BuChE

	AChE	BuChE
Location	Basement membrane at cholinergic synapses, erythrocytes	Soluble form in plasma; also in liver and elsewhere
Substrate specificity	ACh and closely related compounds	Less specific: butyrylcholine, other esters (e.g. **suxamethonium** and **procaine**)

At fast synapses, such as those at the NMJ and in ganglia, but not at slow ones (cardiac muscle, smooth muscle, glands), AChE hydrolyses the released ACh in about 1 ms.

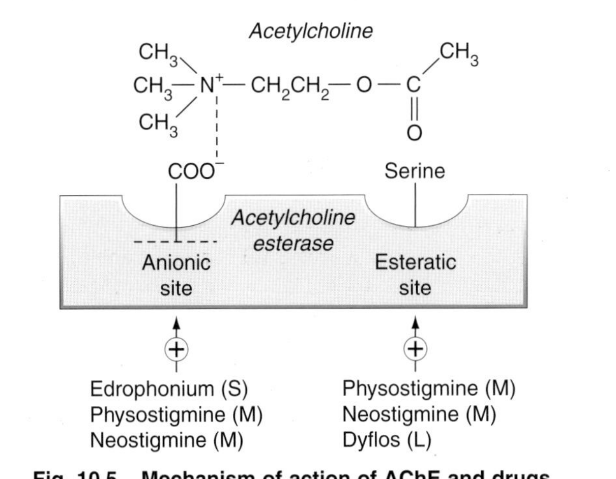

Fig. 10.5 Mechanism of action of AChE and drugs inhibiting it. Duration of drug action: short (S), medium (M) or long (L).

Anticholinesterases

Anticholinesterases inhibit cholinesterase. There are three main groups, the differences in their duration of action depending on how they interact with AChE (see Fig. 10.5).

- ***Short acting:*** simple reversible association with enzyme (e.g. edrophonium)
- ***Medium duration of action:*** interact with the serine hydroxyl at the active site to give a carbamylated product, which is only slowly hydrolysed (e.g. **neostigmine,** physostigmine, **pyridostigmine**)
- ***Irreversible:*** irreversibly phosphorylate the serine hydroxyl group. Most are organophosphate compounds with generalised toxic effects. Ecothiopate has a more or less selective action on postganglionic parasympathetic receptors and has been used in glaucoma. Parathion is used as an insecticide and its toxic effects may sometimes be seen clinically.

The action of the 'irreversible' anticholinesterases can be reversed, at an early stage, by the cholinesterase reactivator **pralidoxime**, which has such a high affinity for the phosphate group that it can effectively extract the blocking group.

Pharmacological actions and unwanted effects

Enhancement of cholinergic transmission results in:

- **autonomic effects**, including bradycardia, hypotension, excessive secretions, bronchoconstriction, GI tract hypermotility and decreased intraocular pressure
- **action at the neuromuscular junction**, causing muscle fasciculation and increased twitch tension; an excessive rise in ACh concentration may produce depolarisation block
- action in CNS: drugs crossing blood–brain barrier can activate muscarinic receptors; they can cause respiratory failure and loss of consciousness (antagonised by atropine).

Clinical uses of the anticholinesterases

- **Ophthalmic:** eyedrops to treat glaucoma (**physostigmine**).
- **Musculoskeletal**
  - —myasthenia gravis: **neostigmine, pyridostigmine**
  - —reversal of non-depolarising neuromuscular block: **neostigmine**.

11 Noradrenergic transmission

Noradrenergic neurons in the periphery are postganglionic sympathetic neurons. The cell bodies lie in sympathetic ganglia and most have long axons with a series of varicosities strung like beads along the branching terminal network. The varicosities are the sites where synthesis and release of noradrenaline (NA) occurs. After release, NA acts on adrenoceptors in various target organs; these include vascular smooth muscle, gland cells and cardiac cells.

TRANSMISSION AT THE NORADRENERGIC VARICOSITY WITH SUMMARY OF DRUG ACTION

High concentrations of NA are present in the varicosities, the NA being held in dense-cored storage vesicles from which it is released by Ca^{2+}-mediated exocytosis triggered by a nerve action potential. (The vesicles are produced in the cell body and pass down to the varicosities.) Figure 11.1 depicts the events at the junction of the noradrenergic varicosity with vascular smooth muscle.

The action of the released NA is short lived because there is rapid re-uptake into the varicosity and then into the storage vesicles; any NA not taken up is metabolised. Termination of the action of NA, therefore, differs from that of acetylcholine, which is hydrolysed after release.

NA is a catecholamine, as are adrenaline and isoprenaline. Differences in the responses to these three in different tissues led to the understanding that there were types of adrenoceptors: α and β, and several subtypes. The relative potencies of the three catecholamines on these are:

- α_1 and α_2 subtype: adrenaline = NA >> isoprenaline
- β_1 subtype: isoprenaline > adrenaline = NA
- β_2 subtype: isoprenaline = adrenaline > NA

Subtypes of the α and α_2 receptors have been identified, as has a β_3 subtype (see p. 34).

The term 'sympathomimetic' refers to the action of agents that mimic—to a greater or lesser degree—the actions of NA or adrenaline.

Many clinically important drugs act by modifying noradrenergic transmission, notably those that act as agonists and antagonists on β-adrenoceptors. (The recommended international drug name for adrenaline is epinephrine and for noradrenaline is norepinephrine.)

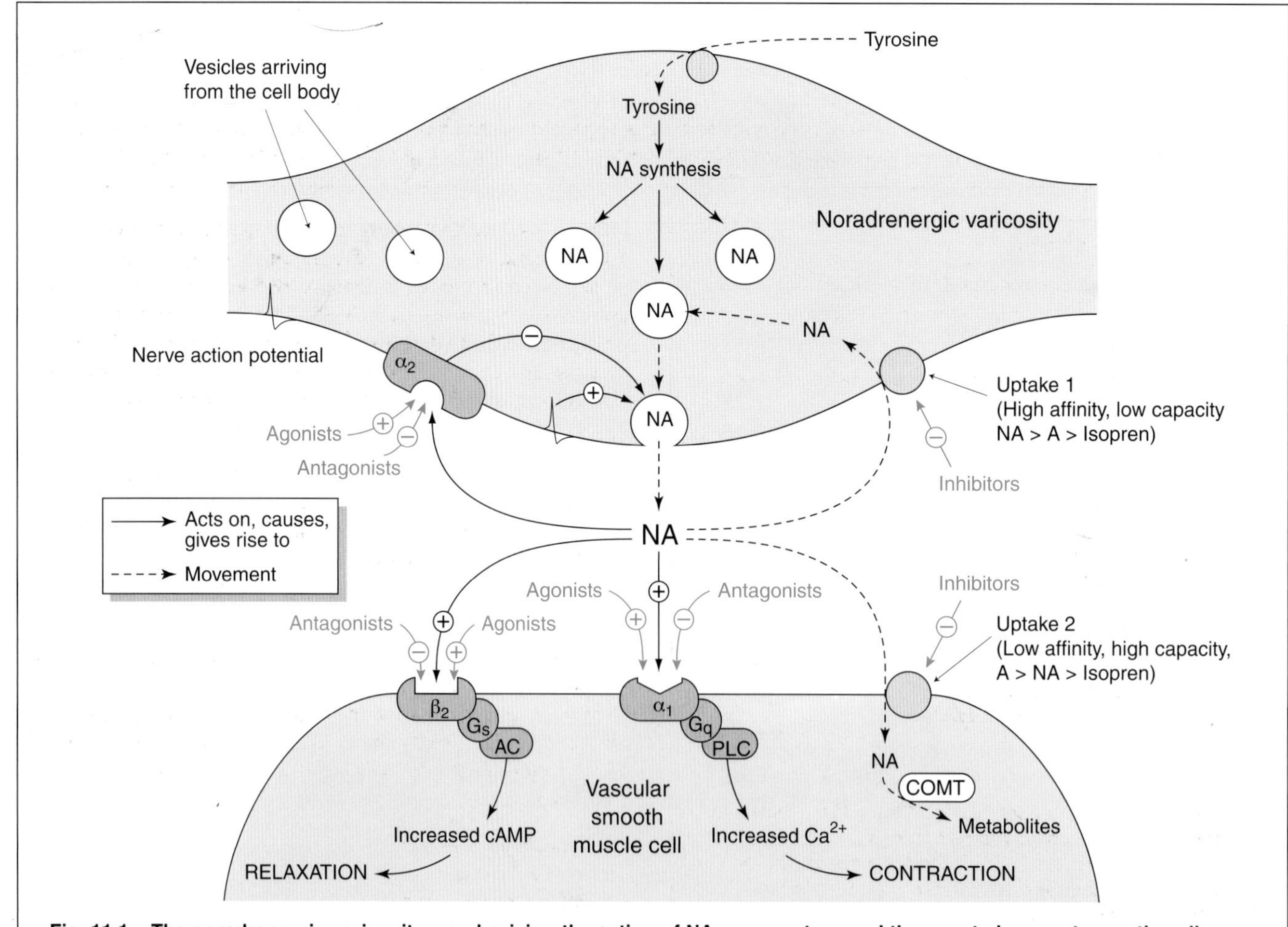

Fig. 11.1 The noradrenergic varicosity, emphasising the action of NA on receptors and the events in a postsynaptic cell. (A, adrenaline; Isopren, isoprenaline; PLC, phospholipase C; AC, adenylate cyclase; G, G protein.)

THE ACTION OF DRUGS ON ADRENOCEPTORS

Many drugs that act on adrenoceptors have selective effects on the various receptor subtypes. Figure 11.2 summarises these. More details on α- and β-adrenoceptors follow below.

Alpha-adrenoceptor agonists and antagonists

Figure 11.3 shows lower part of a varicosity and the events and drugs modifying α-adrenoceptor action.

Alpha agonists

The main α agonists that are of value clinically are epinephrine (adrenaline) and norepinephrine (noradrenaline); others are shown in Figures 11.2 and 11.3.

Pharmacological actions

- At α_1-adrenoceptors:
  - — contraction of the smooth muscle of blood vessels (causing increase in blood pressure), uterus, the sphincters of the GI tract, the bladder sphincter and the radial muscle of the iris
  - — glycogenolysis in liver cells
- At α_2-adrenoceptors:
  - — inhibition of NA release
  - — inhibition of lipolysis.

Mechanism of action

Stimulation of α_1-adrenoceptors results in G-protein-mediated activation of phospholipase C (PLC) with generation of the second messengers IP_3 and DAG. IP_3 increases intracellular Ca^{2+}, which activates the contractile mechanism in smooth muscle cells. DAG activates protein kinase C (PKC), which phosphorylates various proteins; there are various isoforms of PKC with multiple intracellular actions. The α_2-adrenoceptors inhibit adenylate cyclase: this leads to reduction in cAMP, which would otherwise enhance Ca^{2+} influx with the passage of the nerve action potential. They also inhibit opening of Ca^{2+} channels directly and promote opening of K^+ channels.

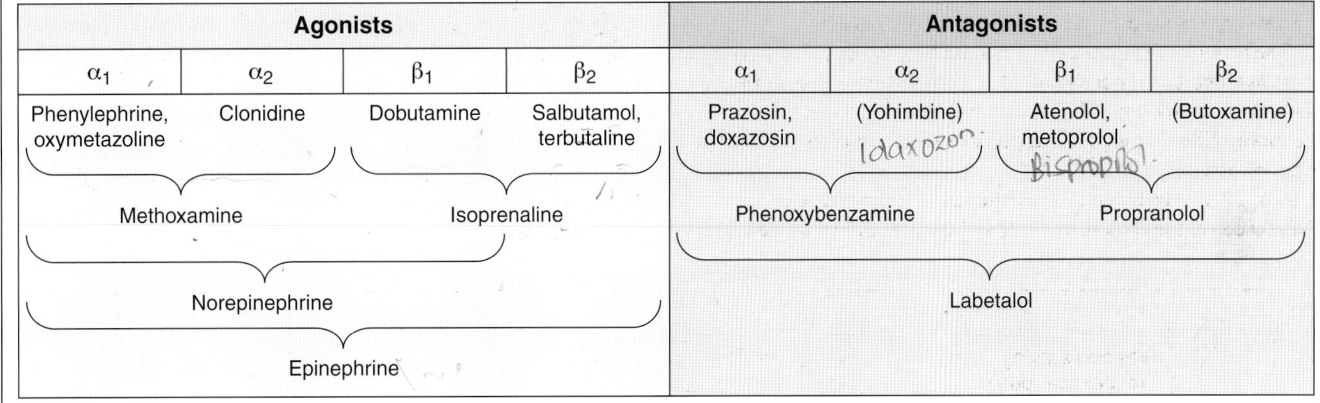

Fig. 11.2 Some examples of drugs that act mainly on particular subtypes of adrenoceptors. Drugs not used clinically are given in parentheses. Note: the names norepinephrine and epinephrine are now used for the *drug* forms of NA and adrenaline, respectively.

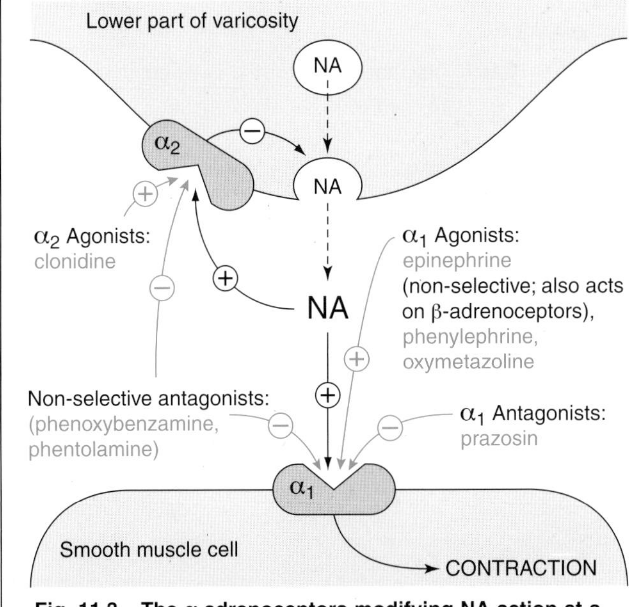

Fig. 11.3 The α-adrenoceptors modifying NA action at a noradrenergic varicosity. The main clinically useful agonist and antagonist drugs are shown, with drugs that are rarely used given in parentheses. NA release is modulated by autoinhibitory feedback of NA on α_2-adrenoceptors. Note: epinephrine is the name now used for the drug form of adrenaline.

Unwanted effects

The main adverse effects with the various α_1 agonists are:

- **epinephrine**: hypertension, increased heart rate (a β-adrenoceptor effect) with possibility of dysrhythmias (though reflex bradycardia can occur)
- **phenylephrine**: increased blood pressure, reflex bradycardia.

Alpha antagonists

The main α antagonists used clinically are the α_1-selective agents **prazosin,** doxazosin, terazosin. Others are the non-selective α-antagonists **phenoxybenzamine** (irreversible, binds covalently to the receptor) and phentolamine. Labetalol blocks both α- and β-adrenoceptors. Ergot alkaloids are antagonists/partial agonists at α-adrenoceptors.

Pharmacological actions

The main actions are:

- a fall in blood pressure
- a rise in heart rate owing to reflex cardiac β-adrenoceptor response to the fall in blood pressure
- decreased tone of the smooth muscle at the bladder neck.

Mechanism of action

Alpha antagonists act by blocking the effect of endogenous mediators (and exogenous agonists) on the relevant receptors by competitive inhibition.

Unwanted effects

Most unwanted effects are extensions of the pharmacological actions: increased heart rate, postural hypotension, congestion of the nasal blood vessels. Some agents can cause impotence.

Beta-adrenoceptor agonists and antagonists

Beta agonists

The main β agonists that are used clinically include the β_2-selective agents **salbutamol,** terbutaline, **salmeterol** and the β_1-selective agent **dobutamine.** Isoprenaline and **epinephrine** stimulate both β_1- and β_2-adrenoceptors (Fig. 11.4).

Pharmacological actions

- At β_2-adrenoceptors:
  - dilatation of bronchioles and arterioles
  - relaxation of the bladder detrusor muscle and of the ciliary muscle of the eye
  - glycogenolysis
- At β_1-adrenoceptors: increase in the rate and force of the heart
- At β_3-adrenoceptors: lipolysis.

Agents with actions on β_1-, β_2- and β_3-adrenoceptors will have a mixture of the effects given above.

Mechanism of action

The cellular action depends on the signal transduction mechanism. Beta-adrenoceptor activation results mainly in G-protein-mediated activation of adenylate cyclase with increase of cyclic AMP, which in turn activates protein kinase A (PKA). In smooth muscle, PKA phosphorylates and inactivates myosin light chain kinase and thus reduces the contractile action. In the heart, PKA phosphorylates Ca^{2+} channels, increasing the inward Ca^{2+} current and thus the force of contraction (see Ch. 19). The cardiac effects of dobutamine are less potent than those of the other β_1 agonists.

Unwanted effects

The main unwanted effects are extensions of the pharmacological effects, mainly cardiac dysrhythmias with the β_1 agonists and tremor and peripheral vasodilatation with the β_2 agonists.

Beta antagonists

The main β antagonists used clinically are **atenolol** and **propranolol** (both β_1 selective), **alprenolol** (non-selective, partial agonist), labetalol (non-selective, also acts on α-adrenoceptors).

Pharmacological actions

The β antagonists have limited action in normal individuals at rest; the main actions are seen in pathological conditions. These include:

- an antihypertensive effect, which is caused by reduced cardiac output, decreased release of renin, central decrease of sympathetic action
- an antianginal effect, which is caused by slowing of the heart rate and thus decreased metabolic demand.

Mechanism of action

The β antagonists act by blocking the effect of endogenous mediators (and exogenous agonists) on the relevant receptors, most acting as competitive antagonists.

Unwanted effects

The main unwanted effects are extensions of the pharmacological actions. Some are unpleasant but not critical for the patient:

- cold extremities
- fatigue.

Some are particularly important in the presence of other diseases:

- bronchoconstriction: this is potentially life threatening in asthmatic patients and clinically undesirable in patients with other respiratory problems (e.g. emphysema)
- slowing of heart rate: this can cause heart block in patients with coronary disease
- cardiac failure can occur in patients with heart disease
- decrease of the warning sympathetic response to hypoglycaemia in diabetic patients.

Table 11.1 summarises the cardiovascular effects of the catecholamines.

Table 11.1 Cardiovascular effects of the catecholamines

	Norepinephrine	Epinephrine	Isoprenaline
Diastolic BP	↑	↓	↓
Systolic BP	↑	↑ (moderate)	↓
Heart rate	↓ (reflex)	↑	↑

BP, blood pressure

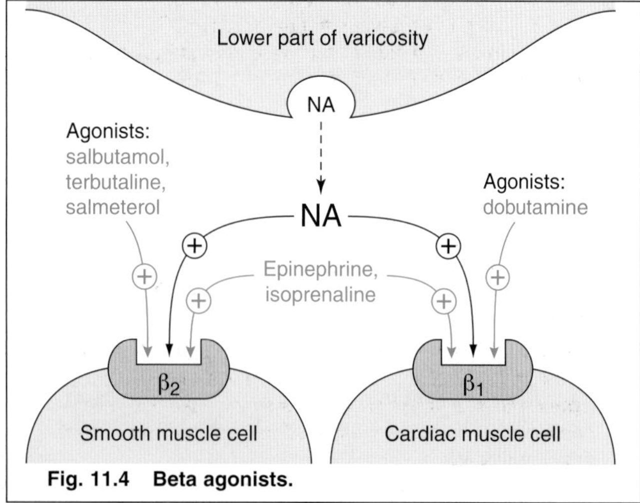

Fig. 11.4 Beta agonists.

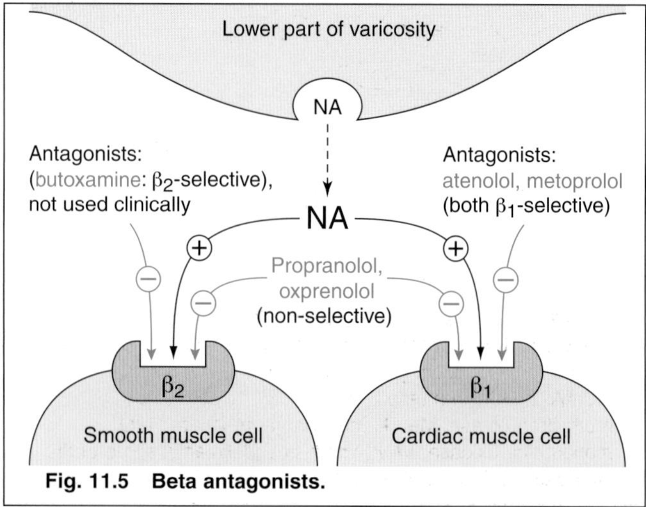

Fig. 11.5 Beta antagonists.

EVENTS IN THE VARICOSITY AND THE ACTION OF DRUGS

Figure 11.6 summarises events in the varicosity and action of drugs thereon.

Pharmacological actions

Uptake 1 inhibitors cause an increase in the effects of NA because they interfere with the main method for terminating NA action, namely the uptake mechanism. For most of the drugs specified in the figure, this action is subsidiary to their main pharmacological effect. Thus **cocaine** is a local anaesthetic, while **phenoxybenzamine** is mainly an α-antagonist. The main actions of the other inhibitors are clear from their names.

Indirectly acting sympathomimetic amines (IASA, e.g. ephedrine) have similar (but weaker) actions to NA on receptors. They are taken up by Uptake 1 then into the vesicle by exchange with NA, which in turn is released from the varicosity by exchange with IASAs at Uptake 1. Actions in the CNS include increased alertness, decreased appetite.

Carbidopa reduces peripheral sympathetic activity when used as an adjunct to levodopa in the treatment of Parkinsonism. It does not cross the blood–brain barrier.

Methyldopa is taken up by an amino acid transporter and acted on by the NA-producing enzymes to give, within the vesicle, methylnoradrenaline, which is released as a false transmitter. It acts mainly on α_2-adrenoceptors, thus reducing further the release of NA. It has antihypertensive action by this effect and also by postsynaptic action on central neurons.

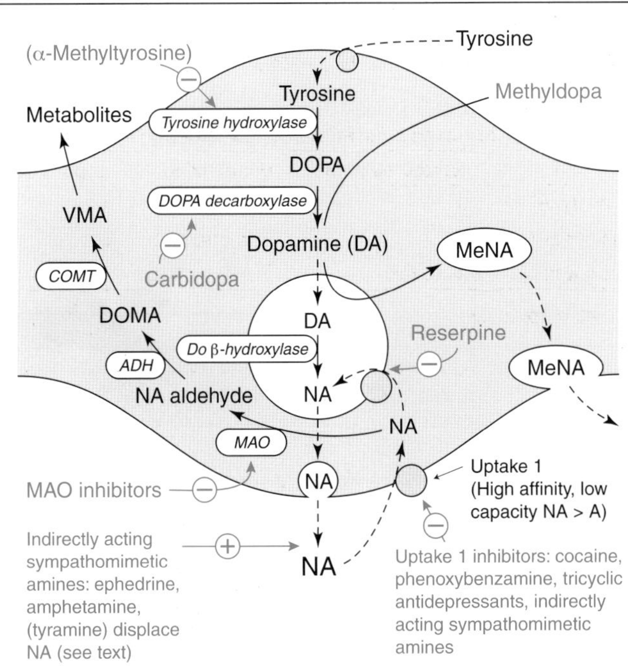

Fig. 11.6 Diagram of a varicosity. The sites of action of drugs are shown; those agents that are not used clinically are given in parentheses. (ADH, aldehyde dehydrogenase; DOMA, dihydroxymandelic acid; COMT, catechol-*O*-methyltransferase; MeNA, methylnoradrenaline; MAO, monoamine oxidase; VMA, vanillylmandelic acid; some of the later steps in NA metabolism take place outside the neuron.)

α-Methyltyrosine inhibits the rate-limiting enzyme in NA synthesis, tyrosine hydroxylase. It has had a use in the treatment of pheochromocytoma, a catecholamine-secreting tumour that causes episodes of serious hypertension.

Guanethidine (not shown) also depletes NA in the vesicle. It was used as an antihypertensive agent but is no longer used for this purpose.

6-Hydroxydopamine (not shown) is used as an experimental tool and is taken up into the varicosity and destroys it. It is not used clinically.

Reserpine inhibits uptake of NA into the vesicle; it is used mainly as an experimental tool.

Clinical use and pharmacokinetic aspects of drugs affecting adrenoceptors

Agonists

- **Epinephrine** (adrenaline) is given s.c. or i.v. for anaphylactic shock and i.v. in cardiac arrest; it can be included in local anaesthetic preparations to delay absorption by vasoconstriction.
- The β_2-selective agonists are given by inhalation to treat the immediate phase of asthma.
- **Salbutamol** and terbutaline have a <30 min onset and are short acting (4–6 h) while salmeterol is longer acting (12 h). Salbutamol or terbutaline may be given s.c. for severe attacks.
- **Salbutamol** or ritodrine may be used to inhibit preterm labour.
- **Dobutamine** (β_1 selective) may be given in heart block while electrical pacing is being organised.
- **Phenylephrine** and **oxymetazoline** are given intranasally to reduce nasal congestion.

Antagonists

- **Prazosin** (α_1 antagonist) is used orally to treat hypertension; it is metabolised in the liver and has a half-life of 4 h.
- **Phenoxybenzamine** (non-selective antagonist, also inhibits Uptake 1) can be used to treat pheochromocytoma; it is given orally and has a half-life of 12 h.
- **Atenolol** (half-life 6 h) and metoprolol, alprenolol, propranolol (half-lives 3–4 h) are β-adrenoceptor antagonists used for hypertension, angina and cardiac dysrhythmias.
- **Timolol** is used in eyedrops to treat glaucoma
- Labetalol (α and β antagonist) is used to treat hypertension in pregnancy; it is given orally and has a half-life of 4 h.

Clinical use of drugs affecting varicosal events

- **Carbidopa**, given orally, is used as an adjunct to decrease the peripheral sympathetic activity of levodopa.
- **Ephedrine** is an indirectly acting sympathomimetic used as a nasal decongestant; it was used to treat asthma but other drugs are safer.

12 Other peripheral mediators: 5-hydroxytryptamine and purines

In this chapter we deal with two mediator/neurotransmitter systems: 5-hydroxytryptamine (5-HT; serotonin) and the purines. The two systems act in both the periphery and the central nervous system (CNS).

5-HYDROXYTRYPTAMINE

5-HT occurs in the gastrointestinal tract, blood vessels and platelets and the CNS. In the CNS, it is found especially in the midbrain raphe nucleus, and it is implicated in the control of appetite, sleep, vomiting and mood and in the descending control of pain inputs (Ch. 41). In the periphery, it is concerned with microvascular control and influences the sensitivity of pain fibres. Substantial amounts are also found in platelets, where it has an important role in platelet aggregation; it also serves as an inflammatory mediator. Most of the 5-HT in the body is, however, found in the enterochromaffin cells in the mucosa of the stomach and intestine, where it influences gut motility. 5-HT function is abnormal in affective disorders and anxiety and it is overproduced by tumours of enterochromaffin cells (carcinoid syndrome).

Synthesis, storage, release and metabolism of 5-HT

5-HT is synthesised from dietary tryptophan (Fig. 12.1) and is stored in granulated vesicles, much like noradrenaline. 5-HT neurons have specific 5-HT reuptake transporters, which are important targets for the SSRI antidepressant drugs (Ch. 39). Reuptake is the main mechanism for terminating 5-HT action. Platelets lack tryptophan hydroxylase and are unable to synthesise 5-HT; therefore, they accumulate it by active uptake from the blood (especially in the intestinal circulation where 5-HT concentration is high). 5-HT's actions are quickly terminated by degradation and reuptake. Much of the 5-HT released into the circulation by enterochromaffin cells will be deaminated by hepatic monoamine oxidase (MAO.) 5-HT that survives first-pass liver metabolism is taken up by endothelial cells in lung blood vessels and subject to further MAO action. Sequential metabolism by aldehyde dehydrogenase yields the major metabolite, 5-hydroxyindoleacetic acid (5-HIAA). 5-HT neurotransmission is enhanced by MAO inhibitors and this contributes to their antidepressant activity. (Ch. 39).

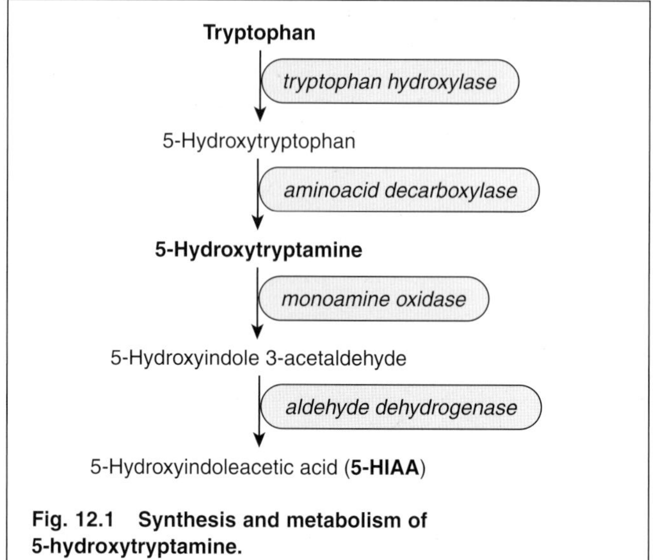

Fig. 12.1 Synthesis and metabolism of 5-hydroxytryptamine.

5-HT receptors

There are seven families of 5-HT receptors (5-HT$_{1-7}$) containing at least 14 members (see Table 12.1) and their activation leads to widespread effects sometimes in opposite directions. Most of the receptor subtypes are found in brain, with overlapping distributions. Except for the 5-HT$_3$, ligand-gated ion channel receptor, they are all G-protein coupled.

Migraine

The aetiology of the visual disturbances, headache and other symptoms of migraine is still not well established, both abnormal neuronal discharge and changes in cerebral blood flow being implicated, The increase in the urinary excretion of 5-HIAA during a migraine attack, and the useful clinical benefits obtained by

Table 12.1 The roles of 5-HT receptors

Receptor	Transduction	Effects	Clinically useful drugs
1A, 1B, 1D, 1E, 1F	$G_{i/o}$ protein activation; inhibits adenylate cyclase, increases neuronal K^+ permeability, inhibits Ca^{2+} conductance	Neuronal inhibition, presynaptic inhibition, behavioural effects, constriction of cerebral blood vessels (1D)	**Sumatriptan**, eletriptan (1B/1D agonists) and **ergotamine** (partial agonist) are used for migraine. **Buspirone** (1A agonist) for anxiety (Ch. 37)
2A, 2B, 2C	G_q activation; phospholipase C and A_2 activation; formation of inositol trisphosphate and diacylglycerol	Neuronal excitation, smooth muscle contraction (vascular, gastrointestinal tract, bronchiolar), platelet aggregation (2A): cerebrospinal fluid secretion (2C)	**Ketanserin**, **methysergide** (2A antagonists) for migraine; **olanzepine**, **risperidone** (2A antagonists) for schizophrenia, Ch. 38. (LSD's psychotomimetic actions are due to activation of 2A receptors)
3	Ligand-gated cation channel	Neuronal excitation, emesis (central and peripheral components), effects on gut motility and secretion	**Ondansetron** and granisetron are antagonists used as antiemetics (Ch. 26)
4	G_s activation and stimulation of adenylate cyclase	Increased peristalsis, neuronal excitation in central and enteric nervous system, intestinal secretion	**Metoclopramide**, **cisapride**, **zacopride** are agonists stimulating peristalsis and can be used in heartburn
5A, 5B, 6, 7	G_s activation of adenylate cyclase by 6 and 7; 5 not established	Not well established	None

modification of 5-HT mechanisms, however, point to a role for 5-HT in the pathogenesis. 5-HT-mediated vasoconstriction may contribute to the early visual effects and inflammatory vasodilatation to the later effects. The beneficial effects of 5-HT_2 antagonists may relate to inhibition of the early vasoconstriction and the effectiveness of 5-HT_1 receptor agonists (sumatriptan and others) to constriction of cranial blood vessels. Dihydroergotamine and other ergot alkaloids have additional effects on α-adrenoceptors (Ch. 11). **Sumatriptan** is administered subcutaneously for an acute attack and is effective in up to 95% of patients. **Methysergide**, used to prevent migraine headaches, is a potent 5-HT_2 antagonist. 5-HT_3 antagonists have also been shown to be effective in migraines. (Other drugs used for migraine are β-blockers (Ch. 11), non-steroidal anti-inflammatory drugs (Ch. 15), Ca^{2+} channel blockers (Chs 18 and 19) and some antiepileptic (Ch. 40) and antidepressant (Ch. 39) drugs.)

PURINES

The purine adenosine and the purine nucleotide ATP act as mediators and neurotransmitters, interacting with specific receptors in a wide range of tissues. ATP is stored in synaptic vesicles and released from nerves as either a primary transmitter or a co-transmitter. Adenosine is not stored in vesicles but can be released by nerve endings and other cell types; it also is formed by the breakdown of ATP in the extracellular space by ectoATPases and other enzymes. Adenosine acts as a neuromodulator rather than neurotransmitter. It reaches high concentration in hypoxic tissues and is an important mediator of reactive hyperaemia. It is quickly removed from the circulation due to rapid uptake into cells (especially endothelial cells) and by the action of adenosine deaminase. This is consistent with its role as a local hormone. An intravenous dose works only for about 10 seconds.

Receptors for purines

For historical reasons, adenosine receptors are referred to either as P_1 or A (adenosine) receptors and ATP receptors as P_2 (Table 12.2). Adenosine receptors are subclassified as A_1, A_{2A}, A_{2B} and A_3. These are G-protein-coupled receptors; A_1 couples to G_i or G_o, to inhibit adenylate cyclase, open K^+ channels or inhibit Ca^{2+} channels. A_2 couples to G_s to stimulate adenylate cyclase, A_3 couples to G_i and G_q.

Methylxanthines are adenosine receptor antagonists and the CNS stimulant action of caffeine can be attributed to inhibition of A_2 receptor activation (Ch. 41).

There are subtypes also of P_2 receptors, the main ones being P_{2X} (ligand-gated cation channel); P_{2Y} (G_q-protein coupled, activating phospholipase C) and P_{2T} (G_i-protein coupled, activated mainly by ADP and found particularly in platelets, where it has a role in thrombosis). Several subtypes of P_{2X} and P_{2Y} receptors have been identified. Receptors for adenosine and ATP are widely distributed throughout neurons and peripheral tissues. P_{2X} receptors are found mainly on excitable cells (neurons and smooth muscle).

Important actions of adenosine and ATP are listed in Table 12.2.

Clinical aspects

Adenosine is used ony in the treatment of supraventricular tachycardia (Ch. 17).
Theophylline (a methylxanthine) is a phoshodiesterase inhibitor used in the treatment of asthma (Ch. 24); it has, as a side effect, CNS stimulation (Ch. 42), which is at least partly due to antagonism at adenosine receptors.
Dipyridamole (another phosphodiesterase inhibitor) interferes with the cellular uptake of adenosine and this contributes to its inhibition of platelet aggregation (Ch. 22) and its vasodilator action.

Table 12.2 Purine mediators and receptors

Mediator	Tissue	Effect	Receptor	Mechanism
Adenosine	Smooth muscle	Vasodilatation, hypotension	A_2	Adenylate cyclase activation
		Vasoconstriction (kidney), bronchoconstriction	A_1	Inhibition of adenylate cyclase
	Cardiac muscle	Slowed atrioventricular conduction, reduced force of contraction, slowed pacemaker activity	A_1	Inhibition of Ca^{2+} channels, increased K^+ permeability
	Neurons	Inhibition of transmitter release (reduced glutamate excitotoxicity)	A_1	Inhibition of Ca^{2+} entry
		Decreased excitability	A_2	Increased K^+ permeability, hyperpolarisation
		Stimulation of pain fibres (e.g. pain of angina)	A_2	
	Mast cells	Release of mediators (bronchoconstriction)	A_3	Stimulation of phospholipase C, inhibition of adenylate cyclase
	Platelets	Inhibition of aggregation	A_2	Adenylate cyclase activation
ATP	Smooth muscle	Relaxation (blood vessels, gut)	P_{2Y}	Increased K^+ permeability
		Contraction	P_{2X}	Depolarisation, Ca^{2+} entry
	Endothelial cells	Endothelium-dependent vasodilatation	P_{2Y}	Nitric oxide release (Ch. 14)
	Neurons	Fast synaptic transmission	P_{2X}	Depolarisation due to Na^+ entry through integral ion channel
ADP	Platelets	Increased aggregation	P_{2T}	Inhibition of adenylate cyclase

13 Other peripheral mediators: peptides

Peptides (<50 amino acid residues) and proteins outnumber non-peptides as mediators within the body. In the nervous system peptides are frequently found as co-transmitters (e.g. neuropeptide Y with noradrenaline).

Synthesis and storage

Peptide mediators are produced by the splitting of precursor proteins, synthesised in the usual manner by mRNA coding in ribosomes, and stored in secretory vesicles. Precursor proteins may give rise to several peptide mediators: the particular peptides generated from the precursor in any given tissue depending on the tissue's complement of peptidases (e.g. proopiomelanocortin, Fig. 13.1). Peptide mediators have important actions in many systems and are of necessity considered in several other chapters (e.g. opioid peptides in Ch. 41, cytokines in Ch. 15).

Mechanism of action

Small peptides and chemokines generally interact with G-protein-coupled receptors, whereas other cytokines and growth factors work via tyrosine kinase receptors.

Pharmacokinetic aspects In general, peptides are poorly absorbed by oral administration and are quickly broken down by peptidases. Unlike other mediators, reuptake is not an important mechanism for termination of peptide action. They do not readily cross the blood–brain barrier. Antagonists produced by amino acid substitution are likely to have pharmacokinetic properties similar to the native peptide. Accordingly, drug companies seek to produce non-peptide antagonists with improved pharmacokinetic properties. Relatively few non-peptide drugs interacting with these receptors are yet available, **morphine analogues** and **losartan** being examples. Inhibition of peptide breakdown is another potential strategy for drug development. (**Kelatorphan,** which has analgesic actions by slowing the breakdown of enkephalins, is an example.)

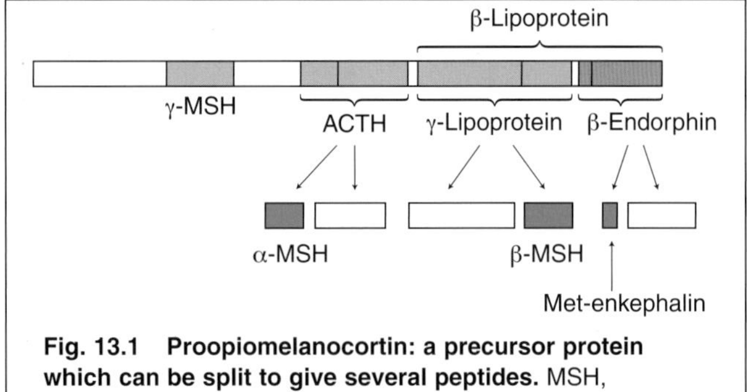

Fig. 13.1 Proopiomelanocortin: a precursor protein which can be split to give several peptides. MSH, melanocyte-stimulating hormone.

Clinical aspects

Peptides may be administered as replacement therapy where natural production is impaired (e.g. insulin, clotting factors, growth hormone) and antibodies can be used to combat foreign proteins (e.g. antivenins). Recombinant methods now allow peptides to be produced in larger quantities by bacteria rather than being extracted from animal tissues. Recombinant technology has also allowed 'human' insulin to be used rather than animal insulins. Selected peptides and antagonists are listed in Table 13.1.

Table 13.1 Selected peptide mediators and clinically useful drugs

Mediator	Receptor	Agonists	Clinical uses of agonists	Antagonists	Clinical uses of antagonists
Angiotensin II, III	AT_1, AT_2			Saralasin, losartan (AT_1 selective)	Hypertension
Bradykinin	B_1, B_2			Icatibant	Liver cirrhosis
Calcitonin gene-related peptide	CGRP receptor			$CGRP^{8-37}$	
Neuropeptide Y (NPY)	Y1–Y5				(Potential anti-obesity)
Somatostatin	sst_{1-5}	Octreotide	Acromegaly, gastro-intestinal tumours		
Cholecystokinin	CCK_A, CCK_B			Lorglumide	Gut disorders
Vasoactive intestinal peptide, VIP	VIPR1, 2				(Specific tumour treatment)
Corticotrophin-releasing factor, CRF	CRF_1, CRF_2			Experimental	
Endothelins	ET_A, ET_B			Bosentan	Pulmonary artery hypertension
Opioid peptides, enkephalins, endorphin	μ, δ, κ, ORL	Morphine fentanyl	Analgesics	Naloxone, naltrexone	Opioid overdose
Oxytocin	OT		Induction of labour	Atosiban	Preterm labour
Vasopressin	V_1, V_2	Desmopressin, felypressin	Diabetes insipidus, vasoconstrictor	Experimental	
Tachykinins (SP etc.)	NK_1, NK_2, NK_3			Experimental	
Glucagon	Glucagon receptor		Hypoglycaemia, cardiac stimulant	Experimental	Potential use in type 2 diabetes
Insulin	Insulin receptor	Insulins	Diabetes mellitus	None	

14 Other peripheral mediators: nitric oxide

Nitric oxide (NO) is produced widely in the body and has important roles as a mediator in the cardiovascular and nervous systems and in the host's defence against pathogenic organisms.

Biological and pathophysiological actions

NO is a transmitter in both the central and peripheral nervous systems, playing a part in appetite control in the former and gastric emptying in the latter. NO is thought to be identical with endothelium-derived relaxing factor (EDRF) and has a role in the control of regional blood flow.

Under- or overproduction of NO has been implicated in various clinical conditions. Essential hypertension may be associated with a decrease in NO generation, and animal studies suggest that impairment of NO production might also predispose to atherogenesis. Increased NO generation may underlie the hypotension associated with septic shock and is implicated in glutamate excitotoxicity (Ch. 33). Dysfunction of the widely distributed nitrergic nerves may lead to a number of disorders in the gastrointestinal, genitourinary and vascular systems (e.g. impotence).

NO has opposing actions in inflammatory diseases. Initially, NO derived from constitutive nitric oxide synthase (NOS, see below) appears to protect against the actions of proinflammatory mediators by inhibiting white cell activation and platelet aggregation, and by inducing vasodilatation. In contrast, NO from iNOS (see below) contributes to many aspects of chronic inflammation.

NO generation underlies the action of the nitrovasodilators, such as glyceryl trinitrate.

Synthesis and breakdown

NO is synthesised by the oxidation of arginine (Fig. 14.1). There are three isoforms of NOS.

Endothelial NOS (eNOS) Found also in other tissues, including platelets and cardiac myocytes.

Neuronal NOS (nNOS) Some brain neurons and many peripheral (nitrergic neurons) possess nNOS.

eNOS and nNOS are referred to as constitutive enzymes, that is, they are present continuously in the cells and their activity can be rapidly modified, especially by receptor-induced rises in $[Ca^{2+}]_i$ and activation of calmodulin.

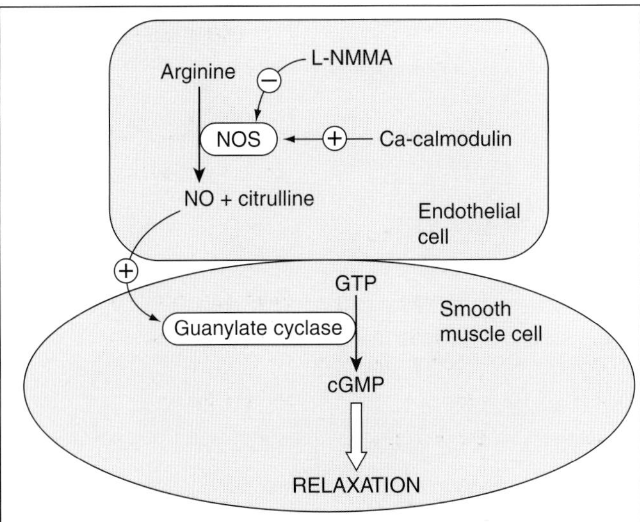

Fig. 14.1 Synthesis of nitric oxide (NO) and generation of cGMP. NOS, nitric oxide synthase; L-NMMA, L-N^G-monomethyl-L-arginine.

Inducible NOS (iNOS) This, in contrast, is not normally expressed but its synthesis in macrophages can be induced by bacterial lipopolysaccharides and cytokines such as interferon γ, produced in response to infection. iNOS can also be induced in neutrophils and vascular smooth muscle. iNOS activity is not regulated by Ca^{2+} and its induction is inhibited by glucocorticoids. Activated macrophages produce NO in large quantities and for long periods (up to 48 h).

Nitric oxide itself is short acting due to oxidation to nitrite/nitrate and to binding to the haem of haemoglobin. It can, however, form longer lasting nitrosothiols, e.g. nitrosoglutathione and nitrosohaemoglobin, which can release NO over a longer period.

Actions

NO inhibits platelet adhesion and aggregation, monocyte adhesion and migration, and smooth muscle and fibroblast proliferation. NO contributes to the cytotoxic activity of immune cells. In smooth muscle cells, activation of cGMP-dependent protein kinases results in Ca^{2+} sequestration and relaxation (Figs 14.1 and 19.2). Smooth muscle relaxation also results from a NO-induced increase in K^+ permeability and resultant hyperpolarisation.

The brain contains the highest activity of NOS found in any tissue. The rapid diffusion of NO through nervous tissue permits actions on many neurons over a wide area. Accordingly, within the brain, NO is generally regarded as a general modulator of neuronal function rather than as a neurotransmitter. In the peripheral nervous system, however, NO has widespread action as a transmitter in nitrergic nerves.

NOS is inhibited by substrate analogues such as N^G-monomethyl L-arginine (L-NMMA). L-NMMA administration causes widespread vasoconstriction and an increase in blood pressure, suggesting that continuous production of NO normally maintains resistance vessels in a dilated state.

Mechanism of action

NO binds to the haem moiety of soluble guanylate cyclase, leading to activation of the enzyme and enhanced synthesis of guanosine monophosphate cGMP (Fig. 19.2). NO, at physiological concentrations, also reversibly inhibits cytochrome *c* oxidase (complex IV) and thus regulates cellular respiration. Excessive NO synthesis, however, can cause neurotoxicity, tissue injury, inflammation and cardiovascular dysfunction through its direct effects on proteins and DNA, as well as through the formation of reactive nitrogen species, notably peroxynitrite ($ONOO^-$) by reaction with superoxide. Peroxynitrite also degrades to form the highly cytotoxic hydroxyl radical.

Clinical aspects

- **Glyceryl trinitrate** and isosorbide mononitrate are nitrovasodilators that act by generating NO (Chs 19 and 20).
- **Sildenafil** (Viagra) is used to treat erectile dysfunction; it specifically inhibits the phosphodiesterase (type V) that breaks down cGMP produced by NO in the corpora cavernosa.
- NO itself, administered by inhalation, produces pulmonary vasodilatation, which is of benefit in some types of lung disease (e.g. respiratory distress syndrome).

15 Inflammation and anti-inflammatory drugs

The term **acute inflammatory reaction** refers to the local events which occur in response to a disease-causing organism (pathogen). It consists of *immunologically specific* reactions (see Ch. 16) superimposed on *innate* (non-immunological) reactions. These reactions have survival value but if inappropriately deployed, as occurs in many diseases, they are deleterious. It is, therefore, important to understand the mediators which control these responses since many drugs currently used or in development are directed at influencing the generation and/or action of these mediators.

The *innate acute inflammatory reaction* involves both vascular events (vasodilatation, increased permeability of the postcapillary venules, exudation of fluid) and cellular events. The *cells* involved are (a) white blood cells (neutrophils, monocytes, lymphocytes, natural killer lymphocytes), which accumulate in the area of inflammation and are activated, some to ingest microorganisms or kill infected cells, some to release mediators, and (b) tissue cells (vascular endothelial cells, mast cells, macrophages). The mediators derived from cells include eicosanoids, cytokines, histamine, neuropeptides (see Ch. 13) and many others; those derived from plasma include complement components and components of the kinin cascade such as bradykinin.

The eventual outcome can be resolution and healing (possibly with scarring) or — if the pathogen or eliciting agent persists — the development of a *chronic inflammatory reaction.*

MEDIATORS OF INFLAMMATION AND THE DRUGS AFFECTING THEM

Eicosanoids and platelet-activating factor

Eicosanoids (prostanoids, leukotrienes) and platelet activating factor are generated from phospholipids and are implicated in many physiological and pathological processes. Many drugs target steps in their production (Fig. 15.1). An important enzyme is cyclooxygenase (COX), which occurs in two main forms: COX-1, a constitutive enzyme expressed in most cells and involved in tissue homeostasis, and COX-2, which is induced in inflammatory cells. A COX-3 enzyme has been described.

Bradykinin

Bradykinin is a nonapeptide clipped out of a plasma α-globulin. Its actions in inflammation are:

- vasodilatation (mediated by released nitric oxide (NO) and prostaglandin I_2 (PGI_2)
- increased vascular permeability
- stimulation of pain nerve endings (this is potentiated by PGs).

Histamine

Histamine is released from mast cells by a complement component C3a or, in type I hypersensitivity, by an antigen–antibody reaction on the cell surface.

Nitric oxide

Most inflammatory cells express the inducible form of NO synthase when activated by cytokines. NO dilates blood vessels, increases vascular permeability and stimulates PG release.

Cytokines

Cytokines are a large family of peptide mediators that are released or generated in inflammatory and immune reactions and which control

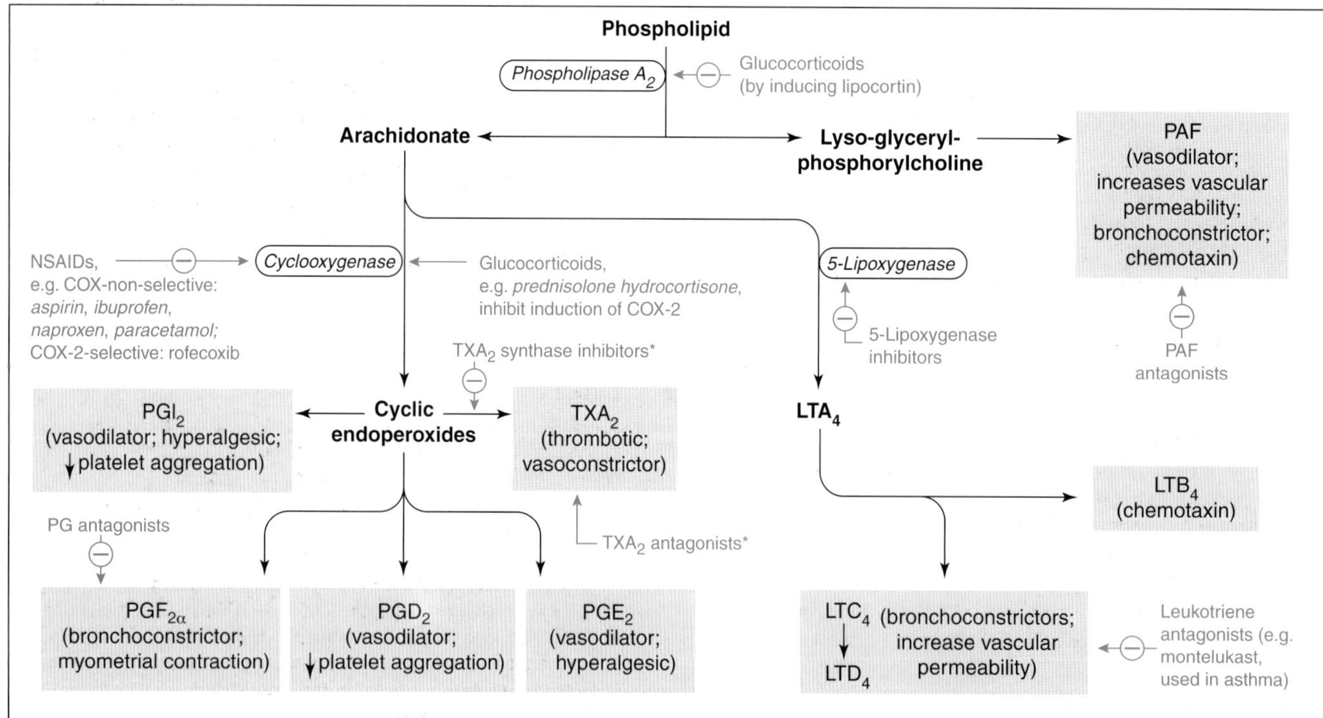

Fig. 15.1 The mediators derived from arachidonate — prostanoids, leukotrienes and platelet-activating factor — provide sites for anti-inflammatory drugs to act. (PG, prostaglandin; LT, leukotriene; TX, thromboxane; PAF, platelet-activating factor.) Important drugs are in italic. *Potential antiplatelet agents.

the actions of inflammatory and immune cells by autocrine or paracrine mechanisms. They include interleukins (e.g. IL-2, Ch. 16), chemokines (mediators that attract and activate motile inflammatory cells such as polymorphs, macrophages), colony-stimulating factors, growth factors (Chs 4 and 49) and many others.

Anti-inflammatory drugs

The principal anti-inflammatory agents are:

- the **glucocorticoids** (Chs 25 and 28)
- the **non-steroidal anti-inflammatory drugs** (NSAIDs).

Others are:

- antirheumatoid drugs (Ch. 16)
- drugs used in the treatment of gout.

NSAIDS

Examples of COX non-selective are: **aspirin, ibuprofen, indometacin**, **piroxicam**, naproxen, **paracetamol**, diclofenac, diflunisal. Examples of COX-2 selective are **rofecoxib**, celecoxib.

Pharmacological actions

Anti-inflammatory actions. NSAIDs reduce those aspects of inflammation in which the COX-2 products have a role, namely vasodilatation, which facilitates increased permeability of the postcapillary venules. Some are strongly anti-inflammatory (e.g. indometacin), some moderately so (e.g. ibuprofen). Some have little anti-inflammatory effect (e.g. paracetamol).

Analgesic actions. NSAIDs reduce pain caused by tissue damage or by inflammatory mediators that act on nerve endings (bradykinin, 5-hydroxytryptamine; see Ch. 41). The action is indirect in that the NSAIDs decrease the production of PGs, which sensitise the nerve endings to these pain-producing mediators.

Antipyretic actions. NSAIDs reduce fever. Body temperature is controlled by a hypothalamic 'thermostat' which ensures that heat production and heat loss are in balance around a set-point. Fever occurs when interleukin-1, an inflammatory mediator, generates, in the hypothalamus, E-type PGs that disturb the hypothalamic thermostat, elevating the set-point. NSAIDs interrupt the synthesis of the relevant PGs.

Mechanism of action

All NSAIDs act mainly by inhibiting COX, some being more potent on COX-1 than COX-2 (e.g. aspirin, piroxicam); others showing little or only moderate selectivity. More COX-2 selective agents are rofecoxib and celecoxib.

With most agents, the effect is reversible; the exception is aspirin, which causes irreversible inactivation of the enzymes and thus its action persists after it has been metabolised.

Pharmacokinetic aspects

NSAIDs are usually given orally. Naproxen and indometacin can be given by rectal suppository, piroxicam by i.m. injection or suppository, diclofenac i.m., i.v. or as rectal suppository. Some have short half-lives of 1–4 h (aspirin, paracetamol ibuprofen); some have rather longer half-lives (e.g. naproxen 14 h, celecoxib 13h); some have very long half-lives (piroxicam 45 h). Note that aspirin's action lasts longer because it acetylates the COX enzymes.

Unwanted effects

Adverse effects (largely due to COX-1 actions) are frequently reported, particularly if large doses are taken over a long period.

Gastrointestinal disturbances are the commonest. Locally produced PGs inhibit acid secretion in the stomach, have a cytoprotective effect by stimulating mucus and bicarbonate secretion and cause vasodilatation. NSAIDs decrease the synthesis of PGs and thus can cause mucosal damage and bleeding. The risk is greatest with piroxicam, less with naproxen and diclofenac, less still with ibuprofen and least with the COX-2 inhibitors. **Misoprostol**, a PG derivative, can prevent NSAID-induced mucosal damage in patients with a peptic ulcer who need to take non-selective NSAIDs.

Skin reactions are fairly common, particularly with sulindac.

Adverse renal effects occur because NSAIDs decrease local renal PG levels. These PGs increase blood flow and promote natriuresis. NSAIDs can produce reversible renal insufficiency by decreasing PG-induced compensatory vasodilatation, an effect more serious in conditions such as liver disease or heart failure. Long-continued NSAID consumption can result in significant renal damage: chronic nephritis and papillary necrosis.

Bone marrow depression and liver disorders are less frequent. Toxic doses of paracetamol, sometimes taken in suicide attempts, can cause potentially fatal liver damage.

A particular type of encephalitis (Reye's syndrome) can be precipitated by aspirin in children with viral infections so aspirin is now no longer used in children. Aspirin may cause **bronchospasm** in some individuals. NSAIDs are contraindicated in asthma and rofecoxib in some cardiac conditions.

DRUGS USED FOR GOUT

Gout is a chronic disease caused by overproduction of purines. Crystals of sodium urate precipitate in the joints evoking an inflammatory response.

Allopurinol reduces uric acid synthesis by competing with xanthines for xanthine oxidase. It is given orally, has a half-life of 2–3 h and is excreted in the urine. It is used only for long-term therapy; it can exacerbate the acute attack.

Colchicine inhibits migration of neutrophils into the joint by binding to tubulin. It is given orally and is excreted in the GI tract and the kidney. Its peak effect is in 1 h. It can both relieve and prevent an acute attack but can cause GI tract disturbances.

Probenecid acts on the proximal tubule of the nephron to increase uric acid excretion. It is given orally and its peak effect is in 3 h. It is used only to prevent attacks.

NSAIDs (diclofenac, naproxen, piroxicam, but not ibuprofen) are used for the pain of the acute attack.

Clinical uses of NSAIDs

- Analgesia e.g. in musculoskeletal pain, dysmenorrhoea, postoperative pain, cancer metastases to bone.
  - —short-term analgesia: **ibuprofen**, naproxen
  - —non-inflammatory pain (e.g. headache): **paracetamol**
  - —chronic pain: diflunisal; **piroxicam**.
- Anti-inflammatory action in rheumatoid arthritis and other connective tissue disorders: ibuprofen or naproxen to start with, longer-acting agents (e.g. **piroxicam**) if necessary. Higher dosage and long-term use means more likelihood of unwanted effects. COX-2 inhibitors are used mainly in patients with high risk of GI tract toxic effects.
- Fever reduction: **paracetamol**.
- (Note: aspirin is now used mainly as an antiplatelet agent in cardiovascular disease.)

16 Drugs affecting immune responses

The inflammatory/immune response is a specific biological mechanism for dealing with invading parasites. It is superimposed on the innate (non-immunological) response (see Ch. 15) to make it more efficient and more *specific*. The immune response consists of two phases: an **induction phase** and an **effector phase**, the latter consisting of an *antibody-mediated* component and a *cell-mediated* component. Various cytokines control these phases. The key cells are the *lymphocytes* of which there are two main types, B cells and T cells. (A third type, natural killer lymphocytes, participate in innate immune responses.) There are several subtypes of T cells. Precursor T cells (ThP) give rise to Th0 cells (not shown in figure), which can be stimulated to develop into helper T cells (Th). The cytokine interleukin-2 (IL-2) drives the differentiation of Thp and Th1 cells (see figure). On first exposure to antigen, memory B cells and T cells are produced; these speed up the response when that antigen is encountered again.

- **Th1** cells activate and participate in the pathway to **cell-mediated immunity**.
- **Th2** cells activate the pathway to **humoral (antibody-mediated) immunity** by stimulating the proliferation of B cells that mature to plasma cells (P) which generate antibodies. (But note that not all B cell responses are dependent on interaction with Th2 cells).

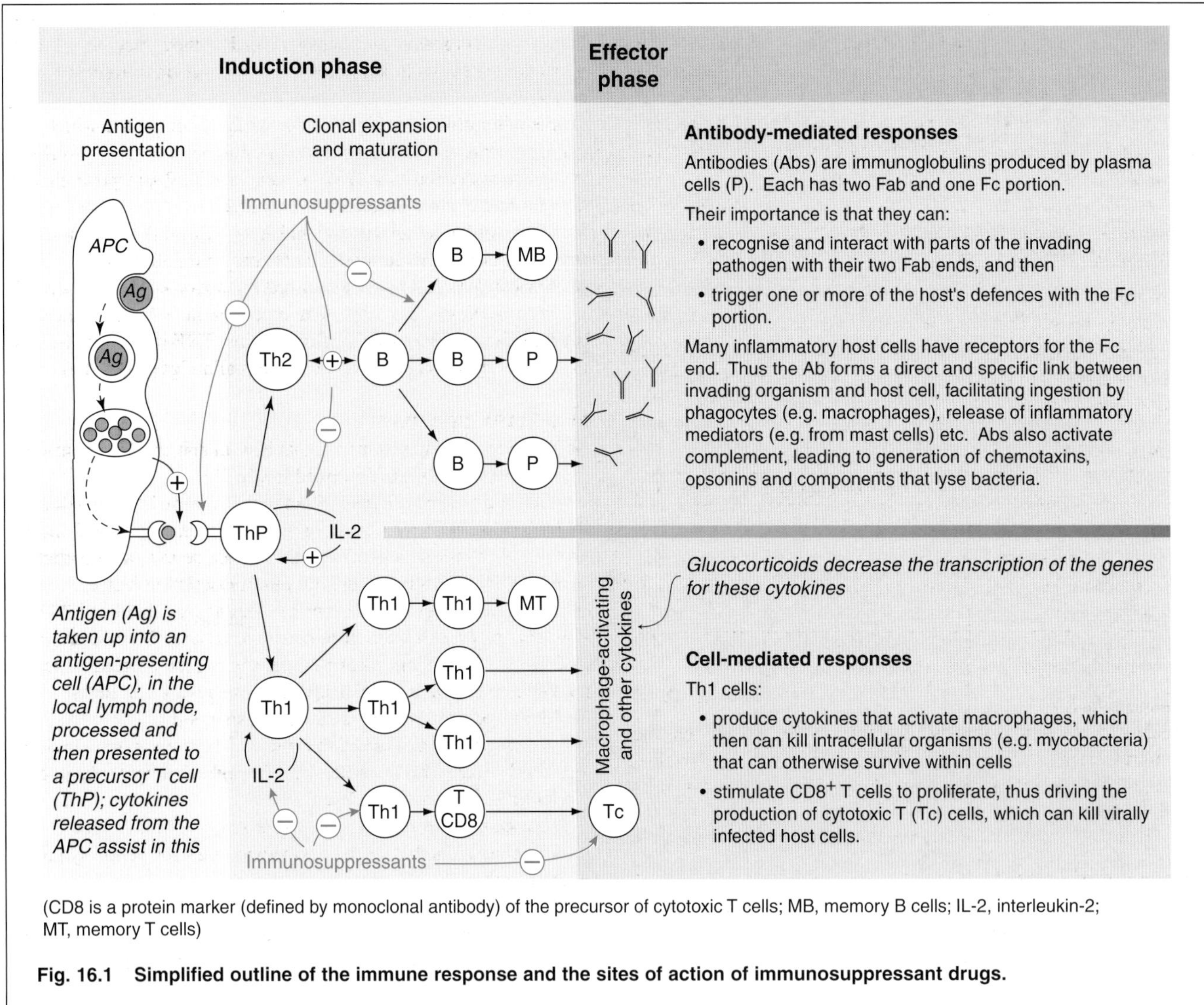

(CD8 is a protein marker (defined by monoclonal antibody) of the precursor of cytotoxic T cells; MB, memory B cells; IL-2, interleukin-2; MT, memory T cells)

Fig. 16.1 Simplified outline of the immune response and the sites of action of immunosuppressant drugs.

Pathophysiology

Immune responses, meant for defence, can themselves cause damage if inappropriately triggered and many diseases are caused by, or have a component of, inappropriately induced immune/inflammatory reactions. Some are associated with Th1 responses (e.g. rheumatoid arthritis, multiple sclerosis, aplastic anaemia, insulin-dependent diabetes). The Th1 pathway is also involved in allograft rejection. Inappropriate Th2 responses are implicated in various allergic (hypersensitivity) conditions. The term **autoimmune disease** is applied to conditions in which the immune response is directed against the body's own tissues.

DRUGS USED FOR UNWANTED IMMUNE REACTIONS

Antihistamines

Histamine is a mediator in both acute inflammation (Chs 15 and 24) and the immediate hypersensitivity response. In the latter, a non-noxious antigen (e.g. grass pollen) evokes a special type of immunoglobulin (IgE), which fixes to mast cells. On subsequent contact with that antigen, the mast cell releases various mediators including histamine. Examples of immediate hypersensitivity reactions are hay fever and urticaria.

Pharmacological actions of histamine

There are two main types of histamine receptor, H_1 and H_2, and antihistamine drugs can target each receptor type.

H_1 receptor activation causes vasodilatation, increased permeability of postcapillary venules, contraction of smooth muscle other than that in the blood vessels (e.g. bronchospasm; Ch. 24). It is these actions that are relevant in immediate hypersensitivity responses.

H_2 receptor activation causes stimulation of gastric secretion and increase in cardiac rate and output. The use of drugs acting at H_2 receptors is described in Ch. 26.

H_1 receptor antagonists

Pharmacology and pharmacokinetics

All H_1 receptor antagonists are competitive at H_1 receptors but some are also sedative or are muscarinic receptor antagonists; their duration of action varies.

Table 16.1 Examples of H_1 receptor antagonists

	Dimenhydrinate	Promethazine	Cetirizine
Sedation	++	++	–
Antimuscarinic effect	++	++	–
Duration of action (h)	4–6	12	12–24
Anti-emetic effect	+	+	–

Unwanted effects

The sedative CNS actions may be unwanted in some situations, and the antimuscarinic effects (dry mouth, blurring of vision, constipation, urine retention) are always unwanted. GI tract disturbances are common.

Antirheumatoid agents

The drugs used are termed **d**isease-**m**odifying **a**nti**r**heumatoid **d**rugs (DMARDs); they alleviate symptoms of rheumatoid arthritis (RA) but do not stop the progress of the disease.

Glucocorticoids (Ch. 28) decrease transcription of the genes for IL-2 and the macrophage-activating cytokines. They are used in RA and also as immunosuppressants.

Sulfasalazine is often a first choice agent. Given orally, it is split into sulfapyridine and salicylate in the bowel. Common side effects are GI tract disturbances, malaise and headache. It can cause skin lesions and low white cell count.

Gold compounds include **auranofin** and sodium aurothiomalate. These cause the symptoms and signs of RA to decrease slowly over 3–4 months. Auranofin is given orally, sodium aurothiomalate by deep i.m. injection. The compounds concentrate in the tissues, particularly in the joints. The half-life is initially 7 days but gradually increases.

Unwanted actions include skin rashes, blood dyscrasias, peripheral neuropathy and encephalopathy; they occur in 30% of patients treated with aurothiomalate but are less frequent with auranofin.

Penicillamine is a highly reactive thiol compound which can chelate metals and also substitute for cysteine in cysteine disulfide. It is given orally and about 75% of patients with RA respond, though the effects are not seen for several months

Chloroquine is an antimalarial drug (Ch. 48) that can cause remission of RA. Given orally, it acts only after 30 days.

Anticytokine agents. These target the action of tumour necrosis factor α (TNF-α), an important mediator in RA. Examples are **infliximab** (a monoclonal antibody against TNF-α) and **etanercept** (a TNF receptor joined to the Fc domain of an IgG molecule).

Immunosuppressants

Main action of immunosuppressants is to inhibit clonal expansion.

Glucocorticoids are described in Ch. 28.

Ciclosporin, tacrolimus. Both drugs act mainly by selective inhibition of IL-2 gene transcription. Both bind with and inhibit proteins that would normally activate calcineurin, a phosphatase necessary for activation of the relevant transcription factors.

Ciclosporin is given orally or i.v. and has a half-life of 24 h; it accumulates in high concentration in the tissues. Tacrolimus has a half-life of 7 h. Main *unwanted effect* is nephrotoxicity, which is common and severe with ciclosporin, less so with tacrolimus.

Rapamycin inhibits IL-2 signal transduction.

Azathioprine, cyclophosphamide. These are cytotoxic drugs also used in cancer chemotherapy (Ch. 49). Cyclophosphamide is particularly toxic to lymphocytes.

Mycophenolate mofetil has a selective action on T and B cell proliferation by inhibiting an enzyme necessary for purine synthesis in these cells.

Antilymphocyte immunoglobulins bind to proteins on the lymphocyte surface, exposing the complement-binding site on their Fc portions. Complement is activated and lyses the cell.

Clinical uses of H_1 receptor antagonists

- Immediate hypersensitivity reactions such as hay fever, insect bites, urticaria, drug allergies: **cetirizine** (does not cross blood-brain barrier so avoids sedative actions).
- Sedation (e.g. **promethazine** (Ch. 36)).
- Motion sickness: **dimenhydrinate** (muscarinic receptor antagonism useful (Ch. 26)).

Clinical use of immunosuppressants

- Inhibition of rejection of transplanted organs and tissues.
- Suppression of graft-versus-host disease in bone marrow transplants.
- Treatment of various conditions that have an autoimmune component, e.g. rheumatoid arthritis.

17 Cardiac rhythm and dysrhythmias

Antidysrhythmic drugs are agents that are used to treat disorders of heart rate and rhythm termed dysrhythmias. The normal regular contractions of the heart are initiated and controlled by a specialised conducting system; dysrhythmias occur when the function of this is deranged. To understand the action of the antidysrhythmic drugs it is necessary to understand the actions of this conducting system.

The specialised conducting system in the heart

A heart beat is initiated in the sinoatrial (SA) node by the pacemaker potential. This triggers an impulse, the action potential, which passes across the atrial muscle to the atrioventricular (AV) node and then, via the Purkinje fibres, through the ventricles—coordinating the contraction of the cardiac muscle. The cardiac action potential has a long duration and long refractory period (Fig. 17.1) and differs from one part of the heart to another. The prolonged activation of Ca^{2+} channels during the action potential plateau in the ventricles maintains Ca^{2+} entry, which is essential for the prolonged contraction required for the effective ejection of blood during systole.

The action of the SA node is controlled by autonomic activity.

Pathophysiology

Clinically important dysrythmias include:

- *Tachycardia (rapid heart beat)*
  - —in the atria ('supraventricular' tachycardias): paroxysmal tachycardia, flutter and fibrillation. In atrial fibrillation (the commonest dysrhythmia), the contraction of the muscle is fast, uncoordinated and ineffective; not all impulses get through to the ventricles, resulting in a very irregular heart rate.
  - —in the ventricles: tachycardia, torsades de pointes (a particular type of tachycardia) and fibrillation (the last frequently fatal).
- *Bradycardia (slow heart beat) and heart block* The latter is due to damage to the AV node or conducting tissue, causing the ventricles to beat at a slower, and often irregular, rate driven by pacemaker activity in the ventricular conducting tissue; an external pacemaker rather than drug therapy is usually required.

Myocardial ischaemia is a common cause of dysrhythmias, which can also be precipitated by reperfusion after an infarction.

The proximal cause of dysrhythmias can be:

- *Abnormal pacemaker activity* Ischaemia-induced depolarisation or increased sympathetic activity can cause pacemaker activity to be initiated at an ectopic focus in atria or ventricles.
- *Early or delayed after-depolarisation (EAD, DAD)* These can act as triggers for the generation of abnormal impulses or extra beats.
  - —DADs. The action potential in non-pacemaker cells does not have a phase 4 depolarisation (Fig. 17.1) but these cells can become ectopic foci of action potential generation if a phase 4-like after-depolarisation occurs. This is associated with increased $[Ca^{2+}]_i$ which can be produced by some drugs (cardiac glycosides, noradrenaline).
  - —EADs. These can arise during phases 2 and 3 of the action potential and can themselves trigger propagated action potentials. They occur when repolarisation is delayed and the action potential is abnormally long: as occurs during bradycardia. EADs can be produced by class III antidysrhythmic drugs.
- *Re-entry* Under normal circumstances, the refractory period of the muscle prevents the action potential re-invading the tissue it has just traversed. If, however, there is damage that allows unidirectional propagation, a continuous cycling of the action potential may occur (circus rhythm) (Fig. 17.2). This is more likely in depolarised tissue where Ca^{2+} channels rather than Na^+ channels produce slowly propagated action potentials with a longer refractory period. Re-entry provides an abnormal site for cardiac excitation.

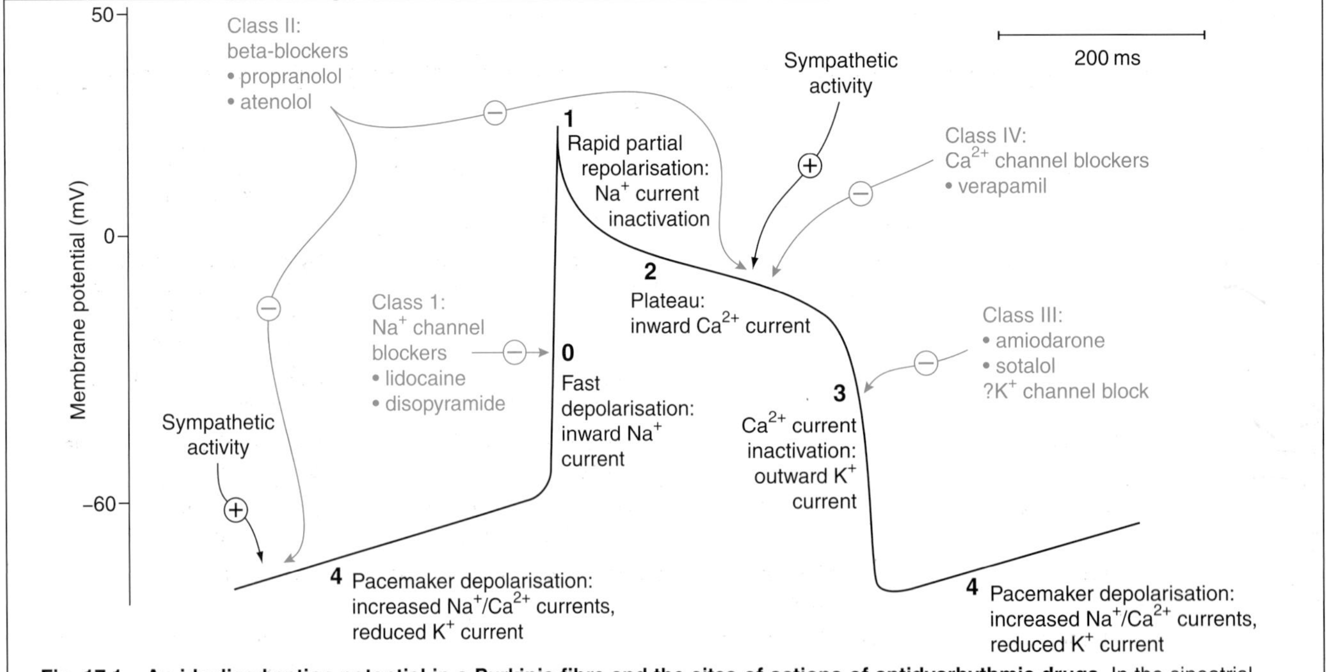

Fig. 17.1 An idealised action potential in a Purkinje fibre and the sites of actions of antidysrhythmic drugs. In the sinoatrial node, an action potential is triggered when the pacemaker potential reaches a critical threshold (approx. –60 mV).

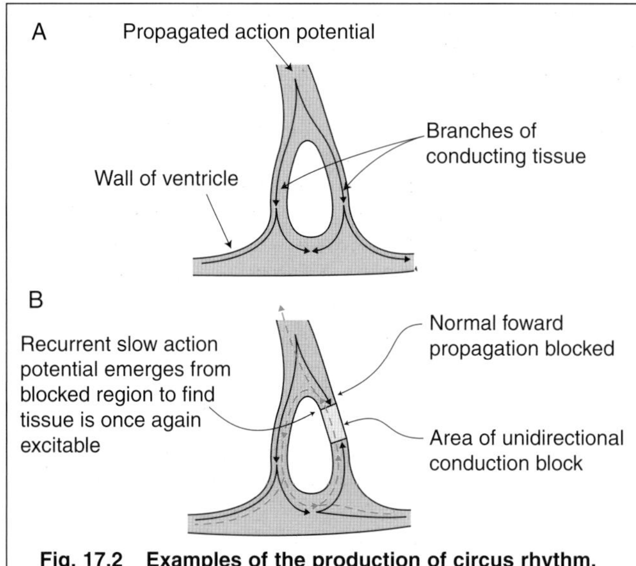

Fig. 17.2 Examples of the production of circus rhythm. A shows the normal conduction pattern. B shows unidirectional block and re-entry.

Antidysrhythmic drugs

Actions and mechanisms of action

Most drugs act on the ion channels involved in the various stages of action potential generation and propagation; some act on the sympathetic control of the heart (Fig. 17.1 and Table 17.1).

All class I drugs show use-dependence, binding preferentially to Na^+ channels in their activated (open) or inactivated states. The block is thus more pronounced at rates above normal (when the channels spend more time in these states) or in depolarised tissues, where recovery from inactivation is delayed. Class I drugs dissociate at different rates from the channel, resulting in different degrees of use-dependence and leading to subdivision of the class into Ia, Ib, and Ic; Ib drugs dissociate rapidly, Ia drugs less rapidly (Ic drugs are not clinically useful).

Amiodarone has class III actions and also blocks Na^+ channels and β-adrenoceptors. These multiple actions may explain its particular efficacy. **Sotalol** has actions in classes II and III. **Adenosine** activates adenosine (A_1) receptors (Ch. 12) in the heart to exert the same cardiac effects as acetylcholine interacting with muscarinic receptors. Its short duration of action reduces the likelihood of side effects. Digoxin has direct effects on myocardial contraction due to its inhibition of the Na^+/K^+ATPase (Ch. 20), which include increased excitability; this may, in fact, cause the conversion of atrial flutter to fibrillation. However, by increasing vagal action on the heart, it blocks AV conduction and usefully reduces ventricular rate.

Pharmacokinetic aspects

Lidocaine is given i.v. following myocardial infarction. It is rapidly metabolised by the liver and so is ineffective orally owing to first-pass metabolism; by the same token it has a short half-life (2 h). **Propranolol** has a half-life of about 4 h with significant first-pass metabolism: its antidysrhythmic activity is maintained by an active metabolite. **Amiodarone** is extensively bound in tissues and only slowly eliminated; its half-life is 10–100 days. **Verapamil** is orally active and has a half-life of 6–8 h. **Adenosine** is given i.v. to terminate supraventricular tachycardia and acts for only 20–30 s due to rapid uptake into erythrocytes and subsequent metabolism.

Unwanted effects

Antidysrhythmics generally have a narrow therapeutic index. As most antidysrhythmics are metabolised by the cytochrome P450 system, pharmacokinetic interactions involving enzyme induction or inhibition may be clinically significant. The Ca^{2+} channel blockers should be avoided in heart failure because of reduction in contractility. Class II drugs should not be used in asthmatic patients because of exacerbation of bronchoconstriction. Amiodarone has important adverse effects, not only triggering torsades de pointes (shared with other class III drugs) but also exhibiting thyroid and pulmonary toxicity.

Table 17.1 The mechanism of action, the electrophysiological actions and clinical uses of selected antidysrhythmic drugs

		Example	Mechanism of action	Electrophysiological actions	Clinical use
Vaughan Williams classification	Class Ia	Disopyramide	Na^+ channel block	Reduced rate of depolarisation of action potential, increased ERP, decreased AV conduction	Ventricular fibrillation, especially associated with myocardial infarction
	Class Ib	Lidocaine			
	Class II	Propranolol, atenolol	β-Adrenoceptor antagonism	Slowed pacemaker activity, increased AV refractory period	Dysrhythmia prevention in myocardial infarction; paroxysmal atrial fibrillation due to sympathetic activity
	Class III	Amiodarone, sotalol	K^+ channel block	Increased action potential duration and increased ERP	Atrial fibrillation; ventricular fibrillation
	Class IV	Verapamil	Ca^{2+} channel block	Decreased APD, slowed AV conduction	Supraventricular tachycardias; atrial fibrillation
Not classified by system		Adenosine	K^+ channel activation	Slowed pacemaker activity, slowed AV conduction	Given i.v. for supraventricular tachycardias
		Digoxin	K^+ channel activation (vagal action)	Slowed AV conduction (block)	Atrial fibrillation
		Magnesium chloride	? Ca^{2+} channel block		Ventricular fibrillation; digoxin toxicity

APD, action potential duration; AV, atrioventricular; ERP, effective refractory period.

18 Blood pressure control and hypertension

The cardiovascular system is regulated by complex mechanisms, the main variable under control being the arterial blood pressure, which is the driving force for the flow of blood through the systemic circulation. The diagram below gives a rough outline of the principal *homeostatic factors* controlling the arterial pressure. The arterioles play the major role in determining the *peripheral resistance* and also regulate the relative blood flow through individual organs. The *cardiac output* depends on the stroke volume (SV) and the *heart rate*. The main factors affecting the SV are the *plasma volume* and the *venous return*; the heart rate is controlled primarily by the sympathetic nerves (which increase the rate) and the parasympathetic nerves (which decrease the rate). Enter the maze below from the CNS, then follow the downward arrow, concentrating on the black text. Paracrine factors influencing the blood pressure are not shown. The boxes give the main antihypertensive drugs.

Vasodilatation involves an increase in cyclic AMP and is brought about partly by adrenaline acting on β_2-adrenoceptors. (A decrease in sympathetic tone can also produce vasodilatation.) Vasodilator paracrine agents include nitric oxide (which increases cyclic GMP), adenosine, prostaglandin I_2 and local accumulation of metabolites. Inflammatory mediators also cause vasodilatation.

Vasoconstriction involves an increase in intracellular Ca^{2+} and is brought about primarily by noradrenaline (NA) released from sympathetic nerves acting on α_1-adrenoceptors (for more detail, see Ch. 11). Other endogenous factors include angiotensin II and local endothelin.

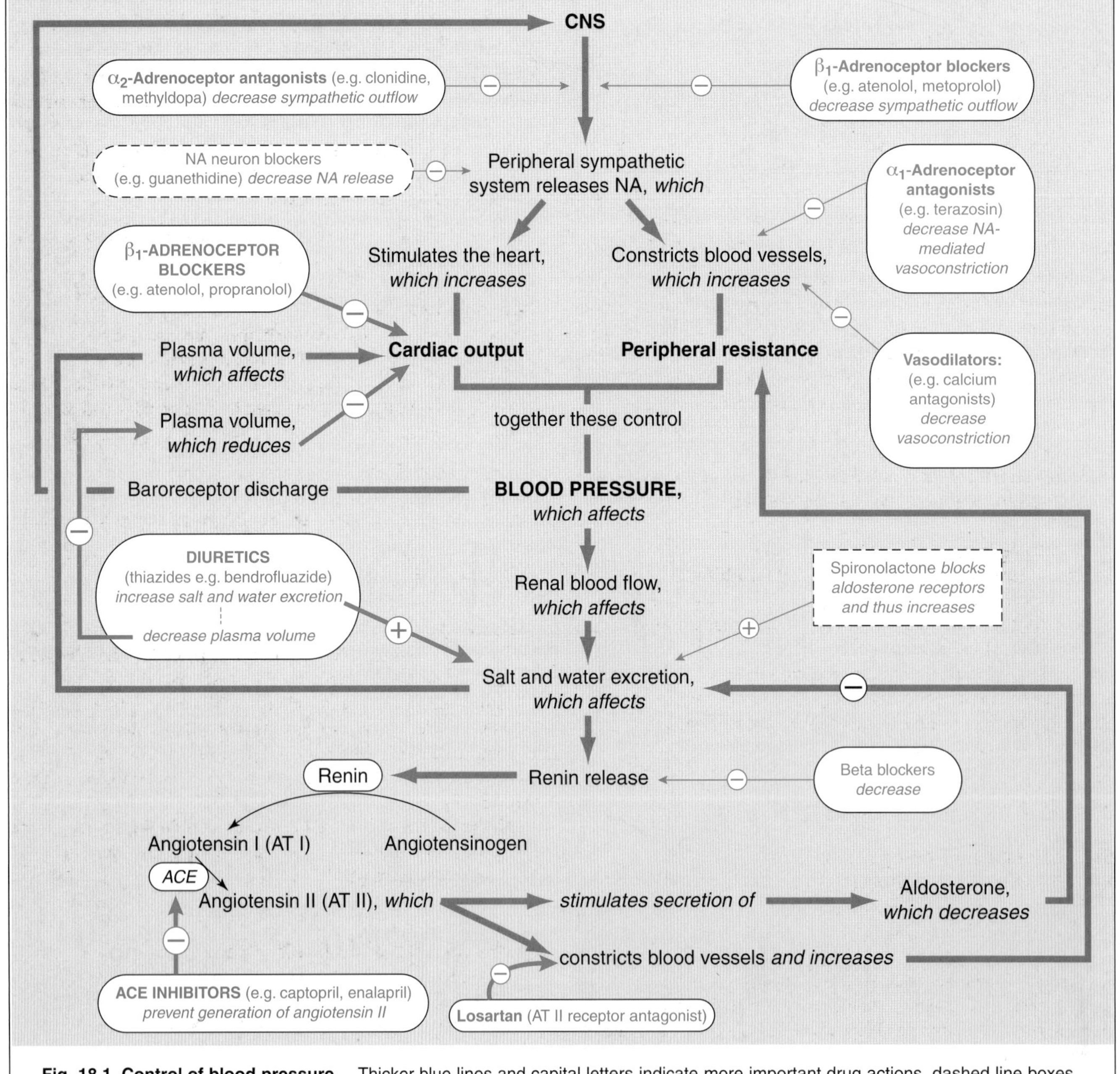

Fig. 18.1 Control of blood pressure. Thicker blue lines and capital letters indicate more important drug actions, dashed line boxes the less important drugs. (ACE, angiotensin-converting enzyme; NA, noradrenaline.)

PATHOPHYSIOLOGY

The main pathological condition affecting the vascular system is hypertension (high blood pressure). This can be caused by renal disease, endocrine disorders or phaeochromocytoma (a catecholamine-secreting tumour; rare), but in most patients the cause is unknown and the hypertension is termed 'essential' (for archaic and mistaken reasons). From Figure 18.1, it is clear that a profusion of factors influences the arterial pressure and theoretically any one or more of them could be implicated in the pathogenesis of hypertension. However, the evidence is that the kidney and/or the sympathetic nervous system play key roles. If hypertension is not treated, coronary thrombosis, stroke or kidney failure may supervene.

ANTIHYPERTENSIVE DRUGS

The main agents used are:

- the **thiazide diuretics** (Ch. 25); actions relevant to the treatment of hypertension are outlined below
- **β-adrenoceptor antagonists** (see Ch. 11); actions relevant to the treatment of hypertension are outlined here
- **calcium antagonists**; these are covered in Ch. 19; actions relevant to the treatment of hypertension are outlined below
- agents affecting the **renin–angiotensin system** (details below).

A thiazide or a beta blocker is used initially; if one of these is ineffective, an angiotensin-converting enzyme (ACE) inhibitor or calcium antagonist is added.

Other drugs that can be used include:

- drugs acting centrally or peripherally on noradrenergic transmission: prazosin, terazosin, clonidine, methyldopa, α-methyltyrosine (aka: metirosine); these are dealt with in Ch. 11
- vasodilators (covered briefly below)
- the ganglion-blocking drug trimetaphan (mentioned in Ch. 10), used only for controlled hypotension during surgery.

Thiazide diuretics

Examples: **bendroflumethiazole, hydrochlorothiazide**.

Actions relevant to hypertension:

- increase in salt and water excretion and thus reduction of extracellular fluid volume
- decrease in cardiac output through reduced plasma volume
- reduction in peripheral resistance (an as yet unexplained effect)
- increase in renin release (which may counteract some of the above effects on the blood pressure).

Thiazides have antihypertensive actions when used alone and also potentiate the action of other antihypertensive drugs.

Beta-adrenoceptor antagonists

Examples: **atenolol, metoprolol**.

Actions relevant to hypertension:

- decrease in cardiac output
- decrease in sympathetic activity by an action in the CNS
- decrease of renin release, which reduces the generation of angiotensin (AT) I and II and thus decreases AT II-induced vasoconstrictor activity and aldosterone-induced salt and water reabsorption.

Calcium antagonists

Examples are: **nifedipine, amlodipine,** diltiazem.

The calcium antagonists block Ca^{2+} entry through Ca^{2+} channels. Action relevant to hypertension is the inhibition of depolarisation-induced Ca^{2+} entry into cardiac and vascular smooth muscle. The vasodilator effect reduces arterial pressure. They cause flushing and ankle oedema; the absence of more serious unwanted actions is a recommendation for their use as antihypertensives.

Drugs acting on the renin–angiotensin system

The sequence of events is outlined in Figure 18.1. (AT III, a breakdown product of AT II, also stimulates aldosterone secretion; not shown.)

The release of renin, a proteolytic enzyme, is stimulated by:

- decreased blood flow through the kidney
- reduced Na^+ concentration in the distal tubule
- β-adrenoceptor agonists

The renin–angiotensin system tends to increase blood pressure by:

- the vasoconstrictor action of AT II (partly through augmentation of NA release)
- the aldosterone-mediated retention of salt and water, which leads to increased extracellular fluid volume. The raised plasma volume increases cardiac output.

These effects can be decreased by ACE inhibitors (see below) and by AT II receptor antagonists (e.g. **losartan**).

ACE inhibitors

Examples: **captopril** and **enalapril**; there are many others.

ACE inhibitors cause a fall in blood pressure, more marked in hypertensive individuals, especially if diuretics are also being given. They are given orally: enalapril (a prodrug) once a day and captopril (which is itself active) twice a day. They are excreted in the urine.

Main unwanted effects

- a dry cough
- hypotension (initially; particularly in the presence of diuretics).

Contraindications

Renovascular disease, pregnancy.

Vasodilators

Various vasodilator agents have been used as antihypertensives (and are sometimes still so used in special circumstances).

Minoxidil is a K^+ channel activator which relaxes vascular smooth muscle by hyperpolarising the plasma membrane, thus preventing Ca^{2+} entry through voltage-dependent Ca^{2+} channels. It is used with a β-adrenoceptor antagonist and a diuretic for very severe hypertension.

Hydralazine relaxes arterioles, causing a fall in blood pressure and reflex tachycardia. It is sometimes used as an adjunct to beta-blocker/diuretic therapy.

Clinical uses of ACE inhibitors

- Hypertension.
- Heart failure.
- As part of the postcardiac infarction treatment.

19 Cardiac blood flow, angina and myocardial infarction

The coronary arteries supply blood to the heart muscle. Blood flow only occurs during diastole and is markedly affected by metabolites, adenosine being the main vasodilator. Other factors less important in the control of the coronary vessels are the sympathetic nerves, circulating catecholamines, and mediators from purinergic, nitrergic and peptidergic neurons.

Pathophysiology of the coronary circulation

The main pathological condition is *atherosclerosis*, in which atheromatous plaque forms within the arteries; this narrows them and decreases perfusion of the myocardium. Plaque formation is initiated by endothelial damage. A simplified explanation of this process has three steps:

1. Platelets, macrophages and low density lipoprotein (LDL; see Ch. 21) adhere to the damaged endothelium.
2. The macrophages release free radicals; these cause lipid peroxidation of the LDL, which the macrophages then ingest.
3. Macrophages release inflammatory cytokines and growth factors, which cause proliferation of smooth muscle and fibroblasts.

Plaque-mediated decreased perfusion of the myocardium causes *angina pectoris*, which is pain caused by the action on nociceptors of chemicals released from the ischaemic muscle. The pain is usually in the chest, is constricting in type and radiates down the left arm. *Stable angina* occurs with a constant amount of exercise; ceasing exertion at the appropriate moment can prevent its onset. Angina that occurs with decreasing amounts of exertion, finally coming on at rest, is termed *unstable angina* and is an indication that a thrombus has formed on the plaque (Fig. 22.1), which may have ruptured. It can presage infarction. *Variant angina* (rare) is caused by coronary artery spasm.

Complete block of a coronary artery is usually a sudden, often dramatic, event and results in *myocardial infarction*, i.e. death, necrotic or apoptotic (see Ch. 4 for explanation of apoptosis), of the tissue supplied by the vessel. It is a very common cause of death in the developed world.

ANGINA

The therapeutic aims in antianginal therapy are:

1. to reduce cardiac work and, thus, metabolic demand
2. to increase perfusion of heart muscle
3. to prevent mycardial infarction.

This last aim may be achieved by several means (Fig. 19.1). *Lipid-lowering drugs*, particularly **statins**, can inhibit plaque development (see Ch. 22). *Antiplatelet drugs*, especially **aspirin** (Ch. 15) and **platelet glycoprotein receptor antagonists** (see Ch. 22) can reduce the possibility of thrombosis. Aspirin is particularly important in unstable angina (which requires hospitalisation).

In this chapter we concentrate on the first two aims.

Drugs used in angina

- **Organic nitrates** have the first two actions specified under therapeutic aims
- **Calcium antagonists** (calcium channel blockers) have the first two actions specified under therapeutic aims (see Chs 18 and 20); only aspects relevant to angina therapy are dealt with below.
- **β-adrenoceptor antagonists** have only the first action (see Ch. 11 for details; only aspects relevant to angina therapy are dealt with below).
- Nicorandil, a K^+ channel activator, has both actions.

Organic nitrates

Examples: **glyceryl trinitrate (nitroglycerin), isosorbide mononitrate.**

The actions and mechanisms of action of nitrates is explained in Figures 19.1 and 19.2 (see also Ch. 14).

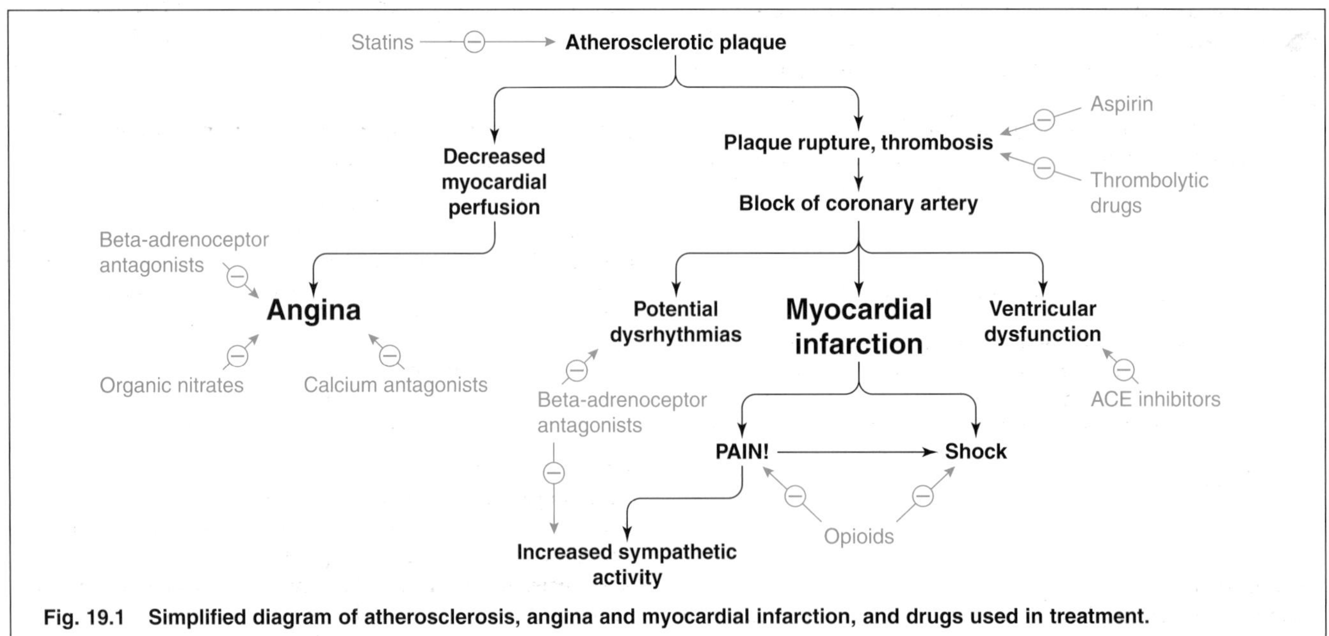

Fig. 19.1 Simplified diagram of atherosclerosis, angina and myocardial infarction, and drugs used in treatment.

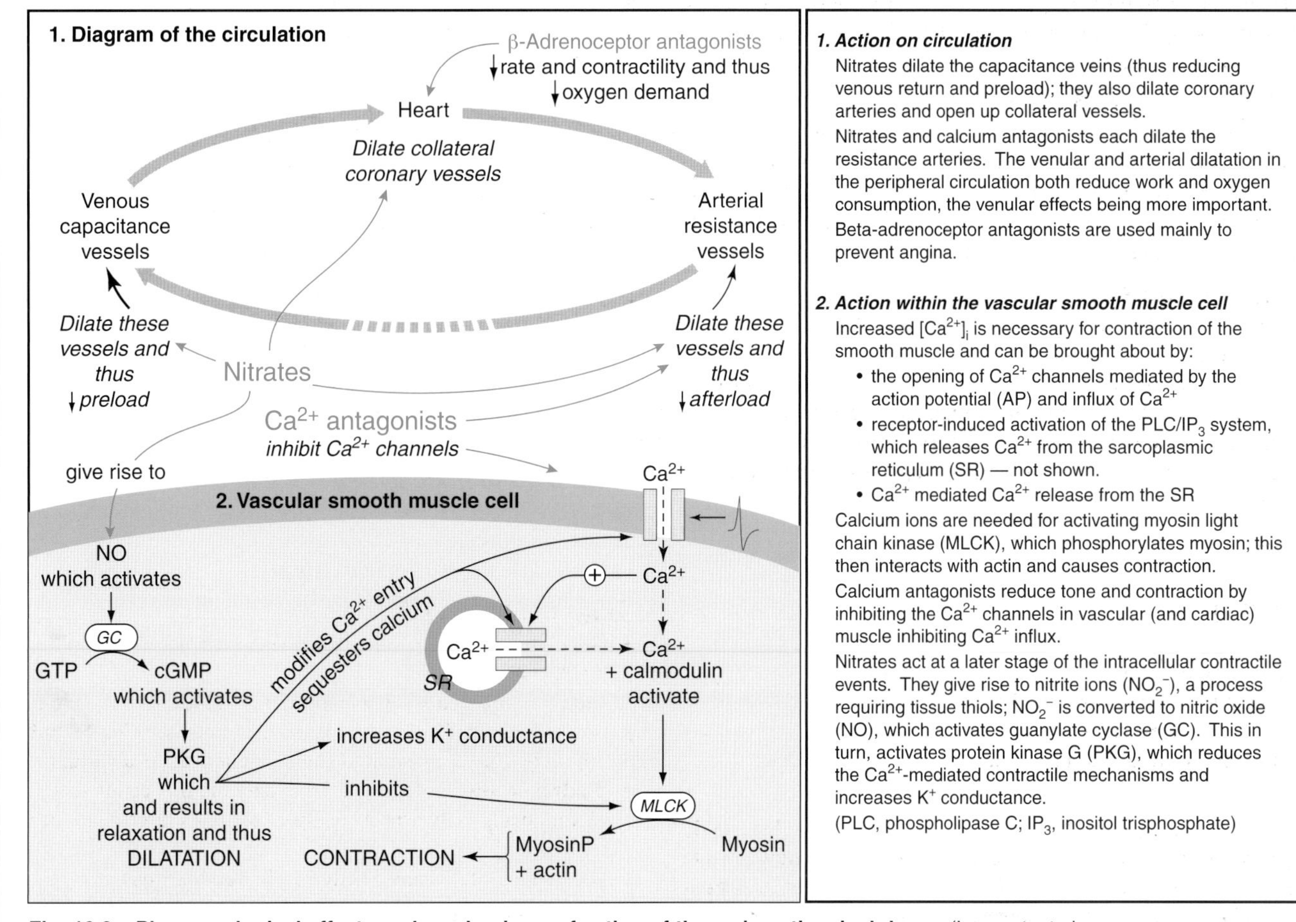

Fig. 19.2 Pharmacological effects and mechanisms of action of the main antianginal drugs. (Larger text size means more important actions.)

Pharmacokinetic aspects

Glyceryl trinitrate can be taken by sublingual tablet or spray, in which case its effects start within minutes and last approximately 30 min. Given by transdermal patch, its action lasts approximately 24 h. It can also be given i.v. It cannot be given orally as it would be inactivated by first-pass metabolism in the liver.

Isosorbide mononitrate is a longer-acting nitrate which is given orally. Its half-life is 4 h. A slow-release preparation is available.

Clinical use of the organic nitrates

- **In the treatment of angina:** glyceryl trinitrate or isosorbide mononitrate is given sublingually to prevent or treat stable angina; glyceryl trinitrate is given i.v. to treat unstable angina.
- **In the treatment of chronic heart failure:** nitrates can be given to decrease venous return and thus reduce preload (Ch. 20).

Unwanted effects

Nitrates can cause headache because of the pronounced vasodilatation, and postural hypotension through the fall in blood pressure. Frequent use of isosorbide mononitrate can cause tolerance through depletion of tissue thiols. The tolerance is short lived, lasting only a day or so after administration of the nitrate is stopped.

Calcium antagonists (calcium channel blockers)

Examples: **nifedipine**, **amlodipine**, verapamil.

Actions and mechanisms of action

Calcium antagonists all act by blocking voltage-dependent L-type Ca^{2+} channels in vascular smooth muscle (see Fig. 19.2) and cardiac muscle. Some are more active on blood vessels; some are more active on the heart.

Actions on blood vessels

Nifedipine and amlodipine act mainly on arterial resistance vessels causing relaxation and vasodilatation (Fig. 19.2).

Actions on the heart

Verapamil acts mainly on the heart, slowing the rate by action on the sino-atrial (SA) and atrioventricular (AV) nodes. It inhibits the slow inward movement of Ca^{2+} during the plateau phase of the cardiac action potential (see Fig. 17.1). It has little useful effect on blood vessels. Verapamil is not used in angina because of the risk of heart failure or heart block from its inhibitory action on AV conduction.

Pharmacokinetic aspects

Calcium antagonists are given orally and are easily absorbed. Nifedipine has a short half-life (approx. 2 h); amlodipine is much longer acting (half-life of approx. 40 h). Verapamil undergoes fairly extensive first-pass metabolism and has a half-life of approx. 4 h.

Unwanted effects

The unwanted effects are extensions of the pharmacological actions. Nifedipine and amlodipine cause reflex tachycardia, headache and flushing due to the vasodilatation. Verapamil can cause constipation, possibly by inhibition of Ca^{2+} channels in intestinal smooth muscle.

Serious adverse effects do not generally occur.

Clinical use of calcium antagonists

- **In the treatment of angina:** amlodipine is used to prevent angina.
- **In the treatment of dysrhythmias:** verapamil, a class IV antidysrhythmic agent, is used to slow the heart in atrial fibrillation; it is also used to prevent supraventricular tachycardias.
- **In the treatment of hypertension:** amlodipine can be used to lower the blood pressure.

Beta-adrenoceptor antagonists

Examples: **atenolol,** metoprolol.

These reduce cardiac work and thus the heart's metabolic demand. Their action in angina is described in Figures 19.1 and 19.2. Other aspects of the pharmacology of beta blockers are covered in Ch. 11.

Cardiac uses of the β-adrenoceptor antagonists

- To prevent angina
- Other uses are given in Chs 11 and 18.

Nicorandil

Nicorandil, a K^+ channel activator with some nitrate-like actions, dilates both arteries and veins. It is given orally and can cause headache, giddiness and flushing.

MYOCARDIAL INFARCTION

Drugs used to treat myocardial infarction

This is a medical emergency requiring hospitalisation. The therapeutic aims are:

1. to alleviate the pain: **opioids** (Ch. 41)
2. to improve oxygenation of the myocardium: **oxygen**
3. to open the blocked artery by reducing thrombus size and limiting its extension:
   - — **thrombolytic drugs** (see Ch. 22) are effective if given within 12 h of onset
   - — **anticoagulants** (Ch. 22)
   - — **antiplatelet drugs** especially aspirin (see Chs 15 and 22)
4. to improve survival: **angiotensin-converting enzyme** (ACE) **inhibitors** (Ch. 20) have been shown to have this effect if given soon after the infarct occurs.
5. to reduce the possibility of re-infarction: **aspirin** (Ch. 15) and **β-adrenoceptor antagonists** (Ch. 11).

20 Cardiac output and cardiac failure

One of the main pathophysiological conditions affecting the heart is *heart failure*. To understand the basis of this and how it is treated it is necessary to understand the mechanism of *contraction* of cardiac muscle and the factors that determine *cardiac output*. In heart failure, the cardiac output is inadequate for bodily needs.

Cardiac contraction

Cardiac contraction requires an increase in intracellular Ca^{2+}, which then activates the contractile mechanism. Figure 20.1 shows the role of Ca^{2+} in contraction, the action of noradrenaline and the sites of action of some drugs.

Cardiac output

The main factors that determine cardiac output include plasma volume, venous pressure, stroke volume and the actions of the sympathetic and parasympathetic nervous systems. The interaction of these factors is shown in Figure 20.2.

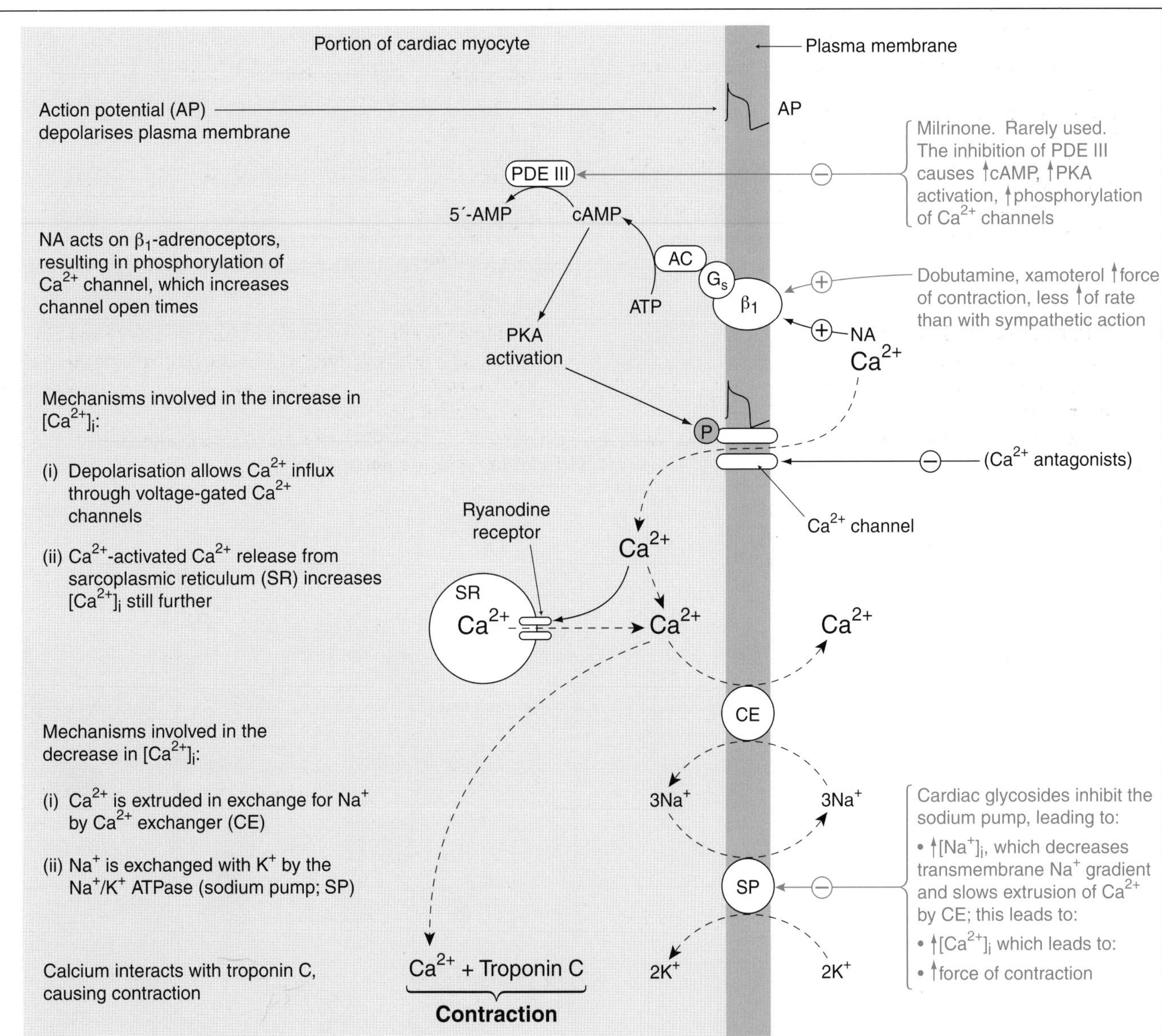

Fig. 20.1 Cardiac contraction, the role of Ca^{2+} and noradrenaline (NA) and the action of drugs. The site of action of the calcium antagonists is shown, *but these are not used for the treatment of heart failure.* AC, adenylate cyclase; G, G-protein; PDE III, phosphodiesterase III; PKA, protein kinase A; →, acts on; →, moves to or is converted to.

Plasma volume
Venous pressure
Venoconstriction
Pre-load (filling pressure)
End-diastolic volume
Input of sympathetic nervous system
Input of parasympathetic nervous system
Stroke volume
Heart rate
Cardiac output

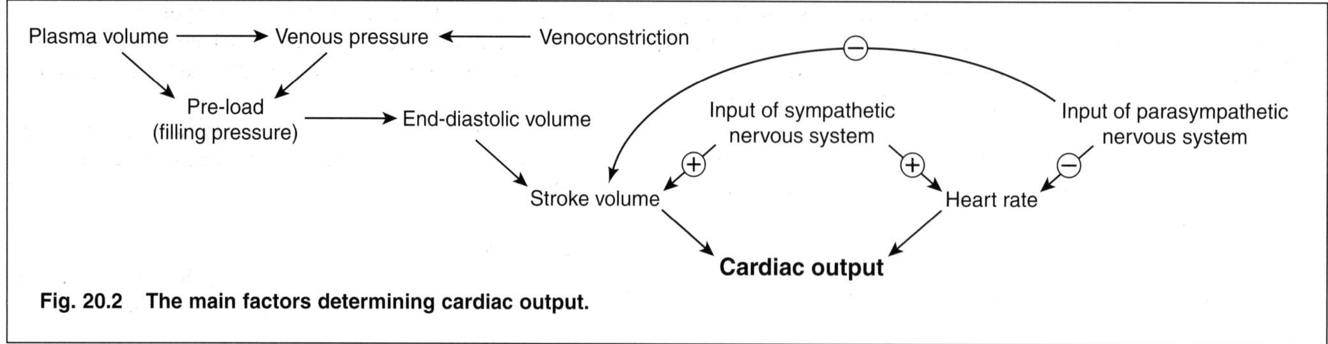

Fig. 20.2 The main factors determining cardiac output.

The autonomic nervous system in the contol of cardiac output

The *sympathetic nervous system*:

- increased force of contraction through effect on Ca^{2+} channels
- increased rate
- increased oxygen consumption (↓ efficiency).

In cardiac failure, increased sympathetic activity increases the vicious cycle of events in that it increases rate and force and increases peripheral resistance, which increases after-load (Fig. 20.3).

The *parasympathetic nervous system*:

- decreased rate and automaticity through the action of acetylcholine on M_2 receptors in nodal tissues increasing K^+ permeability
- decreased force of contraction mainly in atria through inhibition of adenylate cyclase and, therefore, decreased protein kinase A activation and decreased phosphorylation of Ca^{2+} channels.

Cardiac failure

Cardiac failure is essentially a reduction of cardiac output in spite of adequate venous filling, the reduced output becoming insufficient to

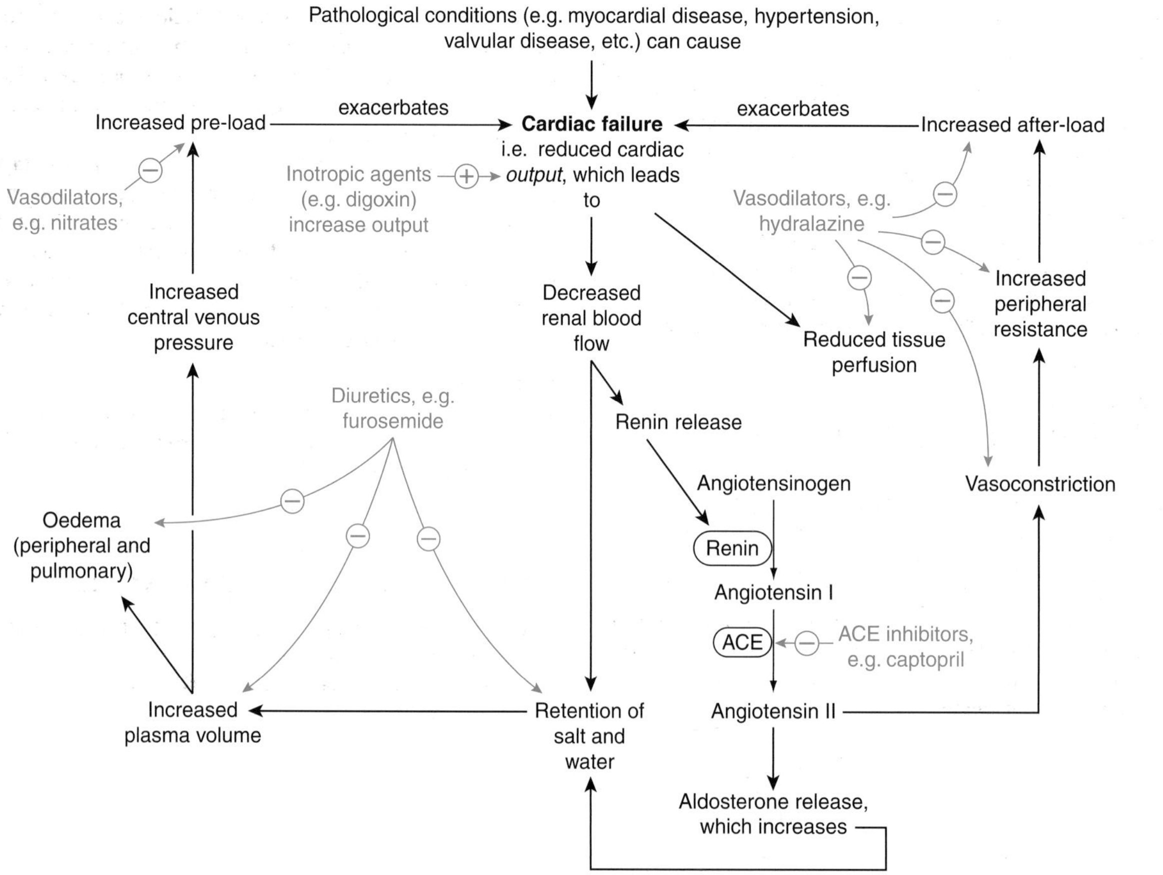

Pathological conditions (e.g. myocardial disease, hypertension, valvular disease, etc.) can cause
Increased pre-load
exacerbates
Cardiac failure
i.e. reduced cardiac output, which leads to
exacerbates
Increased after-load
Vasodilators, e.g. nitrates
Inotropic agents (e.g. digoxin) increase output
Vasodilators, e.g. hydralazine
Increased central venous pressure
Decreased renal blood flow
Reduced tissue perfusion
Increased peripheral resistance
Diuretics, e.g. furosemide
Renin release
Angiotensinogen
Vasoconstriction
Oedema (peripheral and pulmonary)
Renin
Angiotensin I
ACE
ACE inhibitors, e.g. captopril
Increased plasma volume
Retention of salt and water
Angiotensin II
Aldosterone release, which increases

Fig. 20.3 The pathophysiology of heart failure. Some of the main factors involved in heart failure with the action of the principal drugs used in treatment. ACE, angiotensin-converting enzyme.

perfuse the tissues. Cardiac failure can result from several factors, such as myocardial disease, hypertension or valvular disease. The interaction of these factors is shown in Figure 20.3. Note that the factors specified as increasing pre-load (along with increased sympathetic activity) are initially compensatory, maintaining cardiac output. But eventually they, and the factors increasing afterload, result in exacerbation of the situation; and the clinical signs and symptoms of failure become evident.

Drugs used to treat heart failure

Diuretics

Diuretics are dealt with in Ch. 25; only actions relevant for heart failure are given here.

Diuretics are first choice drugs for heart failure; a loop diuretic is usually used (e.g. **furosemide** (frusemide)) though a thiazide (e.g. **bendroflumethiazide** (bendrofluazide)) may be used instead. The action is shown in the chart; essentially they decrease pre-load by increasing salt and water excretion.

Angiotensin-converting enzyme (ACE) inhibitors

Examples are **captopril** and **enalapril**. These are dealt with in Ch. 18; only actions relevant to heart failure are given here.

ACE inhibitors are used with a diuretic if the diuretic alone is not effective. They inhibit formation of angiotensin II and thus reduce not only peripheral resistance (and, therefore, afterload) but also the release of aldosterone. This results in reduction of salt and water retention and, therefore, decreased plasma volume leading to decreased pre-load.

Beta-blockers

Sympathetic nervous systems action increases cardiac contraction; in the early stages of failure this is comensatory. Accordingly, it has been thought that blocking this would worsen the failure. Paradoxically, however, sympathetic *overactivity* can be an exacerbating factor in established cardic failure and in this circumstance the use of β-adrenoceptor antagonists would seem to be logical step. Some light has been shone on this problem because it has been reported recently that beta-blockers (e.g. metaprolol; see Ch. 11) used carefully, along with other agents, can prolong survival.

Digitalis glycosides

The digitalis glycosides are third-line drugs; the main example is **digoxin**.

Pharmacological actions and mechanisms of action

- An increase in the force of contraction without increasing oxygen consumption; this is their main action in heart failure
- A decrease in rate mainly by an action on the vagus, which reduces atrioventricular (AV) conduction; there is an increase in the refractory period in the AV node and the bundle of His (the rate decrease allows for better filling and this, with the increased force of contraction, increases cardiac output)
- An increased possibility of disturbances of rhythm:
  —digoxin inhibits the sodium pump (which normally tends to cause hyperpolarisation by the $3Na^+/2K^+$ exchange), causing depolarisation
  —digoxin increases $[Ca^{2+}]_i$, thus increasing after-depolarisation; if this reaches threshold, an action potential is generated leading to ectopic beats.

Pharmacokinetic aspects

Digoxin is given orally, usually with a loading dose (except in mild failure) and is excreted largely unchanged by the kidney. It has a half-life of 36 h.

Unwanted effects

- dysrhythmias; ventricular fibrillation with high doses
- nausea and vomiting
- confusion
- disturbances in colour vision.

Vasodilators

Vasodilators also have a role in the treatment of heart failure:

- **nitrates** (see Ch. 19 for details): actions relevant to the treatment of heart failure are shown in Fig. 20.3.
- **hydralazine**: only used if it is not possible to use ACE inhibitors (see Fig. 20.3 for site of action; mechanism of action unknown).

Drugs used in acute severe cardiac failure

The term cardiac failure is usually used to refer to chronic congestive cardiac failure. This develops slowly, fluid retention occurring first as indicated by an increase in weight, before actual oedema, breathlessness and decreased exercise tolerance are evident. The cardiac output is, however, sufficient for the patient to pursue most daily activities for several years.

However, the heart can fail more suddenly (e.g. with myocardial infarction), producing all the features of heart failure while the patient is at rest. This is acute severe cardiac failure. **Dobutamine**, a β_1-agonist (see Fig. 11.2), can be used in treatment because its effect on cardiac contractility is believed to be greater than its effect on cardiac rate. Dobutamine effect on the heart also has a place in the treatment of hypovolaemic shock.

Dobutamine

Acute severe heart failure is treated by i.v. infusion with dobutamine; the drug is a β_1-adrenoceptor agonist and increases sympathetic input (Fig. 20.2).

> **Clinical uses of the digitalis glycosides**
>
> - Treatment of chronic heart failure if diuretics and ACE inhibitors are not effective.
> - Treatment of atrial fibrillation (see Ch. 17).

21 Atherosclerosis and lipoproteins

Excessive concentrations of plasma cholesterol associated with low density lipoproteins are important risk factors for atherosclerosis and ischaemic heart disease. To understand how drugs that lower plasma cholesterol concentrations work, it is necessary to know how lipids are handled in the body and to have some acquaintance with dyslipidaemias and the pathophysiology of atherosclerosis.

Lipid transport in the blood

Lipids are insoluble in water and are transported through the blood stream in the form of lipoproteins. These are macromolecular complexes consisting of a central core of hydrophobic lipid (triglycerides or cholesteryl esters) surrounded by a more hydrophilic coat of phospholipids and free cholesterol. Apoproteins embedded in the coat can be recognised by receptors in the liver and other tissues, enabling the particles to bind to the cells.

There are four main classes of lipoprotein, differing in the relative proportion of the core lipids and in the type of apoprotein:

- high density lipoproteins (HDL)
- low density lipoproteins (LDL)
- very low density lipoproteins (VLDL)
- chylomicrons.

In the transport of lipids, each of the above lipoproteins has a specific role and there are different pathways for exogenous and endogenous lipids (Fig. 21.1).

The exogenous pathway

Cholesterol and triglycerides absorbed from the gastrointestinal tract are transported as chylomicrons to the liver and peripheral tissues. Here, a surface-bound lipoprotein lipase on the vascular endothelial

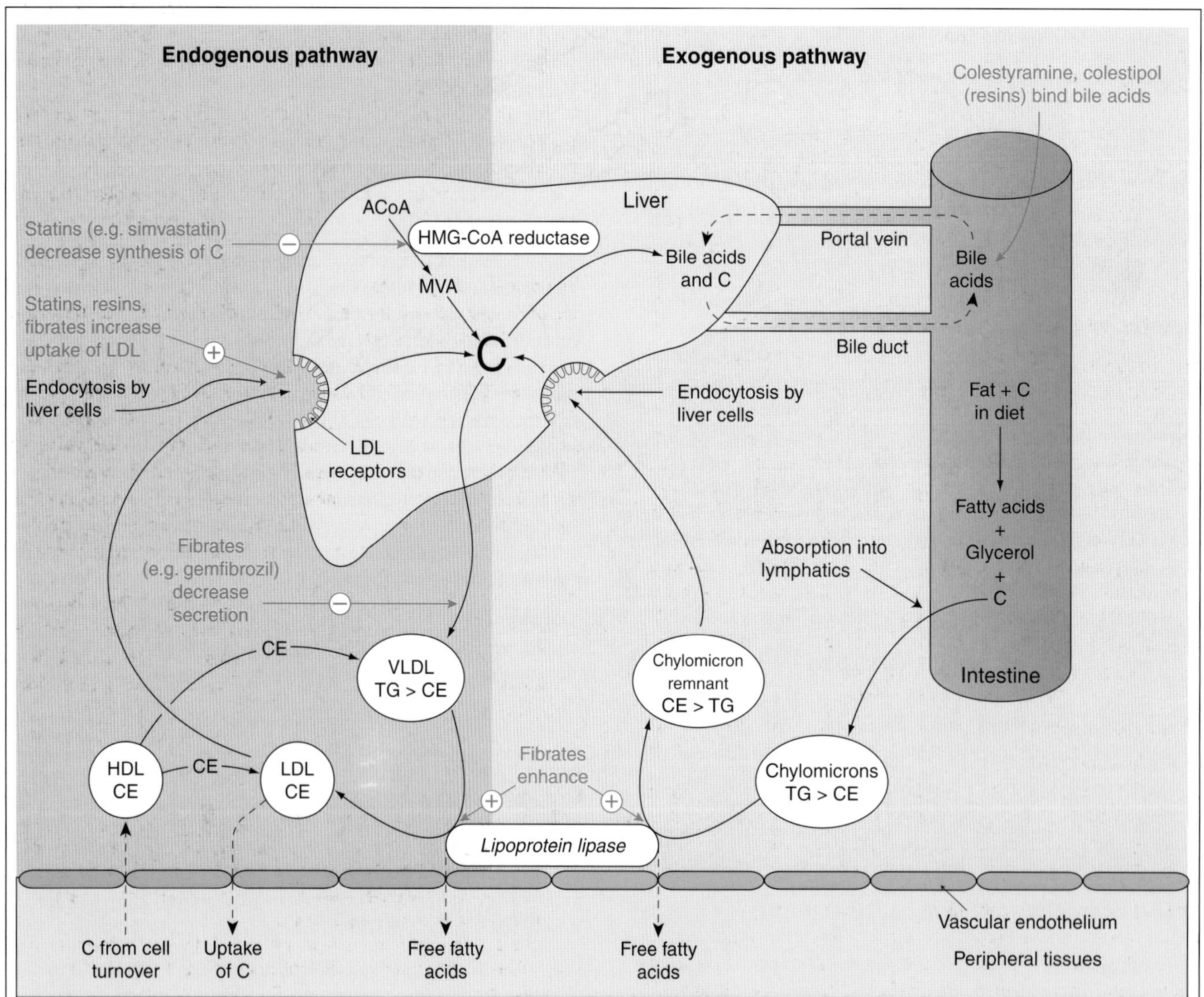

Fig. 21.1 Diagram of the synthesis and metabolism of cholesterol, the transport of lipoproteins in the plasma and the sites of action of lipid-lowering drugs. VLDL are the main carriers of triglycerides to the tissues and thus the main purveyors of free fatty acids. LDL are the main purveyors of cholesterol to the tissues. ACoA, acetyl coenzyme A; C, cholesterol; CE, cholesteryl esters; HMG-CoA, 3-hydroxy-3-methylglutaryl-CoA; HDL, high density lipoproteins; LDL, low density lipoproteins; MVA, mevalonate; TG, triglycerides; VLDL, very low density lipoproteins. HMG-CoA reductase is the rate-limiting enzyme in cholesterol synthesis.

cells hydrolyses the core triglycerides allowing the free fatty acids to be taken up by the tissues. The chylomicron remnants, with the full complement of cholesteryl esters, pass to the liver, where they are endocytosed and the cholesterol liberated to join the hepatic cholesterol pool. The cholesterol (some of which will have been synthesised through the 3-hydroxy-3-methylglutaryl-coenzyme A (HMG-CoA) mevalonate pathway) may enter the endogenous pathway in **VLDL**, be oxidised to bile acids, be stored or be secreted unaltered in the bile.

The endogenous pathway

VLDL, consisting of newly synthesised triglycerides and cholesterol with a small amount of an apoprotein, are synthesised in the liver and then enter the circulation. After apoprotein-mediated binding to cells, the triglycerides are hydrolysed by cell-attached lipoprotein lipase. The released fatty acids enter the tissues but the full complement of cholesteryl esters is retained. The particles pass through a phase in which they are termed intermediate density lipoproteins (not shown in Fig. 21.1) and eventually become **LDL**. LDL are the main carriers of cholesterol, essential for synthesis of steroids and new plasma membrane. There is a strong association between average fat consumption, mean LDL cholesterol concentration and the incidence of ischaemic heart disease.

Cells obtain cholesterol by synthesising receptors for the relevant apoproteins of LDL so that they can take these up by receptor-mediated endocytosis. Some drugs (e.g. statins) reduce the plasma LDL concentration by stimulating the synthesis of these receptors in liver cells. Free cholesterol is taken up from cells by **HDL** particles and then esterified, the resulting cholesteryl esters being transferred to VLDL or LDL particles in exchange for triglycerides (Fig. 21.1).

Dyslipidaemias

Dyslipidaemias (hyperlipidaemias) may be primary (genetic) or secondary to other diseases (e.g. diabetes, hypothyroidism).

Lipoproteins and atherosclerosis

Atherosclerosis is characterised by intimal plaques (Fig. 22.1); these are formed when local damage to the endothelium is followed by deposition of lipoproteins (mainly LDL) and adhesion and activation of macrophages, which generate oxygen radicals that cause lipid peroxidation of the LDL (Ch. 19). The macrophages also produce growth factors that stimulate smooth muscle proliferation and the deposition of extracellular matrix (see Ch. 4). Thrombi can develop on the plaque (see Ch. 22), which narrows the artery and can block it (Fig. 22.1). These are major risk factors for ischaemic heart disease and can result in myocardial infarction (Ch. 19) or stroke.

Lipid-lowering drugs

Several drugs, with different mechanisms of action, can decrease plasma LDL-cholesterol. They are used in conjunction with dietary management and correction of other cardiovascular risk factors.

Statins: HMG-CoA reductase inhibitors

The statins are amongst the most valuable of the drugs introduced in the last decade and are proving to be very important in the treatment of cardiovascular disease. Examples are **simvastatin** and pravastatin. Their main overall effect is to reduce plasma LDL-cholesterol and total cholesterol. They also decrease plasma triglyceride and increase HDL-cholesterol.

Mechanism of action Statins inhibit cholesterol synthesis in the liver by specific, reversible competitive inhibition of HMG-CoA reductase (Fig. 21.1). Falling cholesterol concentrations increase expression of the LDL receptor gene and, hence, augment synthesis of LDL receptors, leading to increased clearance of LDL.

Pharmacokinetic aspects Statins are given orally and are well absorbed. They are extracted by the liver and undergo first-pass metabolism. Simvastatin is inactive until biotransformed in the liver.

Unwanted effects These are mild and include gastrointestinal disturbances, an increase in liver transaminases, rash and insomnia. There is a low incidence of a more severe adverse effect—myositis—and combination with fibrates increases this risk.

Fibrates

Examples of fibrates are **bezafibrate** and gemfibrozil. The main overall effect is a marked reduction in plasma triglyceride but the drugs also decrease LDL-cholesterol and increase HDL-cholesterol.

Mechanism of action These drugs bind to and activate a nuclear transcription factor termed peroxisome proliferator-activated receptor alpha (PPARα), which results in stimulation of the β-oxidation of fatty acids and an increase in lipoprotein lipase synthesis. This latter action leads to greater plasma clearance of triglycerides (Fig. 21.1).

Pharmacokinetic aspects Fibrates are given orally and are well absorbed if given with food; they are metabolised to glucuronate conjugates, which are excreted by the kidney.

Unwanted effects Fibrates may cause a myositis-like syndrome (and combination with statins can potentiate this action) and can increase the risk of gallstones.

Bile acid-binding resins

Examples are **colestyramine** and colestipol. Their overall effect is to decrease LDL-cholesterol.

Mechanism of action These positively charged drugs bind the negatively charged bile acids in the gut inhibiting their absorption, which diminishes the pool of bile acids in the liver. This stimulates the synthesis of bile acids, thus decreasing the hepatic store of cholesterol (which the resins also lower by reducing absorption from the gut). This, in turn, stimulates the synthesis of LDL receptors. As with statins, this increases LDL uptake, reducing the plasma concentration of LDL. There can be some temporary increase in plasma triglycerides.

Pharmacokinetic aspects and unwanted effects The drugs are given orally and as they are not absorbed, systemic adverse effects do not occur. Within the bowel, they interfere with the absorption of fat-soluble vitamins and some drugs. They are likely to produce bloating and dyspepsia.

Clinical uses of lipid-lowering drugs

- **Statins** are used to prevent myocardial infarction and stroke in patients with predisposing conditions and to prevent arterial disease in individuals with high serum cholesterol. Therapy once initiated is usually life long.
- **Fibrates** are used in patients with familial hyperlipidaemia, in which both serum cholesterol and serum triglycerides are raised.
- **A bile acid-binding resin** is used in combination with a statin if this on its own fails to lower serum LDL-cholesterol sufficiently or if a statin cannot be used.

22 Haemostasis and thrombosis

Haemostasis is the arrest of blood loss from damaged blood vessels and is essential to life. During haemostasis a haemostatic plug is formed, the main processes being:

- adhesion and activation of platelets
- activation of clotting factors, leading to blood coagulation (fibrin formation).

Thrombosis is a pathological condition — the formation of a haemostatic plug associated with arterial disease or with stasis of blood in the veins or the atria of the heart. An **embolus** is a portion of a thrombus that breaks away into the circulation. If it derives from a venous thrombus, it may lodge in the lungs; if it comes from a thrombus in the left heart, it may lodge in the brain or other organs.

Therapy to promote haemostasis with procoagulant drugs is rarely employed, but drug therapy of thromboembolic disease (with anticoagulant drugs, antiplatelet agents, fibrinolytic drugs) is extensively used because these diseases are the major cause of death in developed countries.

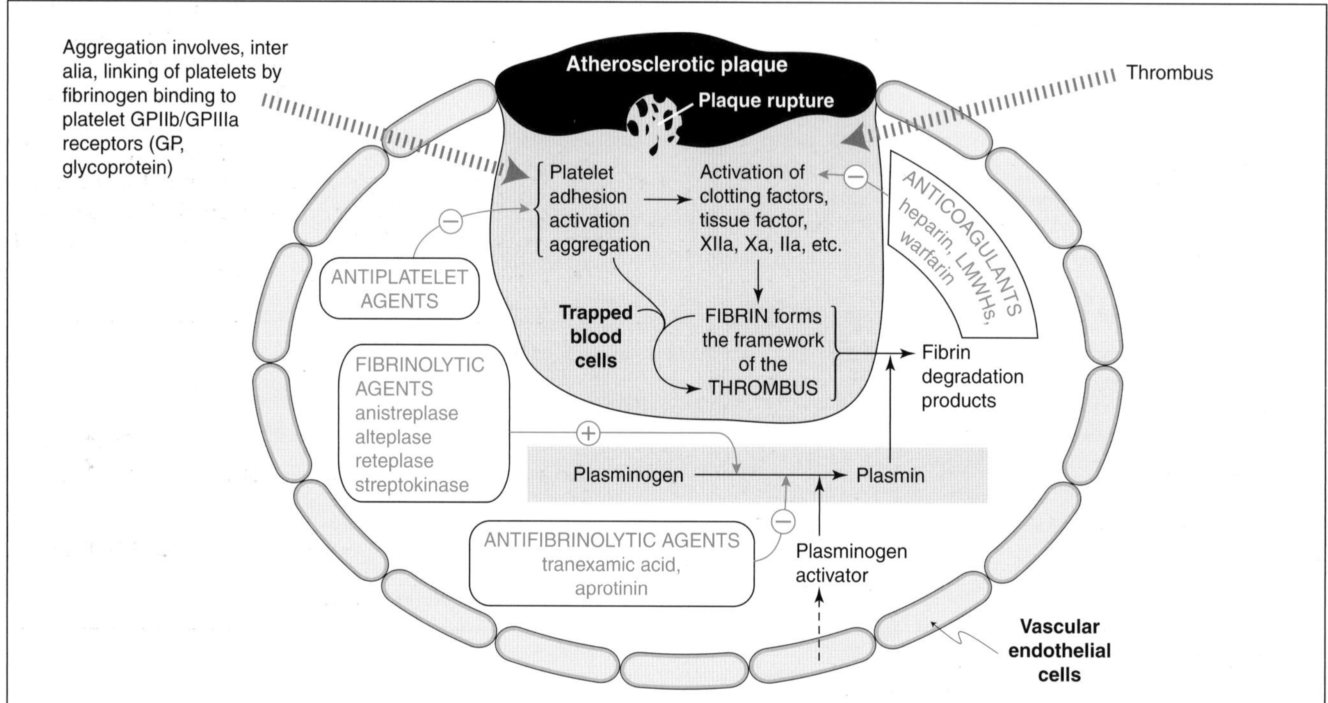

Fig. 22.1 Diagram of a thrombus showing the interaction of the platelet-activation system, the coagulation cascade and the fibrinolytic (thrombolytic) system along with the action of drugs on these systems. (LMWHs, low-molecular-weight heparins.)

PROCOAGULANT DRUGS

Examples: fat-soluble **vitamin K** (phytomenadione), synthetic water-soluble **menadiol**.

Mechanism of action. Vitamin K, when reduced, acts as a cofactor in the post-translational γ-carboxylation of a cluster of glutamic acid (Glu) residues in factors II, VII, IX and X (see Fig. 22.4, below).

Administration and pharmacokinetic aspects. Vitamin K can be given orally, i.m. or i.v. Phytomenadione requires bile salts for oral absorption, menadiol does not. Vitamin K is metabolised in liver and excreted in bile and urine.

DRUGS DECREASING THROMBOSIS

Injectable anticoagulants

Examples: **heparin, low-molecular-weight heparins (LMWHs)**.

Mechanism of action. Heparin accelerates the action of antithrombin III, which inactivates factors XIIa, IXa, Xa and IIa. The drugs are active both in vivo and in vitro.

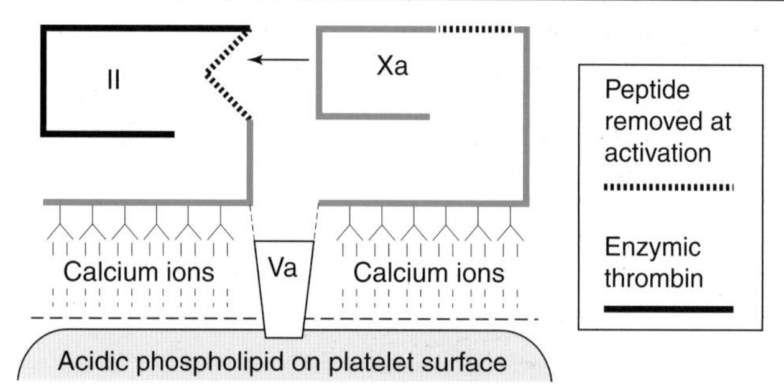

Fig. 22.2 The activation of prothrombin (factor II) by factor Xa. Factor Va complexed with a negatively charged phospholipid surface (both partly supplied by aggregated platelets) forms a binding site for factor Xa and prothrombin. Platelets thus serve as a localising focus. Calcium ions form a bridge between the γ-carboxylated glutamate residues (⅄) and the phospholipid surface. When X is activated it activates prothrombin, liberating enzymic thrombin. (Modified from Jackson C M 1978 Br J Haematol 39:1.)

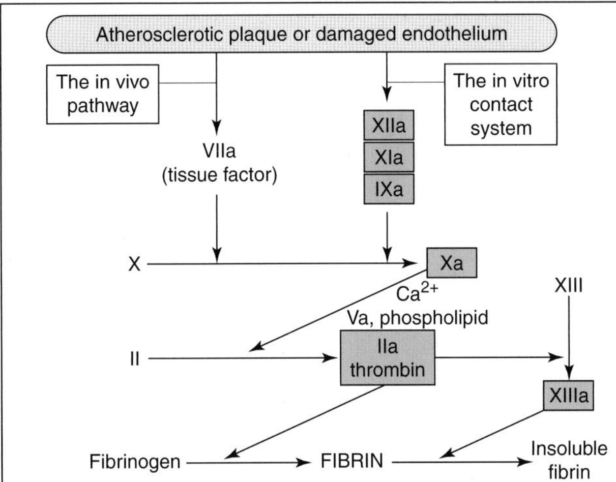

Fig. 22.3 Sites of action of heparin and low-molecular-weight heparins (LMWHs). Heparin (plus antithrombin III) acts on the enzymic forms of the factors (blue boxes). LMWHs act only on Xa.

Administration and pharmacokinetic aspects. Heparin is a sulfated mucopolysaccharide. It is given i.v. (when it acts immediately) or s.c. (acts after 1 h). It has a two-phase elimination: first rapid then slow. The effect is monitored by the activated partial thromboplastin time (APTT). LMWHs (see above) can be given s.c. and have a longer half-life. No blood monitoring is needed. They are eliminated by the kidney.

Unwanted effects The main hazard is bleeding, which can be treated with i.v. protamine sulfate, a strongly basic protein that neutralises heparin. Thrombosis associated with thrombocytopenia occurs rarely.

Oral anticoagulant: warfarin

Mechanism of action. Warfarin inhibits the reduction of vitamin K and thus inhibits the necessary γ-carboxylation of the Glu residues in factors II, VII, IX and X (Fig. 22.4).

Administration and pharmacokinetic aspects. Warfarin is given orally and has a small distribution volume. Onset of effect takes several days because the circulating γ-carboxylated factors have first to be degraded. The effect must be carefully monitored by the prothrombin time. It is metabolised in the liver.

Unwanted effects. Bleeding (into bowel or brain) is the main problem. It is treated by giving natural vitamin K (orally, i.v. or i.m.), fresh plasma or coagulation factor concentrates.

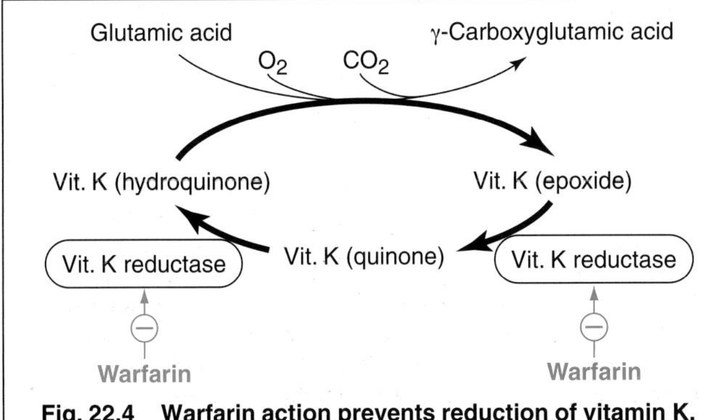

Fig. 22.4 Warfarin action prevents reduction of vitamin K.

Drug interactions. These are important. Some drugs potentiate warfarin, increasing the risk of bleeding (e.g. cimetidine, imipramine, ciprofloxacin, carbenicillin, aspirin, cephalosporins, etc.). Some lessen the anticoagulant action, increasing the risk of clotting (e.g. rifampicin, carbamazepine, etc.).

Antiplatelet agents

The action of antiplatelet agents is summarised in Figure 22.5.

Aspirin irreversibly inactivates cyclooxygenase and alters the balance between thromboxane A_2 (TXA_2), which promotes platelet adhesion and aggregation, and prostaglandin I_2 (prostacyclin), which inhibits it (Ch. 15). Vascular endothelium can synthesise more enzyme but platelets cannot; so platelet TXA_2 is restored only when existing platelets are replaced. Intermittent small doses given orally decrease platelet TXA_2 without significantly reducing endothelial PGI_2.

Platelet aggregation inhibitors. **Clopidogrel** inhibits ADP-induced aggregation; it is given i.v. short term. **Dipyridamole** inhibits platlet phosphodiesterase. **Abciximab** (antibody Fab fragment against the GPIIb/IIIa receptor) blocks the linking of platelets by fibrinogen; it is given by i.v. infusion.

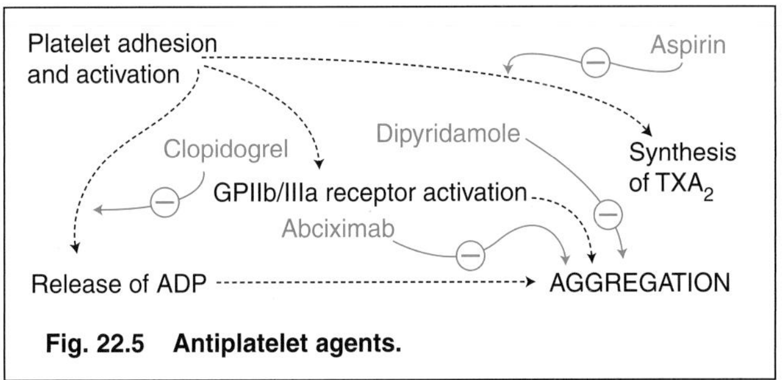

Fig. 22.5 Antiplatelet agents.

Fibrinolytic drugs

Examples and antidotes are given in Figure 22.1. Most have short half-lives and are given i.v., mainly by infusion. The main unwanted effect is bleeding.

Clinical uses of anticoagulants, antiplatelet agents and fibrinolytic drugs

- Anticoagulants are used in venous thromboembolism since the underlying process is predominantly coagulation (fibrin formation) with only a small component of platelet aggregation. **Heparin** or **LMWHs** are used for short-term action and warfarin for prolonged therapy.
- Fibrinolytic agents (e.g. **streptokinase**) plus **aspirin** are used in acute myocardial infarction; the sooner these are given after onset the better.
- **Aspirin** is also used to reduce the risk of occlusive cardiovascular disease in patients who have recovered from myocardial infarction or have unstable angina. Also used in acute thrombotic stroke and after coronary bypass grafting. Platelet aggregation inhibitors and dipyridamole can be additive with aspirin.

23 The haemopoietic system

The term haemopoiesis covers both red blood cell generation (erythropoiesis) and white blood cell generation (leukopoiesis). Normal haemopoiesis requires certain exogenous substances (haematinic agents, e.g. iron, folic acid, vitamin B_{12}) and various endogenous haemopoietic growth substances (e.g. colony-stimulating factors, erythropoietin, intrinsic factor).

Erythropoiesis

The main function of the red blood cells is to carry oxygen.

Pathophysiology

The main disorders of erythropoiesis are the *anaemias*, which are classified according to the changes in the erythrocytes:

- hypochromic, microcytic anaemia (small red cells with low haemoglobin) due to deficiency of iron, the main cause being chronic blood loss
- macrocytic anaemia (large red cells, few in number) due to deficiency of folic acid and/or vitamin B_{12}
- normochromic normocytic anaemia (fewer normal-sized red cells with normal haemoglobin) due usually to acute excessive destruction of red blood cells—'haemolytic anaemia'.

Haematinic agents

Iron

Iron is essential for haemoglobin production. A summary of its distribution in the body, transfer in the plasma, storage, movement between compartments and removal from the body is shown in Fig. 23.1. Iron is readily available for transfer to the plasma from ferritin stores in the liver.

The main preparation of iron is **ferrous sulfate**, given orally. A preparation for deep intramuscular use is **iron sorbitol**.

Unwanted effects. The main unwanted effect is dose-related gastrointestinal disturbance: nausea, epigastric pain, abdominal cramps, diarrhoea . Acute iron toxicity with necrotising gastritis and cardiovascular collapse can occur if large amounts of iron salts are ingested; chronic iron toxicity can follow repeated blood transfusion. Both are treated with an iron chelator: **desferrioxamine**.

Clinical uses of iron salts

- For iron-deficiency anaemia caused by
  - —chronic blood loss, e.g. from excessive menstrual loss, haemorrhoids, etc.
  - —increased need during pregnancy
  - —reduced iron intake or absorption.

Folic acid and vitamin B_{12}

Both folic acid and vitamin B_{12} are essential for DNA synthesis and cell proliferation.

Pathophysiology

Deficiencies of folic acid and/or vitamin B_{12} lead to megaloblastic anaemia in which there are large, fragile, distorted red cells and abnormal precursors in the blood. Vitamin B_{12} deficiency also causes neurological disease.

The principal cause of vitamin B_{12} deficiency is decreased absorption of the vitamin either because of a lack of intrinsic factor (normally secreted by the stomach but missing in pernicious anaemia) or because of conditions that interfere with its absorption in the ileum. As there are large stores in the liver, the results of the deficiency can take a long time to become manifest.

Folic acid deficiency results from dietary insufficiency, often associated with increased demand.

Folic acid

Folic acid (pteridine + *para*-aminobenzoic acid + glutamic acid) is essential for DNA synthesis and cell proliferation.

Actions. Folates, in the tetrahydrofolate (FH_4) polyglutamate form, are cofactors in the synthesis of purines and pyrimidines, being particularly important in thymidylate synthesis (Fig. 23.2).

Pharmacokinetic aspects. Folic acid is absorbed by active transport into intestinal cells where it is reduced by dihydrofolate reductase to FH_4 and then methylated to methyl-FH_4 which passes into the plasma. Eventually extra glutamates are added to give the active polyglutamate form.

Unwanted effects. These do not occur. However, if folic acid alone is given in vitamin B_{12} deficiency, the blood picture may improve but other lesions (e.g. neurological) will not improve.

Vitamin B_{12}

Actions. Vitamin B_{12} is important in reactions that enable folate to function in thymidylate synthesis (Fig. 23.2). The reactions convert 5-methyl-FH_4 (a functionally inactive form of folate carried in the

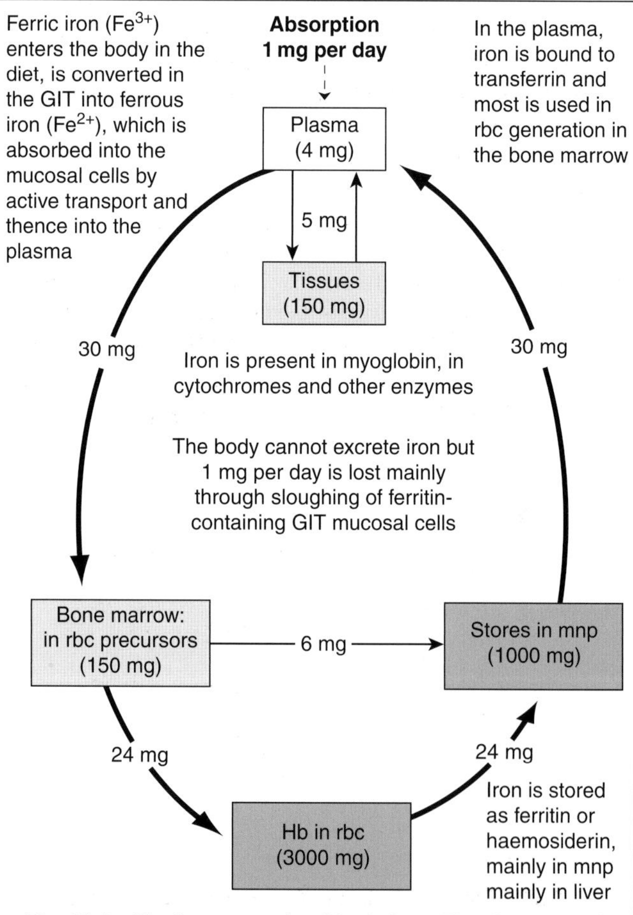

Fig. 23.1 The homeostasis of body iron. The distribution and daily movement between tissues is shown; the darker the colour the higher the concentration of iron. Hb, haemoglobin; rbc, red blood cells; mnp, mononuclear phagocytes; GIT, gastrointestinal tract.

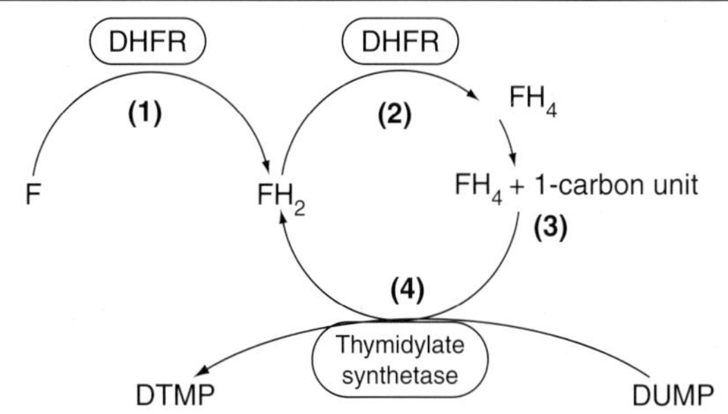

Fig. 23.2 Simplified diagram of the role of a folate in thymidylate synthesis. (1) Folate is reduced to dihydrofolate (FH_2) by dihydrofolate reductase (DHFR). (2) Dihydrofolate (FH_2) is reduced to tetrahydrofolate (FH_4) by DHFR. (3) The FH_4 functions as a carrier of a one-carbon unit, providing the methyl group necessary for (4) the conversion of 2'deoxyuridylate (DUMP) to 2'deoxythymidylate (DTMP) by thymidylate synthetase. During the transfer of the one-carbon unit, FH_4 is oxidised to FH_2, which must be reduced by DHFR to FH_4 (step 2) before it can act again. The thymidylate synthetase action is rate limiting in DNA synthesis. Note that in all the actions of folates it is the polyglutamate form that is most active.

plasma) to the form of folate (FH_4) that can carry the one-carbon unit necessary for the formation of DTMP from DUMP (Fig. 23.2). The mechanism of action is shown in Figure 23.3.

Administration. Vitamin B_{12} is given intramuscularly and is stored in the liver.

Unwanted effects. There are none.

Haemopoietic growth factors

There is continuous generation of erythrocytes and leukocytes from pluripotent stem cells in the bone marrow. Various haemopoietic growth factors are responsible for the division of these cells and the multiplication and maturation of their progeny. Erythropoietin, produced in the kidney, controls red cell production; myeloid growth factors, produced by many cells types, control the production of monocytes and polymorphonuclear leukocytes; interleukins control lymphocyte production and thrombopoietin controls platelet production (Fig. 23.4).

Erythropoietin

Recombinant erythropoietin (**epoietin**) is available for therapeutic use. It can be given intravenously, subcutaneously or intraperitoneally.

Unwanted effects. Include 'flu-like symptoms, a dose-related increase in blood pressure and encephalopathy.

Myeloid growth factors

Recombinant forms of the two main myeloid growth factors are available for therapeutic use. Granulocyte colony-stimulating factor (G-CSF) is available as **filgrastim** and granulocyte–macrophage colony-stimulating factor (GM-CSF) is available as **molgramostim**.

Filgrastim stimulates only polymorphonuclear development; molgramostim stimulates the development of all myeloid cells. Both can be given either i.v. or s.c. Both require specialist administration.

Clinical uses of folic acid and vitamin B_{12}

- Folic acid is used mainly
  —to treat anaemias caused by folic acid deficiency
  —in prophylaxis if there is potential for developing deficiency, as in pregnancy.
- Vitamin B_{12} is used for pernicious anaemia.

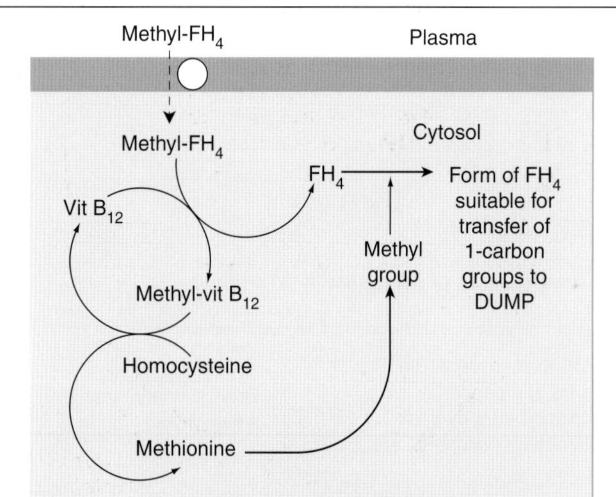

Fig. 23.3 The role of vitamin B_{12} in reactions necessary for the eventual synthesis of thymidylate. Methyl-FH_4 enters cells from the plasma by carrier. The methyl group is transferred to homocysteine to form methionine via vitamin B_{12}, which is bound to a methyltransferase (not shown). Methionine donates the methyl group to FH_4.

Clinical use of haemopoietic growth factors

- Epoietin is used mainly for the anaemia of chronic renal failure.
- Filgastrim is used in some cases of neutropenia.
- Molgramostim is used to shorten neutropenia after procedures such as cancer chemotherapy or autologous bone marrow transplantation.

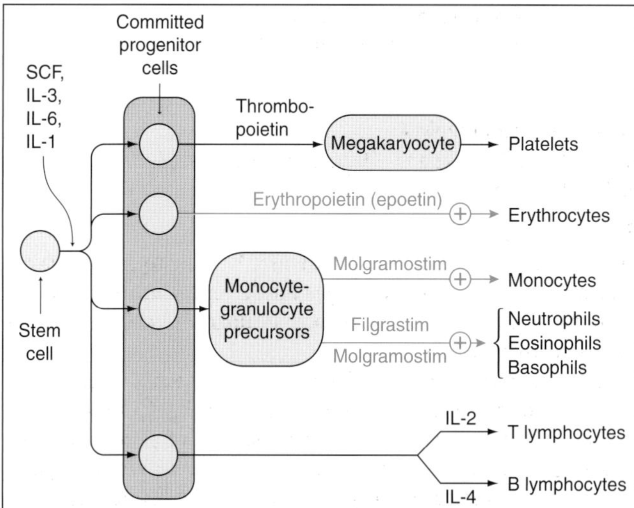

Fig. 23.4 Schematic digram of the growth factors controlling haemopoiesis. IL, interleukin; SCF, stem cell factor.

24 Respiration and asthma

The chief functions of respiration are to supply O_2 and remove CO_2. The main disorders of the respiratory system are *asthma* and *chronic bronchitis* but respiratory depression can be caused by overdosage of most drugs that have a CNS depressive effect.

The control of airway muscle, blood vessels and glands

Airway smooth muscle. The upper airways are constricted by acetylcholine acting on muscarinic M_3 receptors. The lower airways can be constricted by excitatory non-adrenergic non-cholinergic (NANC) transmitters (e.g. inflammatory peptides released from sensory neurons) and are relaxed by inhibitory NANC transmitters (e.g. nitric oxide) and circulating adrenaline acting on β_2-adrenoceptors. Note there is no sympathetic nerve supply to airway muscle.

Blood vessel smooth muscle. These are relaxed mainly by circulating adrenaline.

Glands. Mucus secretion is inhibited by the sympathetic system and is stimulated by the parasympathetic system, by inflammatory mediators and by chemical (e.g. air pollutants) and physical (e.g. cold air) stimuli.

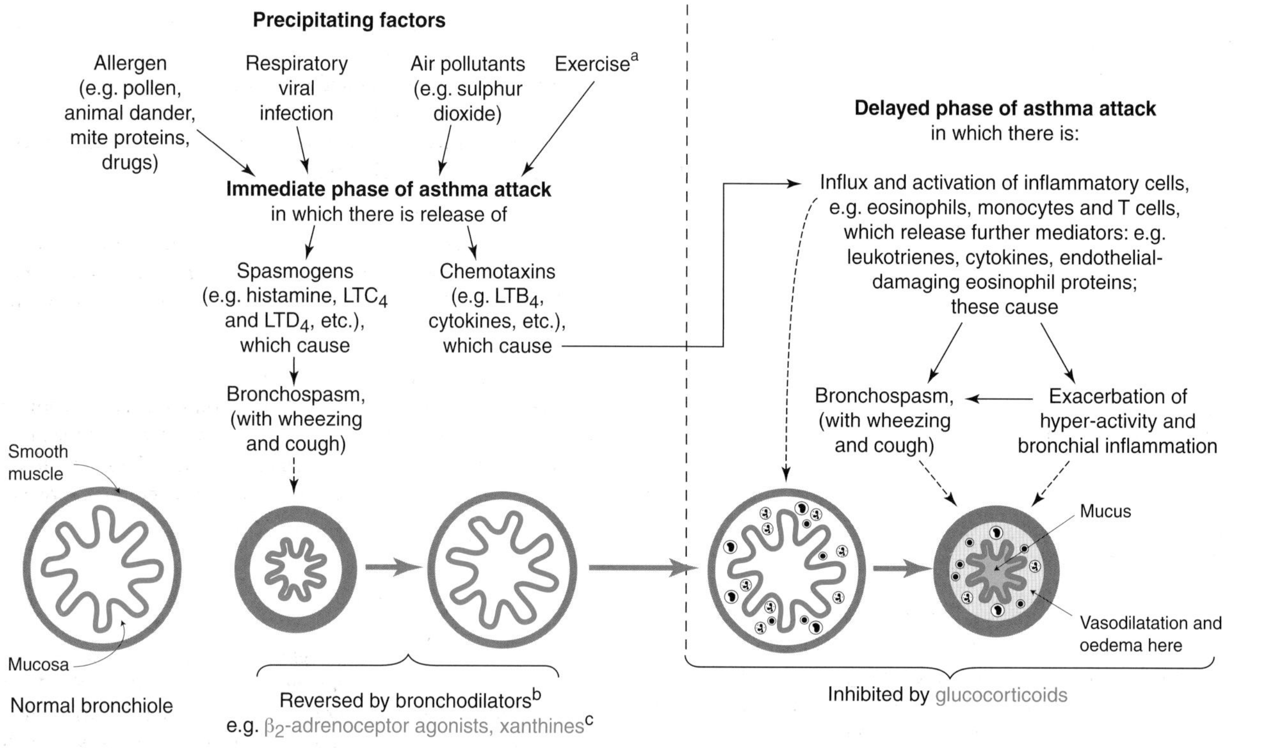

Precipitating factors

Allergen (e.g. pollen, animal dander, mite proteins, drugs)
Respiratory viral infection
Air pollutants (e.g. sulphur dioxide)
Exercise[a]

Immediate phase of asthma attack in which there is release of

Spasmogens (e.g. histamine, LTC_4 and LTD_4, etc.), which cause
Chemotaxins (e.g. LTB_4, cytokines, etc.), which cause

Bronchospasm, (with wheezing and cough)

Delayed phase of asthma attack in which there is:

Influx and activation of inflammatory cells, e.g. eosinophils, monocytes and T cells, which release further mediators: e.g. leukotrienes, cytokines, endothelial-damaging eosinophil proteins; these cause

Bronchospasm, (with wheezing and cough)
Exacerbation of hyper-activity and bronchial inflammation

Smooth muscle
Mucosa
Mucus
Vasodilatation and oedema here

Normal bronchiole

Reversed by bronchodilators[b] e.g. β_2-adrenoceptor agonists, xanthines[c]

Inhibited by glucocorticoids

Both phases can be prevented by cromoglicate, though not in all individuals.
[a]Exercise usually only causes the immediate phase. [b]Muscarinic antagonists may be of some use if there is a component of acetylcholine-induced spasm. [c]Xanthines are second-line drugs. (LT, leukotriene.)

Fig. 24.1 Outline of the genesis of an attack of asthma and the action of anti-asthmatic drugs.

ASTHMA

Asthma is a syndrome in which there are recurrent attacks of reversible airway obstruction—caused by bronchoconstriction and mucus secretion—occurring in response to stimuli that are not in themselves noxious. The underlying condition is essentially a special type of inflammatory reaction, and the asthma attack is characterised by difficulty in breathing *out*, wheezing and cough. The attack can often be treated, in the early stages, by the use of inhaled drugs, but acute severe asthma (*status asthmaticus*) requires hospitalisation. The prevalence of asthma is increasing and it is associated with a rising mortality.

An asthma attack usually (but not invariably) consists of two phases: immediate phase and delayed.

The development of susceptibility to asthma

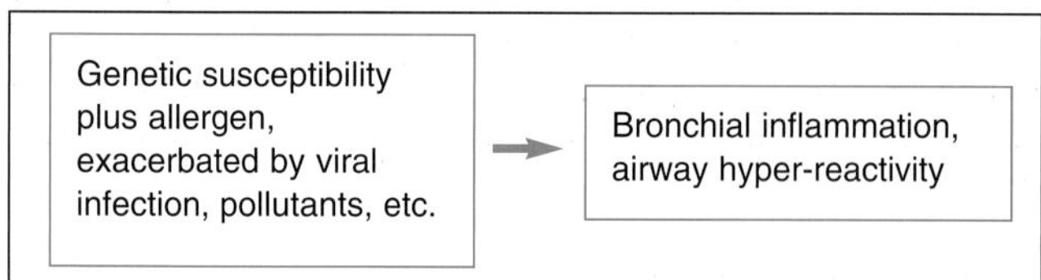

Note that aspirin can precipitate asthma in susceptible individuals.

Drugs used in the treatment of asthma

Two main types of drug are used:

- bronchodilators
- anti-inflammatory agents.

Bronchodilators

Beta-2 adrenoceptor agonists (first-line drugs)

Examples: **salbutamol**, terbutaline (both short acting, peak action in 30 min, duration 4–6 h); **salmeterol** (longer acting, duration 12 h). See Ch. 11 for aspects other than use in asthma.

Mechanism of action. All act as physiological antagonists to the various spasmogenic mediators. They have no effect on the hyperreactivity or inflammatory components.

Pharmacokinetic aspects. Usually given by aerosol inhalation but can be given orally or by injection. Salbutamol can be given i.v. in acute severe asthma. The *short-acting agents* are usually given on an 'as needed' basis and the *longer-acting agents* are used regularly in preventative therapy, often twice daily with a glucocorticoid.

Unwanted effects. The main unwanted effect during asthma treatment is tremor. Other effects that can occur if the drugs are absorbed are given in Ch. 11.

Xanthine compounds (second-line drugs)

Examples: the methylxanthines **theophylline** and aminophylline (theophylline ethylene diamine).

Pharmacological actions. In asthma these are primarily bronchodilators. They also have an excitatory action on the CNS, a stimulatory effect on the rate and force of contraction of the heart and a weak diuretic action.

Mechanism of action. The relaxant action on smooth muscle is probably a result of inhibition of one of the several subtypes of phosphodiesterase, resulting in an increase in cyclic GMP or AMP. The effect of cyclic GMP on smooth muscle is shown in Chs 14 and 18.

Pharmacokinetic aspects. Theophylline is given orally as a sustained-release preparation and acts for ~12 h. It is useful for nocturnal asthma. Aminophylline, which is more soluble, is given by a sloooow i.v. injection (at least 20 min) for acute severe asthma. The xanthines are metabolised in the liver. Half-lives are approximately 8 h but vary widely in different individuals. Drug interactions occur and are important in view of the narrow range of safe plasma concentrations. Some drugs increase the plasma xanthine concentration (e.g. oral contraceptives, erythromycin, ciprofloxacin, cimetidine, some calcium channel blockers), some decrease it (e.g. rifampicin, carbamazepine).

Unwanted effects of the xanthines. The drugs have stimulant effects on the heart and the CNS and cause gastrointestinal disturbances. Note that there is a narrow window between the therapeutic dose and the dose that causes adverse effects.

Muscarinic receptor antagonists (second-line drugs)

The main antimuscarinic agent used for asthma is **ipratropium**. It binds to all muscarinic receptor subtypes. It decreases any acetylcholine-mediated spasm, reduces irritant-induced mucus secretion and increases ciliary clearance of bronchial secretions. It has no preventative action against allergen challenge and no effect on the inflammation within the bronchioles. (See Ch. 10 for more detail.)

Anti-inflammatory agents

Glucocorticoids

Examples used for asthma: **beclometasone dipropionate**, **budesonide**, fluticasone (all given by inhalation), **prednisolone** (given orally), **hydrocortisone** (given i.v. for acute severe asthma). These agents are ineffective for relieving the immediate phase but can reduce the inflammatory component of the delayed phase and are life-saving in acute severe asthma. The mechanism of action is described on p. 40 and in Ch. 28. In summary, they reduce the activation of inflammatory cells as well as the release of cytokines (particularly those generated by Th1 lymphocytes (see Fig. 16.1)) and other inflammatory mediators.

Unwanted effects. Inhaled glucocorticoids may cause thrush (oropharyngeal candidiasis) and voice problems; spacing devices that reduce deposition of the drug in the pharynx and promote deposition in the smaller airways can ameliorate these effects. Systemic adverse effects (Ch. 28) are rare with inhaled agents but can occur with regular large doses of oral agents.

Cromoglicate

Mechanism of action. This is unknown. They have no direct effect on the immediate phase but, given prophylactically by inhalation of an aerosol or powder, can inhibit the development of both phases of asthma in some subjects.

Unwanted effects. Irritation of the upper respiratory tract and, occasionally, hypersensitivity.

Leukotriene receptor antagonists

Leukotriene receptor antagonists are now available (e.g. **montelukast**, used for adding to β-stimulant plus inhaled corticosteroid therapy if necessary, and **zafirlukast**, used for exercise-induced asthma).

Regimen for the treatment of asthma

Mild asthma is usually treated with β_2-agonists taken as required for symptomatic relief. With progressively more severe asthma, inhaled corticosteroids, long-acting β_2-agonists and xanthines are introduced on a prophylactic basis. Oral steroids are used only in severe asthma because of their more serious side effects.

CHRONIC BRONCHITIS

Chronic bronchitis causes coughing, which if long-continued can lead to emphysema (chronic obstructive lung disease). A short-acting **β_2-adrenoceptor agonist** given by inhalation 'as needed' or a muscarinic antagonist given by inhalation regularly may help. **Antitussive drugs** (drugs that relieve cough) include codeine (see Ch. 40) and **pholcodine**. They are used to alleviate dry painful cough (e.g. in cancer of the bronchi, acute bronchitis) but should not be used in asthma and can cause sputum retention in chronic bronchitis.

Drugs used clinically for asthma

- Bronchodilators
  - —β_2-adrenoceptor agonists, e.g. **salbutamol**, as first-line drugs
  - —xanthines, e.g. **theophylline**, (second line)
  - —muscarinic receptor antagonists, e.g. **ipratropium** (second line).
- Anti-inflammatory agents
  - —**glucocorticoids** can be given by inhaler, orally (chronic or severe deteriorating asthma) or i.v. (for severe acute asthma).
  - —**cromoglicate** is used prophylactically.

25 The kidney

The main function of the kidney is the excretion of waste products; it is also important in the regulation of the salt and water content of the body and in acid–base balance. The main active transport mechanism in the renal tubule is the Na^+/K^+ ATPase (the sodium pump) in the basolateral membrane of the tubule cells. All the constituents of the plasma (other than protein) are filtered into the renal tubules at the glomerulus and 75% of the filtrate is reabsorbed isosmotically in the *proximal tubules*, bicarbonate in particular. Some organic acids and bases are secreted into the tubule. Water is absorbed in the *descending limb of the medullary loop* (Henle's loop). In the *thick ascending limb of the loop*, which is impermeable to water, there is active reabsorption of salt via a $Na^+/2Cl^-/K^+$ cotransporter (a symport in which transport of one ion is coupled to that of another) in the luminal membrane. This reabsorption of salt from the filtrate into the cells and from there into the interstitia is a major factor in producing hypertonicity in the interstitia in this area. In the *distal tubule*, more absorption of Na^+ and Cl^- occurs, and K^+ is secreted into the filtrate. The *collecting tubule* and *collecting ducts* have low permeability to both salts and water; here Na^+ reabsorption and K^+ excretion is promoted by aldosterone and passive water absorption promoted by the antidiuretic hormone (ADH). The hypertonicity of the interstitia produced by the reabsorption of salt in the thick ascending loop is the main factor providing the osmotic gradient for ADH-mediated water reabsorption. Normally less than 1% of filtered Na^+ is excreted in the urine.

DRUGS ACTING ON THE KIDNEY

- Diuretics
- Drugs affecting urinary pH (see lower right of Fig. 25.1).
- Drugs that can alter the excretion of organic molecules: e.g. probenecid.

Diuretics

Diuretics are drugs that increase Na^+ (and thus water) excretion by a direct action on the kidney. They do this mainly by reducing the absorption of salt from the filtrate, the increase in water loss being secondary to the increased salt loss.

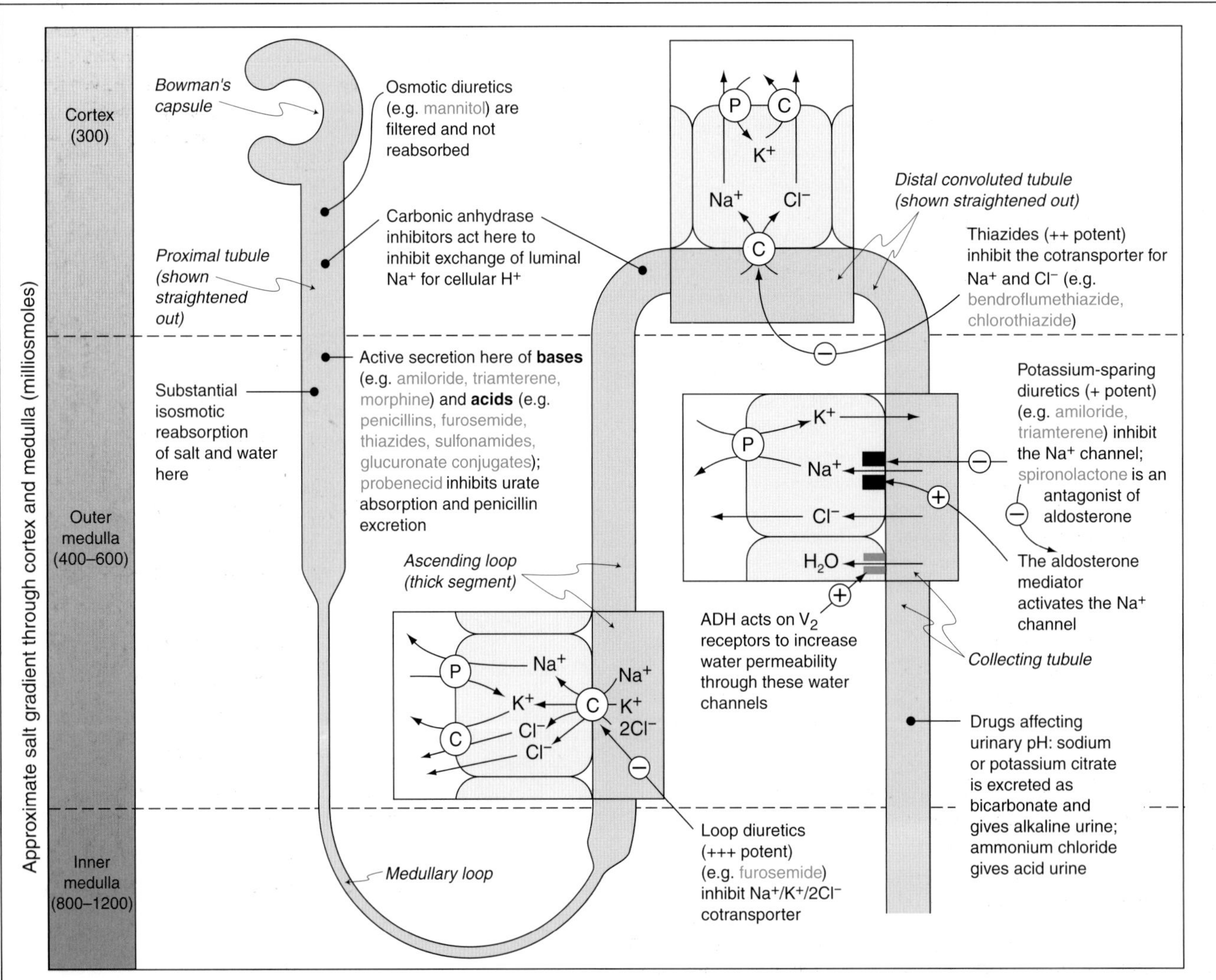

Fig. 25.1 Diagram of the nephron. The movement of ions in the main parts of the tubule, the sites of action of the principal drugs, some of the main agents secreted into the proximal tubule and the range of salt concentration from cortex to inner medulla are shown. (P, Na^+ pump; C, cotransporter)

Loop diuretics

Examples: **furosemide,** torosamide.

Pharmacological actions

- very potent diuretics, causing a profuse flow of urine
- K^+ and H^+ loss
- decreased excretion of uric acid
- increased excretion of Ca^{2+} and Mg^{2+}
- moderate vasodilator effect.

Mechanism of the diuretic action

See the main figure.

Pharmacokinetic aspects

Loop diuretics are given orally or i.v. and are secreted into the proximal tubule. The fraction not secreted is metabolised in the liver. Furosemide has a half-life of 90 min and a duration of action of 3–6 h. Torosamide has longer half-life and duration of action.

Unwanted effects

The main unwanted effects follow the renal actions of the drugs:

- hypokalaemia owing to K^+ loss
- metabolic alkalosis owing to H^+ loss
- depletion of Ca^{2+} and Mg^{2+}
- depletion of the extracellular fluid volume, resulting in hypotension.

High i.v. doses can cause deafness. Nausea and hypersensitivity reactions can occur.

Thiazides and related diuretics

Examples of thiazides: **bendroflumethiazide,** hydrochlorothiazide); examples of the related agents are chlortalidone, xipamide, adipiodone (indapamide).

Pharmacological actions of thiazides and their congeners

- moderately potent diuretic effect (but in diabetes insipidus, thiazides *reduce* urine volume)
- K^+ and H^+ loss
- decreased excretion of uric acid
- decreased excretion of Ca^{2+}
- increased excretion of Mg^{2+}
- moderate vasodilator effect.

Mechanism of the diuretic action

See Figure 25.1.

Pharmacokinetic aspects

Given orally, thiazides and related agents are secreted into the proximal tubule (Fig. 25.1). With most agents, the diuresis starts within 2 h and lasts 8–12 h. Chlortalidone has a longer duration of action.

Unwanted effects of thiazides and related agents

The main unwanted effects are a result of renal actions:

- hypokalaemia due to K^+ loss
- metabolic alkalosis due to H^+ loss
- increased plasma uric acid (gout thus a possibility)

Other unwanted effects include: possible hyperglycaemia (a problem in diabetes mellitus), increased plasma cholesterol (with long-continued use), male impotence (reversible) and allergic reactions. A rare but serious adverse effect is hyponatraemia.

Potassium-sparing diuretics

Examples: **amiloride**, **spironolactone**, triamterene,

These have only limited diuretic action and all act in the distal tubule and collecting tubules, the sites for the control of K^+ homeostasis.

Spironolactone is given orally and is rapidly metabolised to an active metabolite, canrenone. The onset of action is slow. It is an antagonist of aldosterone, inhibiting aldosterone's Na^+-retaining, K^+-excreting effect. Unwanted actions on other steroid receptors can occur, resulting in gynaecomastia, testicular problems and menstrual disorders.

Triamterene, amiloride are both given orally, triamterene having a more rapid onset and shorter duration of action than amiloride. They inhibit Na^+ reabsorption and reduce K^+ excretion.

Unwanted effects. All three agents can cause hyperkalaemia and may cause acidosis.

Osmotic diuretics

Osmotic diuretics (e.g. **mannitol**) are inert compounds that pass into the tubules in the glomerulus and increase the osmotic pressure of the filtrate. They act mainly in the proximal tubule and the overall effect is to increase water excretion. They are usually given i.v. and the principal unwanted effects are a temporary expansion of the extracellular fluid compartment and hyponatraemia, resulting from osmotic extraction of intracellular water.

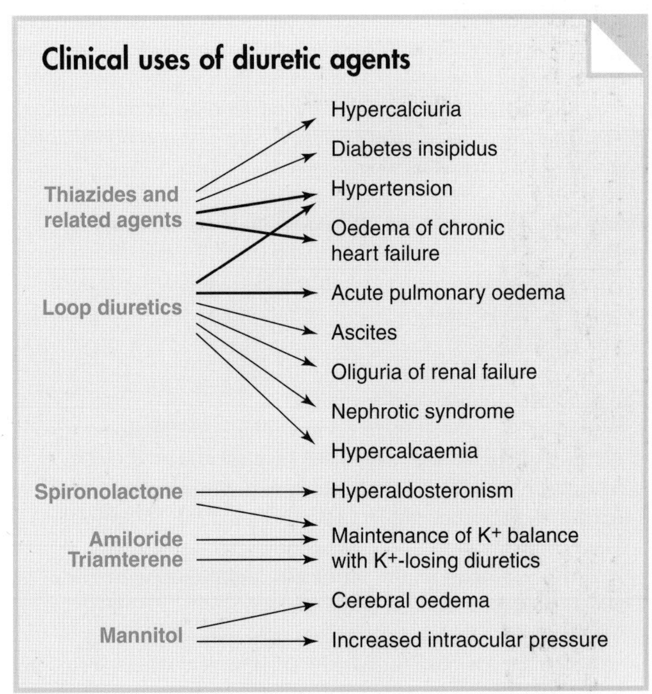

26 The gastrointestinal tract

The main physiological aspects of GI tract function that are of pharmacological importance are gastric acid secretion, the motility of the bowel and the excretion of its contents; the main pathophysiological conditions are peptic ulcer, vomiting, disturbances of excretion (diarrhoea, constipation), gallstones and chronic inflammatory bowel disease (ulcerative colitis, Crohn's disease).

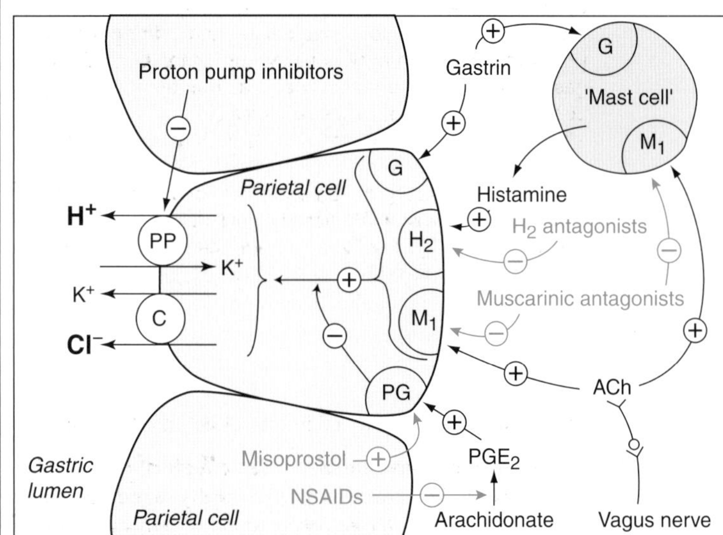

Control of acid secretion

HCl is secreted by the parietal cells within the gastric glands and passes into the stomach lumen producing a pH of ~1. Secretion is stimulated by histamine H_2 receptors, acting via an increase in cAMP within the cell, and by acetylcholine (ACh) and gastrin acting on muscarinic and gastrin receptors, respectively. ACh and gastrin may act directly on the parietal cell (increasing cell $[Ca^{2+}]$) (one-cell hypothesis) or can act indirectly via release of histamine from mast cell-like cells (two-cell hypothesis). Rises in cAMP and $[Ca^{2+}]$ in the parietal cell activate a proton pump (PP), which exchanges H^+ in the cell with K^+ in the lumen of the gastric gland. The cotransporter (C) moves Cl^- into the lumen with K^+. Activation of prostaglandin receptors (possibly EP_3) by PGE_2 inhibits HCl secretion.

Fig. 26.1 Control of acid secretion and drug actions.

GASTRIC SECRETION AND PEPTIC ULCER

Pathogenesis of peptic ulcer

In peptic ulceration the balance between mucosal-damaging processes (secretion of acid and pepsin) and mucosal-protective mechanisms (secretion of bicarbonate and mucus) is altered. The bacillus *Helicobacter pylori* is likely to be a major cause of the swing towards mucosal damage, by increasing gastrin secretion. Non-steroidal anti-inflammatory drugs (NSAIDs) are an additional important cause of gastric ulceration.

Drugs used to treat peptic ulcer, with their mechanisms of action

The main approaches are (i) to reduce acid secretion (this is the most important), (ii) to treat *H. pylori* infection and (iii) to protect the gastric mucosa.

Drugs used to reduce acid secretion

- Histamine H_2 antagonists (e.g. **cimetidine, ranitidine**) or proton pump inhibitors (**omeprazole**) are the most effective agents.
- Selective muscarinic M_1 antagonists (e.g. **pirenzepine**) also reduce acid secretion but less effectively than H_2 antagonists. (There are no clinically useful gastrin antagonists).
- Antacids (e.g. **magnesium trisilicate, aluminium hydroxide**) simply neutralise the acid in the stomach.
- **Misoprostol**, a PGE_2 analogue, not only reduces gastric acid secretion but may also increase bicarbonate and mucus secretion by epithelial cells. Its main use is to counteract the damaging effects of NSAIDs on the gastric mucosa.

Drugs used to treat H. pylori *infection*

H. pylori infection is treated with a combination of a proton pump inhibitor or H_2 antagonist with two antibiotics (**metronidazole, clarithromycin and amoxicillin** are commonly used). **Bismuth chelate**, which has an antibacterial action plus a mucosa-protective effect, is usually part of the therapy.

Drugs used to protect the gastric mucosa

Sucralfate (a complex of aluminium hydroxide and sulfated sucrose) can form complex gels with mucus to enhance its protective effect on the mucosa. Bismuth chelate is also protective.

Pharmacokinetic aspects and unwanted actions

H_2 antagonists are readily absorbed after oral administration. Both cimetidine and ranitidine can inhibit renal tubular secretion of basic drugs. Cimetidine, importantly, can inhibit cytochrome P450 and so potentiate the actions of many drugs including oral anticoagulants, phenytoin and aminophylline. Omeprazole has a half-life of only 1 h but its concentration in the parietal cell canaliculus allows its action to persist for 2–3 days. Most of a sucralfate dose remains in the gut, where it can reduce the absorption of other drugs (e.g. digoxin, tetracycline and theophylline).

Summary of drugs used to treat peptic ulcer

- Histamine H_2 antagonists: **cimetidine,** ranitidine
- Proton pump inhibitors: **omeprazole**
- Antacids: **magnesium trisilicate, aluminium hydroxide**
- Antibacterial agents effective against *H. pylori*: **clarithromycin, metronidazole, amoxicillin, bismuth chelate**
- Mucosal protectants: **sucralfate,** bismuth chelate.

EMESIS AND ANTI-EMETIC DRUGS

Pathophysiology

Vomiting is a complex act involving the coordinated activity of the involuntary muscles of the GI tract and the somatic respiratory and abdominal muscles. It is controlled by two centres in the medulla:

- the vomiting centre
- the chemoreceptor trigger zone (CTZ).

Many stimuli can give rise to emesis (Fig. 26.2)

- input from higher centres, e.g. repulsive sights or smells, pain, emotional factors
- impulses from the labyrinths and/or vestibular nuclei (e.g. in motion sickness, Ménière's disease)
- endogenous blood-borne factors (e.g. in uraemia)
- drugs (e.g. cancer chemotherapy agents); the toxic effects of many drugs result in emesis
- stimuli acting in the pharynx or stomach.

The main receptors involved in the control of vomiting include histamine H_1, muscarinic, dopamine D_2, 5-hydroxytryptamine ($5HT_3$), and possibly opioid receptors.

Anti-emetic drugs

The selection of agents depends on the cause of vomiting and in particular on the relative importance of the vestibular nuclei, CTZ and vomiting centre. Antagonists of histamine, muscarinic, dopamine and $5HT_3$ receptors are used as appropriate.

- H_1 antagonists (e.g. **cyclizine**, **cinnarizine**)
  —effective against vestibular apparatus stimuli and local gut stimuli
  —ineffective against CTZ stimuli
- antimuscarinics (e.g. **hyoscine**)
  —effective against vestibular apparatus stimuli and local gut stimuli
  —ineffective against CTZ stimuli
- D_2 antagonists (e.g. **thiethylperazine**, **domperidone**, metoclopramide)
  —effective against CTZ stimuli
  —ineffective against local gut stimuli
- $5HT_3$ antagonists (e.g. **ondansetron**, granisetron)
  —effective against CTZ stimuli
  —ineffective against local gut stimuli

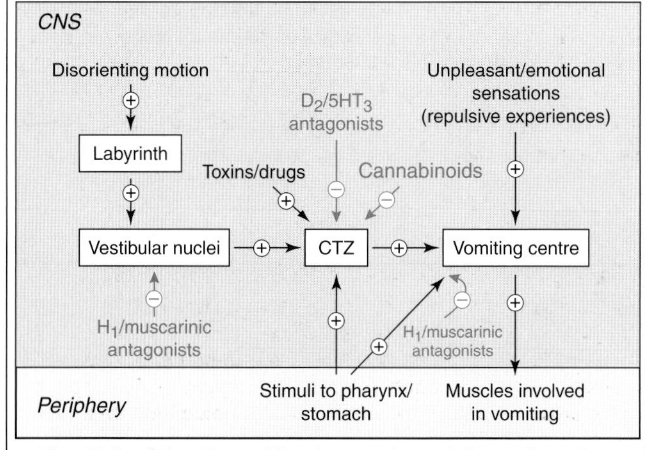

Fig. 26.2 Stimuli resulting in emesis and the action of anti-emetic drugs.

> **Clinical use of anti-emetic drugs**
>
> - $5HT_3$ receptor antagonists (e.g. **ondansetron**): emesis caused by cancer chemotherapy agents (drugs of choice), postoperative and radiation-induced vomiting.
> - Dopamine D_2 receptor antagonists (e.g. **domperidone**, **phenothiazines**): emesis caused by uraemia, radiation, gastrointestinal disorders, viral gastroenteritis (thiethylperazine is the phenothiazine of choice).
> - Muscarinic receptor antagonists (e.g. **hyoscine**): motion sickness (drug of choice)
> - Histamine H_1 receptor antagonists: **cyclizine** (motion sickness), **cinnarizine** (Ménière's disease).
> - Cannabinoids (e.g. nabilone): emesis caused by cytotoxic drugs.

- cannabinoids (e.g. nabilone) inhibit the effect of CTZ stimulants.

Pharmacokinetic aspects and unwanted effects of anti-emetics

Antihistamines and hyoscine can be taken orally to prevent nausea, but once vomiting ensues there is obviously a difficulty in using this route. Transdermal preparations of hyoscine have been developed that circumvent this problem (Ch. 6). Antihistamines and hyoscine cause drowsiness and hyoscine has many other side effects owing to parasympathetic inhibition (e.g. dry mouth, blurring of vision). The D_2 antagonists can be given orally, rectally or parenterally. Important side effects are the extrapyramidal effects on movement and increased prolactin release, resulting in galactorrhoea. GI tract disturbances can occur. Domperidone has fewer extrapyramidal effects because of its reduced penetration of the blood–brain barrier.

OTHER GASTROINTESTINAL CONDITIONS

Diarrhoea

Diarrhoea caused by infectious agents (*Escherichia coli*, *Campylobacter*) will only require the use of antibiotics if severe. Replacement of fluid and electrolytes is essential. Opiates and, less usefully, muscarinic receptor antagonists are used to reduce motility. Of the opiates **loperamide** and **diphenoxylate** are used in preference to **codeine** because they have less CNS action. Opiates also have an antisecretory action.

Constipation

Bulk laxatives (e.g. dietary cellulose (bran) or methylcellulose) are not digested and increase the mass of material in the gut lumen so stimulating peristalsis. Osmotic purgatives (e.g. **magnesium sulfate**, lactulose) are not absorbed and retain water, by osmotic action, in the gut — the increased fluid volume stimulating peristalsis. Stimulant purgatives act by increasing mucosal secretion or by stimulating enteric nerves. Senna is a natural product containing anthracene derivatives that are metabolised by bacteria in the colon to produce the active stimulants.

Gallstones

Non-calcified cholesterol gallstones can be dissolved by oral administration of the bile acids chenodeoxycholic acid and ursodeoxycholic acid, which reduce the synthesis and secretion of cholesterol.

27 Blood sugar and diabetes

Blood glucose concentrations are predominantly under the control of the pancreatic hormones *insulin* and *glucagon*. The pancreatic islets of Langerhans contain B cells, which secrete insulin, and A, D and PP cells, which secrete glucagon, somatostatin and pancreatic polypeptide, respectively. Insulin exerts a major control over the metabolism of carbohydrates, fats and proteins and is the main regulator of blood glucose.

Insulin release is primarily regulated by glucose, though other 'fuels' (fatty acids and amino acids) will also modify release. Change in B cell ATP concentration as a consequence of glucose metabolism is a key factor in insulin release.

Glucagon causes a rise in blood glucose by initiating glycogenolysis and gluconeogenesis and inhibiting glycogen synthesis.

Pathophysiology

Deficient secretion of insulin results in diabetes mellitus, of which there are two types:

- *insulin-dependent diabetes mellitus* (IDDM, type 1 or juvenile onset) in which the B cells have been completely destroyed by an autoimmune process and insulin replacement therapy is essential
- *non-insulin-dependent diabetes mellitus* (NIDDM, type 2 or maturity onset) in which individuals are insulin resistant and fail to secrete sufficient hormone.

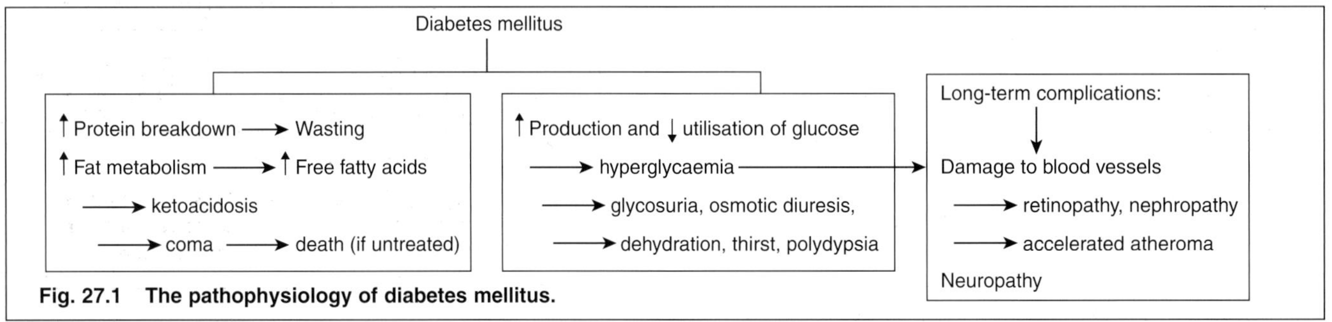

Fig. 27.1 The pathophysiology of diabetes mellitus.

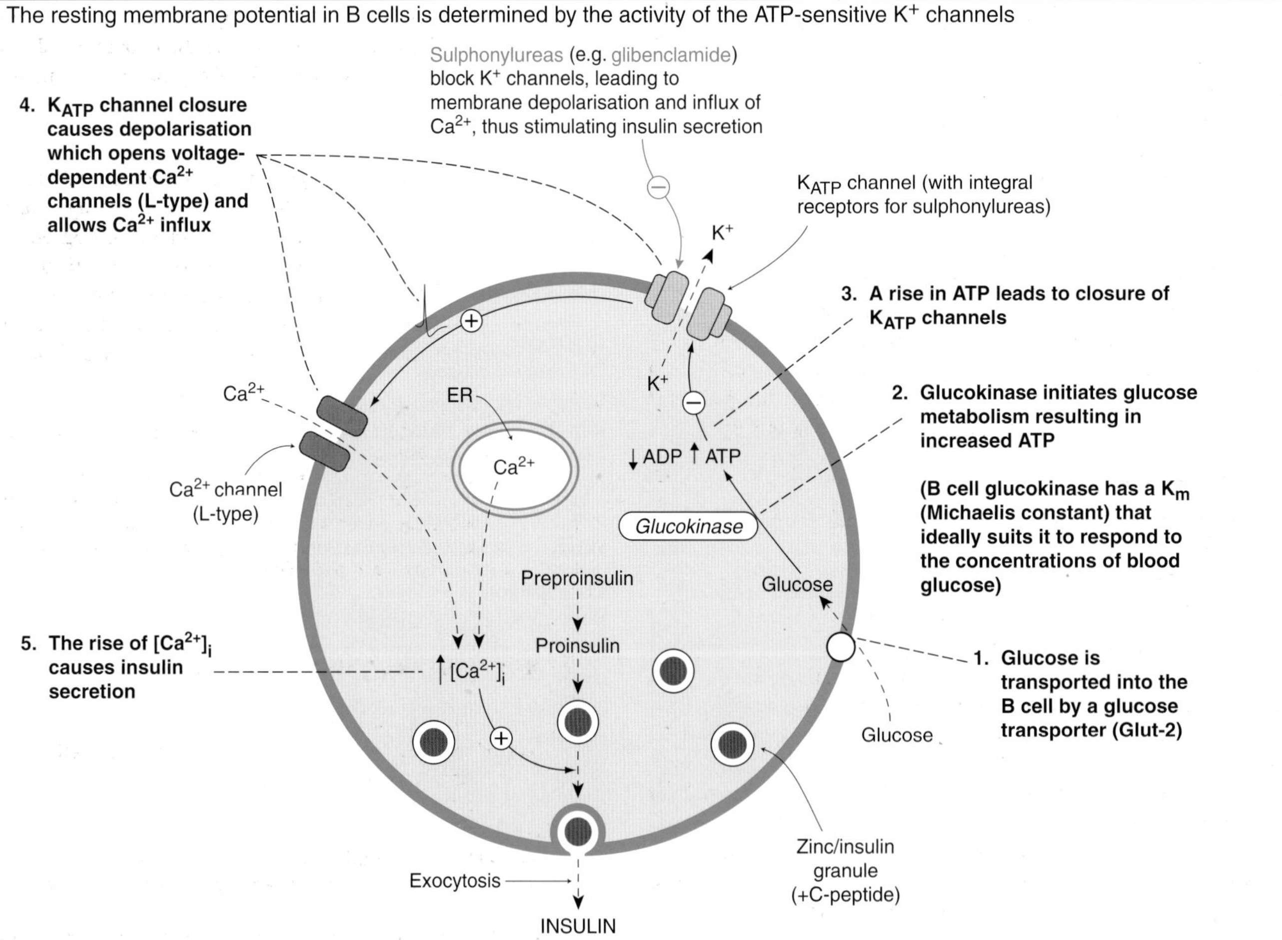

The resting membrane potential in B cells is determined by the activity of the ATP-sensitive K^+ channels

Sulphonylureas (e.g. glibenclamide) block K^+ channels, leading to membrane depolarisation and influx of Ca^{2+}, thus stimulating insulin secretion

4. K_{ATP} channel closure causes depolarisation which opens voltage-dependent Ca^{2+} channels (L-type) and allows Ca^{2+} influx

K_{ATP} channel (with integral receptors for sulphonylureas)

K^+

3. A rise in ATP leads to closure of K_{ATP} channels

Ca^{2+}

ER

K^+

2. Glucokinase initiates glucose metabolism resulting in increased ATP

Ca^{2+}

↓ ADP ↑ ATP

Ca^{2+} channel (L-type)

Glucokinase

(B cell glucokinase has a K_m (Michaelis constant) that ideally suits it to respond to the concentrations of blood glucose)

Preproinsulin

Glucose

5. The rise of $[Ca^{2+}]_i$ causes insulin secretion

↑ $[Ca^{2+}]_i$

Proinsulin

1. Glucose is transported into the B cell by a glucose transporter (Glut-2)

Glucose

Exocytosis

Zinc/insulin granule (+C-peptide)

INSULIN

Fig. 27.2 An outline of the sequence of events in B cells from glucose uptake to insulin release and the action of drugs. ER, endoplasmic reticulum.

- Agonists of α_2-adrenoceptors → hyperpolarisation, inhibited electrical activity → ↓insulin release
- Agonists of muscarinic receptors → Ca^{2+} efflux from ER → ↑insulin release
- Galanin, somatostatin → open K_{ATP} channel, hyperpolarisation → ↓insulin release

DRUGS USED TO TREAT DIABETES

Insulin

The actions of insulin are shown in Figure 27.3. Note that insulin also has a role in the synthesis of the enzymes implicated in glucose metabolism. Insulin receptor substrates (IRSs) activity may initiate the cascade: activation of the RAS (cell growth regulator) system → activation of MAP kinases → DNA transcription → RNA production → enzyme synthesis.

Insulin preparations

- Short acting: **soluble insulin, insulin lispro** (an insulin analogue in which a lysine and a proline residue are interchanged)
- Intermediate acting: **isophane insulin** (a suspension of a complex of insulin with protamine)
- Long acting: **insulin zinc suspension**.

Human insulin, made in bacteria by recombinant DNA technology, has largely replaced insulin extracted from bovine or porcine tissues.

Insulin administration and pharmacokinetic aspects

Insulin is inactive by mouth, owing to the proteolytic action of digestive enzymes, and must be given by injection. Various regimens are used.

Day-to-day control of blood glucose in IDDM. Patients can optimise control of their blood glucose by adjusting the timing of injections and proportions of soluble to long-acting insulin. A typical regimen would be twice daily s.c. injection of soluble insulin (peak effect 2–4 h, duration of action 6–8 h) combined with an intermediate or long-acting preparation. For tight control, soluble insulin or insulin lispro can be given shortly before meals.

Hyperglycaemic emergencies. Soluble insulin is given i.v. (rapid but short action, inactivated in liver and kidney, half-life ~10 min).

Unwanted effects and their treatment

The most important untoward action is hypoglycaemia which occurs if the dose exceeds the requirement for the food intake and/or amount of exercise. An excessively low blood glucose can lead to unconsciousness and possible brain damage. If the patient is conscious, a sweet drink, glucose tablet or snack may suffice. If the patient is unconscious, glucose i.v. or **glucagon** i.m. will be necessary.

Oral hypoglycaemic agents

- **Sulfonylureas:** examples are **tolbutamide**, glibenclamide, glipizide
- Biguanides: The only example is **metformin**
- Acarbose.

Actions and mechanism of action

The sulfonylureas act adequately only in patients with some functioning B cells. They increase appetite and may promote weight gain. They work by binding to the 'sulfonylurea receptor' (SUR) associated with the K_{ATP} channel to inhibit channel opening. Metformin has no effect on insulin release (and, therefore, does not cause hypoglycaemia) but it increases glucose uptake into tissues and inhibits gluconeogenesis. It can cause weight loss. Acarbose inhibits intestinal α-glucosidase, so delaying carbohydrate absorption and reducing the rise in blood glucose which follows a meal.

Pharmacokinetic aspects

Sulfonylureas are well absorbed by mouth and are well tolerated. They bind extensively to plasma albumin and may be displaced by other drugs given concommitantly. Their action is enhanced by reduced renal function associated with age or disease. Tolbutamide has a half-life of 4 h and glibenclamide 10 h; both yield active metabolites. Metformin has a half-life of approx. 3 h. Acarbose is taken with meals.

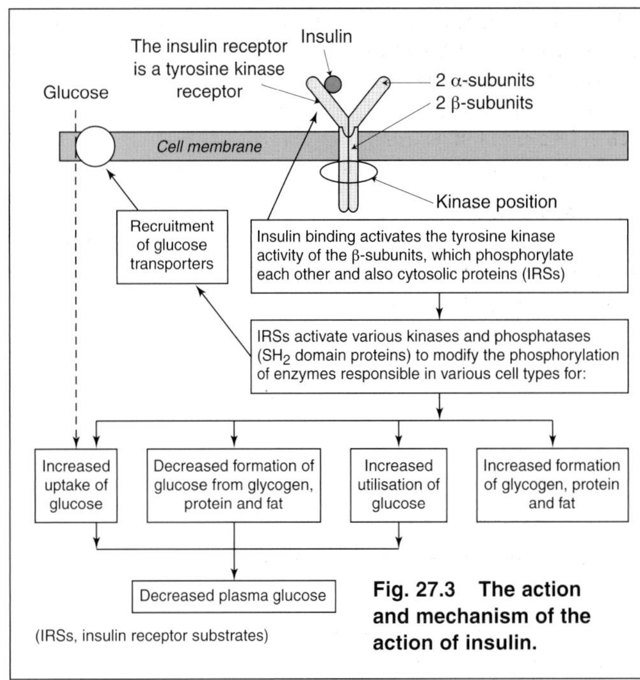

Fig. 27.3 The action and mechanism of the action of insulin.

Unwanted effects

The sulfonylureas can cause hypoglycaemic attacks; this is more likely in the elderly and with the longer acting drugs such as glibenclamide. Agents that inhibit the drug-metabolising enzymes increase the likelihood of hypoglycaemia. Gastrointestinal upsets and skin rashes are seen in a small percentage of patients. Metformin tends to cause anorexia and diarrhoea, and thus weight loss. A rare effect is potentially fatal lactic acidosis. Acarbose causes flatulence.

Newer oral hypoglycaemic drugs

Repaglinide, like the SURs, blocks the K_{ATP} channel. It stimulates insulin secretion, has a rapid onset and is eliminated quickly.

Thiazolidinediones (glitazones; e.g. pioglitazone). Pioglitazone lowers blood glucose very slowly (over months) and enhances the effect of administered insulin. It acts by binding to the peroxisome proliferator-activated gamma (PPARγ) nuclear receptor. Onset is rapid but action is prolonged to 24h by an active metabolite. It causes weight gain and fluid retention.

Summary of drug use in diabetes

- Insulin
  —for life-long treatment of IDDM
  —in treatment of NIDDM if oral drugs become less effective, e.g. during infections or major surgery.
  —different formulations have different durations of action.
- Oral hypoglycaemic drugs
  —in NIDDM if needed as a supplement to dietary control
  —**sulfonylureas** are main agents; effective in 30% of patients
  —metformin is used in obese patients or if sulfonylureas are ineffective
  —acarbose is used in NIDDM not controlled by other drugs

28 The adrenal cortex

The principal adrenal steroids are: the *glucocorticoids* (GC, e.g. hydrocortisone and cortisone) and the *mineralocorticoids* (MC, e.g. aldosterone). Some *sex steroids* (mainly androgens) are also secreted. Synthetic steroids have been developed in which the GC and the MC actions have been separated. Examples are prednisolone (GC > MC), fludrocortisone (MC > GC).

GLUCOCORTICOIDS

GCs are not stored pre-formed but are released when needed. The controlling factors are shown in Figure 28.1. The starting substrate for synthesis is cholesterol.

Pharmacological actions of the glucocorticoids

- *Regulatory*: negative feedback effects on anterior pituitary and hypothalamus (prolonged therapy can cause atrophy of adrenal cortex).
- *Metabolic*
  —carbohydrates: decreased uptake and utilisation of glucose, increased gluconeogenesis (thus tendency to hyperglycaemia)
  —protein: increased catabolism and decreased synthesis
  —fat: permissive effect on the lipolytic hormones
  (These actions are only made use of therapeutically in replacement therapy.)
- *Anti-inflammatory and immunosuppressive*: reduction in chronic inflammation and in autoimmune and allergic reactions; *but* decreased healing and diminution of the protective effects of the inflammatory and immune responses (as in infection). Mediators whose activity is reduced include eicosanoids, platelet-activating factor, many interleukins, cell adhesion molecules, nitric oxide. (These actions are the ones that are most commonly made use of therapeutically.)

Mechanism of action

GCs interact with intracellular receptors belonging to a superfamily that control transcription (Fig. 28.2). The GC/receptor complexes form dimers before entering the nucleus (not shown). Some genes are repressed (i.e. transcription is prevented) some are induced (i.e. transcription is initiated).

For metabolic actions, most of the mediator proteins induced are enzymes, e.g. cyclic AMP-dependent kinase.

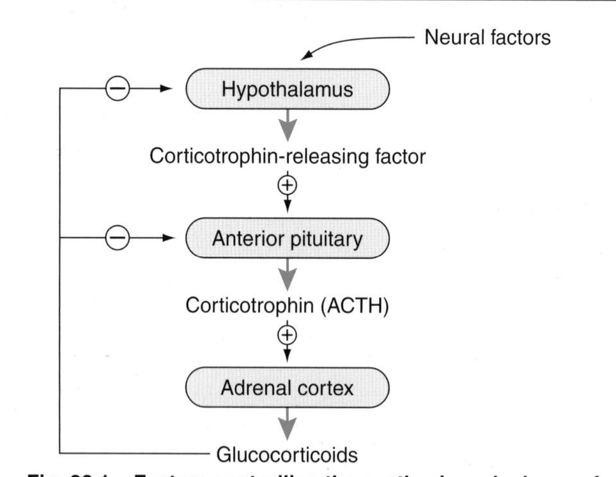

Fig. 28.1 Factors controlling the synthesis and release of glucocorticoids. Blue arrows, releases; black arrows, acts on.

For anti-inflammatory and immunosuppressive actions:

- inhibition of transcription of the genes for cyclooxygenase 2, cytokines (e.g. the interleukins), the inducible form of nitric oxide synthase, etc.
- block of vitamin D_3-mediated induction of the osteocalcin gene in osteoblasts and modification of transcription of the collagenase genes
- increased synthesis of lipocortin 1, which has a role in the negative feedback effects and may have anti-inflammatory actions.

Repression of genes involves inhibition of various transduction factors (AP-1, NFκB).

Main glucocorticoid drugs

Prednisolone, hydrocortisone and **dexamethasone** can be given orally, parenterally or topically. **Beclometasone** is given by inhalation.

Unwanted effects

Unwanted effects of GCs are seen mainly with prolonged systemic use as anti-inflammatory or immunosuppressive agents (in which case all the metabolic actions are unwanted), but not usually with

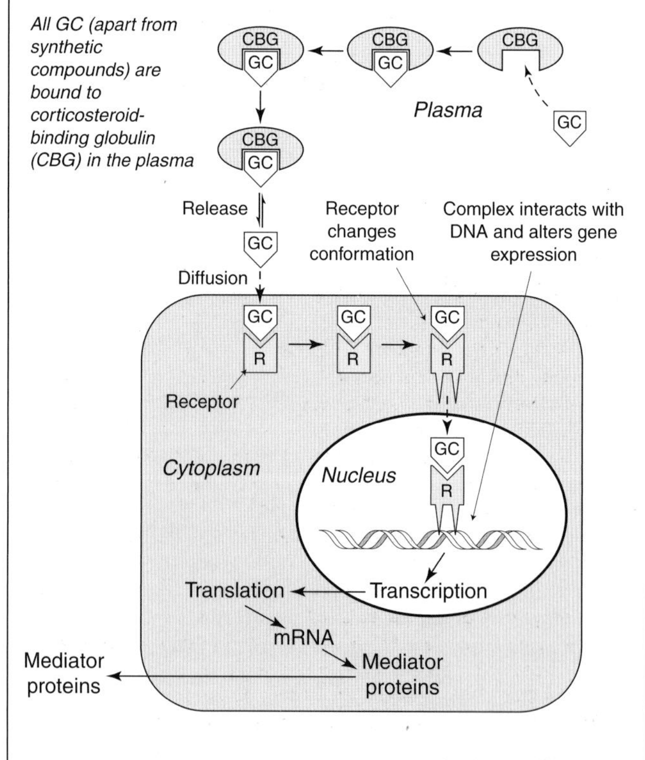

Fig. 28.2 Action of glucocorticoids in cells. R, receptors; GC, glucocorticoid.

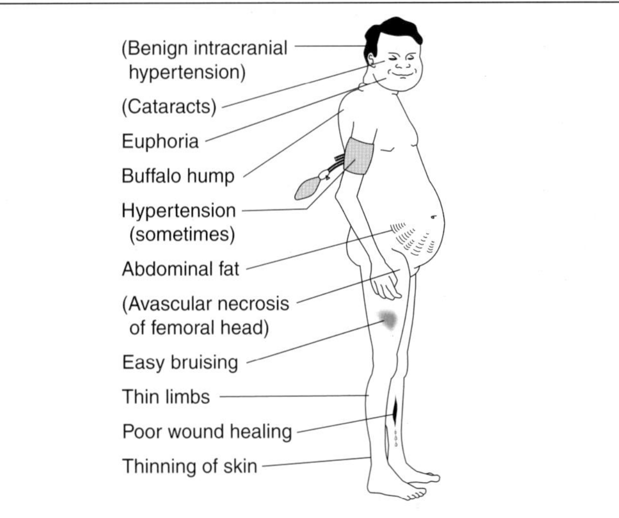

Fig. 28.3 Iatrogenic Cushing's syndrome (less frequent events in parentheses.)

replacement therapy. The most important (with the most common in italics) are:

- *suppression of response to infection*
- suppression of endogenous GC synthesis (the negative feedback effect); after prolonged use the drugs must be withdrawn gradually to prevent the precipitation of adrenal insufficiency
- metabolic actions (see above)
- iatrogenic Cushing's syndrome (see diagram)
- growth suppression in children
- *osteoporosis* (a limitation to long-term therapy).

Clinical uses of adrenal steroids

Glucocorticoids

- Anti-inflammatory/immunosuppressive therapy
  - —in asthma (by inhalation or, in severe cases, systemically)
  - —in hypersensitivity states, e.g. severe allergic reactions to drugs or insect venom
  - —in miscellaneous diseases with autoimmune and inflammatory components, e.g. rheumatoid arthritis and other 'connective tissue' diseases
  - —in various inflammatory conditions of skin, eye, ear or nose (given topically)
  - —to prevent graft-versus-host disease following organ or bone marrow transplantation
  - —in various neoplastic diseases, often in combination with cytotoxic drugs.
- Replacement therapy for patients with adrenal failure, e.g. Addison's disease (an MC will also be necessary).

Mineralocorticoids

- Replacement therapy in adrenal insufficiency (**fludrocortisone** orally with a GC).

Pharmacokinetic aspects

GCs can be given orally, topically, by injection and inhalation. They are metabolised principally in the liver and the metabolites excreted in the urine. The plasma half-lives are short (e.g. 90 min for hydrocortisone) but the main biological effects occur only after 2–8 h because protein synthesis of enzymes and mediators is required. Cortisone is inactive until converted to hydrocortisone.

MINERALOCORTICOIDS

The synthesis and release of the mineralocorticoids is shown in Figure 28.4.

Pharmacological actions

The MCs are critically important for water and electrolyte balance. Aldosterone acts on the distal renal tubules to cause increased Na^+ reabsorption, with concomitant increased excretion of K^+ and H^+.

Mechanism of action

The mechanism of action is the same as that of the GCs (Fig. 28.2) but aldosterone receptors occur virtually only in the kidney. (Spironolactone is a competitive antagonist of aldosterone at these receptors, see Ch. 25).) GCs enter renal cells but are inactivated by an enzyme (11-β-hydroxysteroid dehydrogenase) and thus have little or no action on these receptors (see Ch. 25). The effect of the mediator(s) produced by interaction of the steroid–receptor complex with the DNA is initially to increase the number of Na^+ channels in the apical membrane of the renal cell and later to increase the number of Na^+ pumps in the basolateral membrane.

PATHOPHYSIOLOGY OF THE ADRENAL CORTICOSTEROIDS

- Excess production of endogenous GCs results in *Cushing's disease*. (Prolonged therapy with exogenous GCs can give a similar picture, *Cushing's syndrome*—see Fig. 28.3).
- Decreased GC production results in *Addison's disease* (muscular weakness, low blood pressure, depression, anorexia, loss of weight, hypoglycaemia).
- Excess production of MCs, termed *hyperaldosteronism*, causes marked Na^+ and water retention, with resultant increase in the volume of extracellular fluid, hypokalaemia, alkalosis and hypertension.

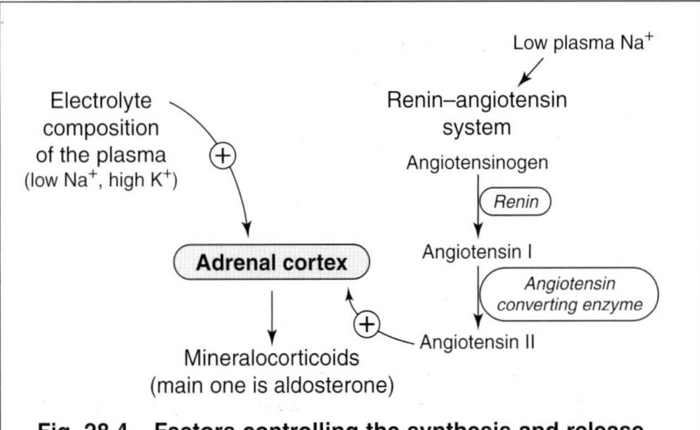

Fig. 28.4 Factors controlling the synthesis and release of mineralocorticoids.

29 The thyroid

The main thyroid hormones are thyroxine (T_4) and triiodothyronine (T_3). They are critically important for normal growth and development and for energy metabolism (see Fig. 29.1 for their regulation). The functional unit of the thyroid is the follicle. Each follicle consists of a single layer of epithelial cells around a cavity, the follicle lumen, which is filled with a thick colloid containing thyroglobulin (TG). The sequence of events in the thyroid is shown in Figure 29.2. Unlike other endocrine secretions, the thyroid retains a store of precursors. More T_4 is released than T_3.

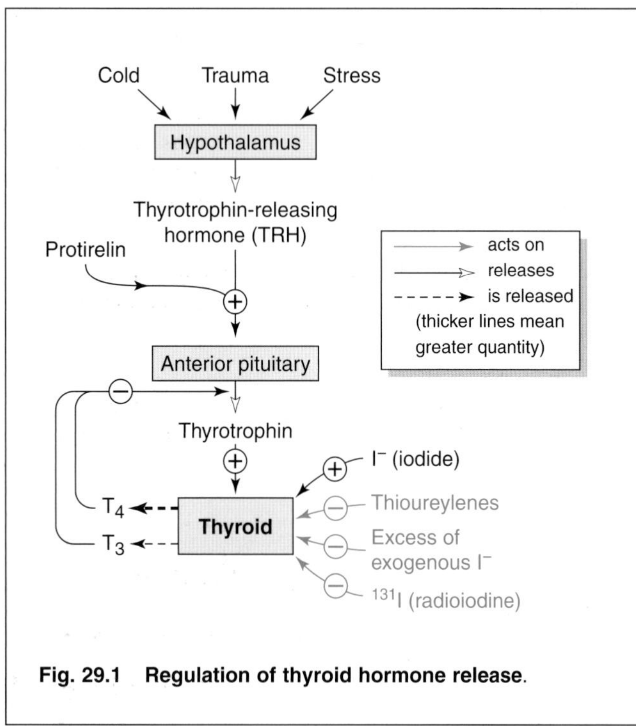

Fig. 29.1 Regulation of thyroid hormone release.

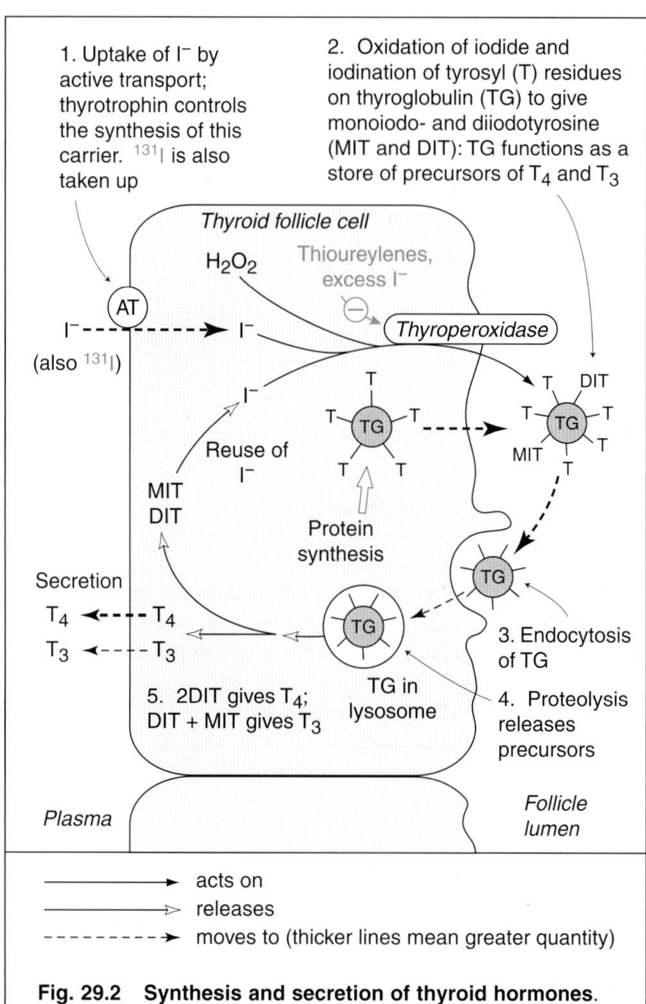

Fig. 29.2 Synthesis and secretion of thyroid hormones.

The action of the thyroid hormones

- *On metabolism*
  - — increased oxygen consumption and increased heat production leading to increase in basal metabolic rate (not in brain and gonads)
  - — increase in metabolism of carbohydrates, fats and proteins by modulation of the action of glucocorticoids, catecholamines, insulin and glucagon.
- *On growth and development*
  Essential for normal growth by
  - — direct action on cells
  - — potentiation of growth hormone.

  Essential for maturation of CNS and for skeletal development.
- *Cellular action:* T_4 is converted to T_3, which binds to specific receptors on DNA. These receptors when unbound, repress basal transcription. T_3 binding activates transcription, resulting in mRNA generation and protein synthesis.

The synthesis and secretion of the thyroid hormones and sites of drug action

The sequence of events leading to the production and release of T_4 and T_3 is shown in Figure 29.2. There is a large pool of T_4 in the body; it has a low turnover rate and is found mainly in the circulation. There is a small pool of T_3 in the body; it has a fast turnover rate and is found mainly intracellularly in the target organs.

Pathophysiology

Hyperthyroidism

Hyperthyroidism (**thyrotoxicosis**) results from overactivity of the thyroid. There is a high metabolic rate, an increase in temperature, sweating, nervousness, tremor, tachycardia, fatiguability and increased appetite; but loss of weight occurs. Main types are:

- *diffuse toxic goitre* (Graves' disease or exophthalmic goitre): caused by an immunological action against the thyrotrophin receptor; patients have protrusion of the eyeballs (exophthalmos) and there is increased sensitivity to catecholamines
- *toxic nodular goitre:* caused by a benign tumour; there is no exophthalmos.

Hypothyroidism

Hypothyroidism is a condition that results from decreased activity of the thyroid; it has several causes. The main types are:

- *Myxoedema*, which is immunological in origin; its manifestations include low basal metabolic rate (BMR), slow speech, deep hoarse voice, lethargy, bradycardia, sensitivity to cold, mental impairment and a thickening of the skin
- *Cretinism* (hypothyroidism in childhood); manifestations are retardation of growth, mental deficiency
- *Hashimoto's thyroiditis*, an autoimmune disease in which there is an immune reaction against TG, can lead to hypothyroidism
- *Radioiodine therapy*-induced hypothyroidism.

Simple, non-toxic goitre

Simple goitre is caused by dietary deficiency of iodine, which causes a rise in plasma thyrotrophic hormone and eventually an increase in the size of the gland. Normal amounts of thyroid hormone are produced, but eventually hypothyroidism may occur.

Drugs used in hyperthyroidism

The main drugs are the thioureylenes (e.g. **carbimazole,** propylthiouracil) and **radioiodine.** Iodide/iodine is also used.

The thioureylenes

Mechanism of action

Thioureylenes act on the thyroid to decrease hormone output (Fig. 29.2).

Actions and pharmacokinetic aspects

The drugs gradually decrease the thyroid hormone output and reduce the signs of thyrotoxicosis over 3–4 weeks.

All are given by mouth. Carbimazole is converted to methimazole (the active compound), which has a half-life of 16 h and causes 90% inhibition of the oxidation of iodine (organification of iodine) within 12 h. The clinical action is delayed until the store of hormones in the follicle lumen has been depleted, which may take several weeks. Propylthiouracil acts a little more quickly because it also inhibits the conversion of T_4 to T_3. The thiourylenes have no effect on the exophthalmos.

Unwanted effects

- Granulocytopenia (rare but serious)
- Rashes (more common)
- Headache, nausea, jaundice and joint pain (occasionally).

Radioiodine

Given orally, ^{131}I is taken up by the thyroid and processed in the same way as I^-, becoming incorporated into TG. It emits both β-particles and X-rays. The X-rays pass through the tissue, but the short range β-radiation causes significant destruction of nearby thyroid cells. Radioiodine has a radioactive half-life of 8 days. It is used in one single dose; its effect on the gland is delayed for 1–2 months and reaches maximum after 4 months.

Hypothyroidism occurs eventually and will need replacement therapy with levothyroxine (synthetic T_4).

Iodide/iodine

Iodide/iodine given orally in high doses temporarily reduces thyroid hormone secretion (mechanism not clear) and decreases the vascularity of the gland.

Other miscellaneous drugs

The **β-adrenoceptor antagonists** decrease signs and symptoms such as tachycardia, dysrhythmias, tremor and agitation. **Guanethidine** eyedrops ameliorate the exophthalmos.

Drugs used in hypothyroidism

The main drugs are **levothyroxine** (T_4) and **liothyronine** (T_3).

The actions and mechanism of action are the same as the natural hormones.

Unwanted effects

The thyroid hormones increase heart rate and output, cause dysrhythmias and the signs and symptoms of hyperthyroidism.

Clinical use of drugs acting on the thyroid

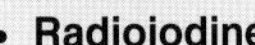

- **Radioiodine**
  —treatment of relapse of hyperthyroidism after thioureylene therapy or surgery
  —as first-line treatment for hyperthyroidism (particularly in the USA); recurrence is rare.
- **Thioureylenes**
  —hyperthyroidism (diffuse toxic goitre); at least 1 year of treatment being necessary; recurrence can occur but is susceptible to further treatment
  —before surgery for toxic goitre
  —as part of the treatment of thyroid storm (very severe hyperthyroidism); carbimazole is preferred.
- **Thyroid hormones**
  —levothyroxine (T_4) is the standard replacement therapy for hypothyroidism.
  —liothyronine (T_3) is used to treat myxoedema coma.

Bone metabolism

Bone is continuously remodelled throughout life, osteoclasts digesting it and osteoblasts laying down new bone (Fig. 30.1). Endogenous factors influencing the process include parathormone (PTH, parathyroid hormone), the vitamin D family, calcitonin and various cytokines. Exogenous factors include diet, exercise and drugs. The action of these factors is closely related to the control of Ca^{2+} homeostasis. Oestrogens, in particular, inhibit bone digestion; glucocorticoids, in pharmacological concentrations, promote it.

The bone remodelling cycle:

Bone resorption

1. The precursor cell releases cytokines (e.g. interleukin-6 (IL-6)) that recruit osteoclasts (OCs). **Parathormone** (PTH) and vitamin D product **calcitriol** promote this; **bisphosphonates** inhibit it
2. OCs digest bone, releasing embedded cytokines particularly insulin-like growth factor (IGF). **Bisphosphonates** and **oestrogens** inhibit this action

Bone formation

3. IGF promotes the differentiation of osteoblasts (OBs) from precursor cells (not shown). Bone morphogenic proteins (BMPs) (osteogenic proteins) promote this; **glucocorticoids** in pharmacological concentrations, inhibit it
4. IGF promotes the action of OBs in secreting osteoid (bone matrix), which consists mainly of collagen but also osteocalcin, phosphoproteins, etc. IGF molecules are embedded in the osteoid. **Glucocorticoids** in pharmacological concentrations inhibit this
5. Mineralisation of the osteoid occurs (i.e. complex calcium phosphate crystals (hydroxyapatite) are deposited)
6. IL-6 released from OBs can recruit OCs (not shown) and the cycle can start again

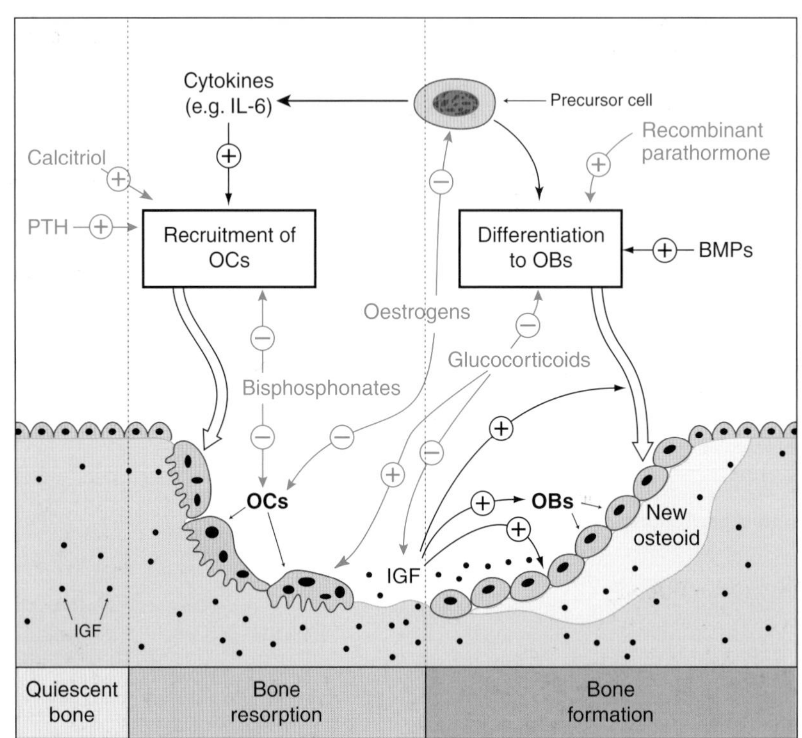

Fig. 30.1 The sequence of events in the bone remodelling cycle and the sites of action of drugs.

Calcium homeostasis

The daily turnover of bone minerals during remodelling includes flux of 700 mg calcium. Cacium influx into the cytoplasm is involved in the signal transduction mechanisms of many cells so plasma Ca^{2+} levels need to be controlled with particular precision. Cytosolic $[Ca^{2+}]$ is about 100 nmol/l and plasma $[Ca^{2+}]$ is about 2.5 mmol/l. The factors controlling plasma $[Ca^{2+}]$ are outlined in Figure 30.2.

Calcitonin

Calcitonin is produced by C cells in the thyroid follicles, its secretion being determined by plasma $[Ca^{2+}]$. It decreases plasma $[Ca^{2+}]$ by the actions shown in Figure 30.2.

Disorders of bone metabolism

Osteoporosis Increased fragility resulting from distortion of the micro-architecture of bone. Main causes are postmenopausal oestrogen deficiency, excessive glucocorticoids or thyroxine.

Rickets Defective bone mineralisation caused by vitamin D deficiency.

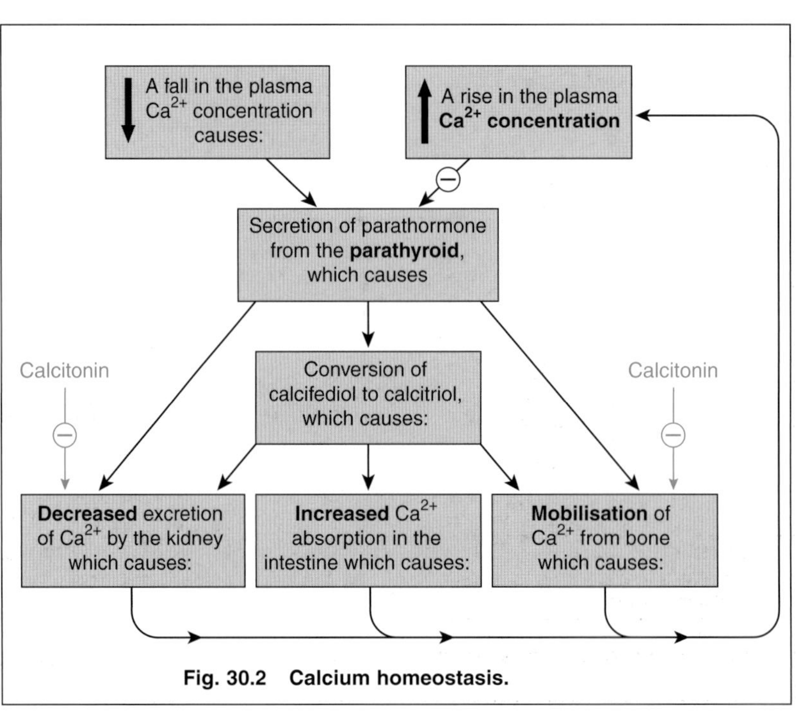

Fig. 30.2 Calcium homeostasis.

Hypocalcaemia Caused by hypoparathyroidism or vitamin D deficiency.

Hypercalcaemia Caused by hyperparathyroidism, some cancers.

Hyperphosphataemia Caused by renal failure.

Drugs used in disorders of bone metabolism

Bisphosphonates

Examples are **disodium etidronate** and **alendronate**.

They reduce bone turnover by attaching to hydroxyapatite crystals, slowing their growth and dissolution, and by inhibiting osteoclasts and stimulating osteoblasts.

Bisphosphonates are given orally (milk impairs absorption) and 50% of the absorbed drug concentrates at sites of bone mineralisation.

Unwanted effects Gastrointestinal disturbances and bone pain.

Clinical use of bisphosphonates

- Paget's disease of bone.
- Malignant hypercalcaemia.
- Postmenopausal osteoporosis (either alone or with oestrogens).
- Glucocorticoid-induced osteoporosis.

The vitamin D family

Vitamin D is a prehormone that is metabolised to give several biologically active substances (Fig. 30.3), the main ones being *calcifediol*, which is the principal metabolite in the plasma (not shown), and the more biologically potent *calcitriol*. These are true hormones.

The vitamin D in the body is derived from:

- dietary ergosterol obtained from plants (gives rise to vitamin D_2)
- cholesterol in the intestinal wall, which gives rise to 7-dehydrocholesterol; this, in the skin, is converted to cholecalciferol (vitamin D_3) by the ultraviolet in sunlight.

Cholecalciferol enters the liver where it is converted to calcifediol (a secosteroid; a steroid in which one of the rings has undegone fission); this, in turn, is converted to calcitriol (also a secosteroid) in the kidney.

Factors controlling the synthesis of calcitriol:

- negative feedback control by plasma calcitriol
- PTH, secretion of this being controlled by the plasma [Ca^{2+}] and the calcitriol level in the blood
- the plasma phosphate concentration (not shown in Fig. 30.3).

Actions The main action is the maintenance of plasma [Ca^{2+}]; this involves:

- increasing Ca^{2+} absorption in the intestine
- mobilising Ca^{2+} from bone
- decreasing renal Ca^{2+} excretion.

Preparations and unwanted effects **Ergocalciferol** (vitamin D_2) is the main drug used. It is given orally and needs bile salts for absorption because it is fat soluble. **Calcitriol** and alfacalcidol are also available; they can be given orally or by injection.

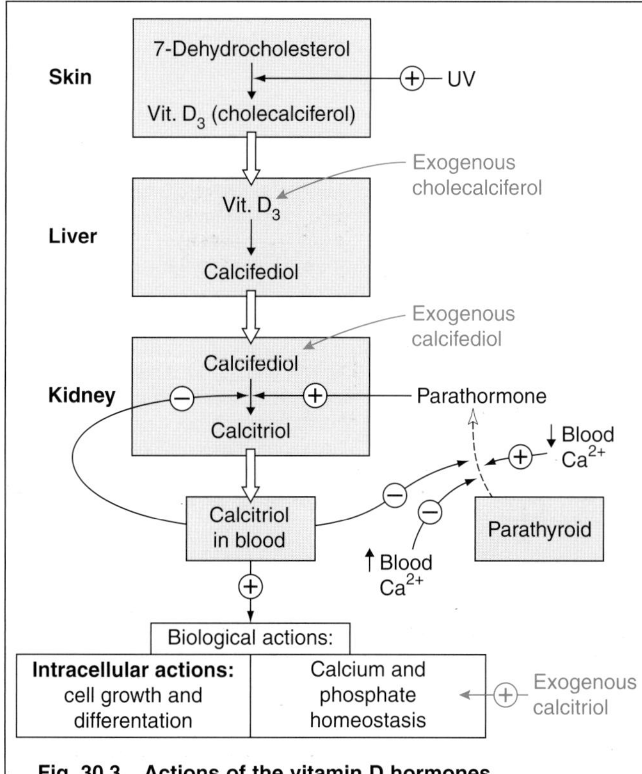

Fig. 30.3 Actions of the vitamin D hormones.

Clinical use of vitamin D

- Rickets.
- Hypocalcaemia of hypoparathyroidism.
- Osteodystrophy of renal failure.

Calcitonin

The peparations for clinical use are salcatonin (synthetic) and calcitonin (natural porcine). They are given s.c. or i.v.

Clinical use of calcitonin

- Paget's disease of bone
- Hypercalcaemia, to lower blood Ca^{2+}.
- As part of the treatment of glucocorticoid-induced osteoporosis.

Calcium salts

Preparations used therapeutically include calcium gluconate, calcium lactate, hydroxyapatite. They are given orally. Unwanted effects include gut disturbances.

Clinical use of calcium salts

- Hypocalcaemia (given orally).
- Hypocalcaemic tetany (given i.v.)
- Postmenopausal osteoporosis (with oestrogen and calcitonin or a bisphosphonate).
- Hyperkalaemia-induced cardiac dysrhythmias.

31 The reproductive system

The control of the reproductive system in both the male and female involves sex steroids from the gonads, hypothalamic peptides and glycoprotein gonadotrophins from the anterior pituitary.

THE FEMALE REPRODUCTIVE SYSTEM

To understand drug action on the female reproductive system it is necessary to be familiar with the events of the menstrual cycle (Fig. 31.1).

Drugs acting on the female system

Oestrogens

The main example is **estradiol**; others are given below.

Pharmacological actions The principal action is contraceptive (discussed below). Other uses are conditional on age and state of sexual maturity. In prepubertal patients, they stimulate the development of the secondary sex characteristics; in adult females with primary amenorrhoea, given with a progestogen, they induce an artificial menstrual cycle. Other effects include some degree of water retention, decreased bone resorption (see Ch. 30) and possibly some mild anabolic actions.

Mechanism of action Oestrogens bind to nuclear receptors in the cells of the target tissues (the reproductive organs and the anterior pituitary), the drug–receptor complexes then bind to steroid-response elements in the DNA and initiate transcription of some genes (e.g. for the synthesis of progesterone receptors) and repress transcription of others.

Pharmacokinetic aspects Oestrogens are well absorbed from the gastrointestinal tract, the skin and mucous membranes. Natural oestrogens are quickly metabolised in the liver, the synthetic non-steroidal oestrogen-like compounds less rapidly.

Unwanted effects these include nausea, salt and water retention and an increased risk of thromboembolism. Administered postmenopausally, oestrogens may cause endometrial thickening

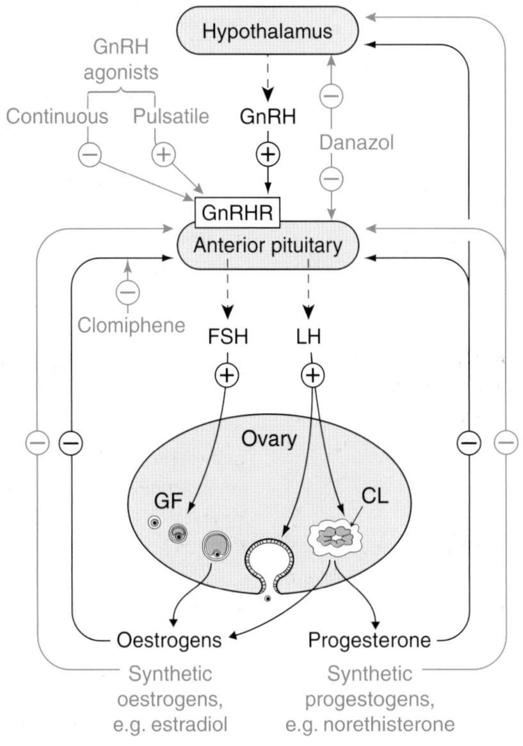

1. The menstrual cycle starts with the onset of menstruation, during which the top layer of the endometrium is shed. When bleeding ceases, the endometrium is regenerated during the rest of the cycle

2. Gonadotrophin-releasing hormone (GnRH) is released from the hypothalamus in pulsatile fashion to act on GnRH receptors (GnRHR) to stimulate release of glycoproteins: follicle-stimulating hormone (FSH) and luteinising hormone (LH) from the anterior pituitary

3. In the initial phase of the cycle, FSH stimulates the development of the Graafian follicle (GF), which contains the ovum

4. FSH stimulates the granulosa cells surrounding the ovum to produce oestrogens (oestradiol, and some oestrone and oestriol), the secretion of which rises till mid-cycle. The oestrogens control the proliferative phase of endometrium renewal (from day 5 or 6 to mid-cycle) and act on the anterior pituitary to reduce gonadotrophin release

5. At mid-cycle, a surge of LH secretion stimulates ovulation

6. Oestrogens promote progesterone receptor synthesis in peripheral target tissues, including the endometrium

7. The ruptured follicle, under the influence of LH, develops into the corpus luteum (CL), which secretes both oestrogen and progesterone

8. The endogenous sex steroids act on nuclear receptors in target tissues, activating transcription of some genes and inhibiting transcription of others

9. Progesterone, acting on oestrogen-induced receptors, stimulates the secretory phase of endometrium regeneration, which prepares it for implantation of the ovum

10. Progesterone acts on the hypothalamus and anterior pituitary, reducing the secretion of GnRH and LH. It also raises body temperature by about 0.5 °C

11. If the ovum does not implant, progesterone secretion ceases, triggering menstruation; in the absence of the negative feedback action the cycle begins again

12. If the ovum implants, progesterone secretion continues and its negative feedback action on hypothalamus and anterior pituitary ensures that another menstrual cycle does not commence. The chorion and later the placenta secrete gonadotrophins (including human chorionic gondotrophin), progesterone and oestrogens; these hormones maintain the pregnancy

Fig. 31.1 Diagram showing the hormonal control of the menstrual cycle and the action of drugs.

unless given with a progestogen. The unwanted effects of contraceptives are given below.

Anti-oestrogens These compete with natural oestrogens for target receptors (e.g. **tamoxifen**, a drug used in breast cancer therapy; see Ch. 49).

Progestogens (progestational hormones) have a mechanism of action similar to that of oestrogen (see Fig. 31.1 and below under contraceptives). **Medroxyprogesterone**, a synthetic compound, can be given orally or by injection. Other progestogens are used in contraception (see below).

Antiprogestogens **Mifepristone** may be used to terminate early pregnancy, acting by sensitising the uterus to abortifacient prostaglandins (see below).

Therapeutic uses of female sex hormones

Female hormones are used for two main purposes: contraception and postmenopausal hormone replacement therapy (HRT). Other uses are less frequent and are mentioned above.

Contraceptive drugs

Contraception can be effected by both oral and injected agents.

The combined pill

The combined pill contains **ethinylestradiol** or **mestranol** with a *progestogen* (e.g. **norethisterone**, **desogestrol**)

Mechanism of action

- Oestrogen suppresses the development of the ovarian follicle by inhibiting FSH release.
- The progestogen prevents ovulation by inhibiting LH release; it also makes the cervical mucus less welcoming to the sperm.
- Together they render the endometrium less suitable for implantation of the ovum.

Unwanted effects These are infrequent but can include weight gain, flushing, mood changes, dizziness and sometimes acne or skin pigmentation and a transient rise in blood pressure. There is some risk of thromboembolism.

The progestogen-only pill

Agents used include **norethisterone** and **levonorgestrol**. The pill is taken every day without a break. The contraceptive effect is mainly through making the cervical mucus unwelcoming to sperm, but the actions on the endometrium cited above may play a part. It is less reliable and irregular bleeding can occur.

Postcoital contraception

Emergency postcoital contraception can be effected with a large oral dose of **levonorgestrol**, with or without an oestrogen, taken within 72 hours of unprotected sex and repeated 12 hours later.

Postmenopausal hormone replacement therapy

A combination of an oestrogen and a progestogen is used for women with an intact uterus, an oestrogen alone in hysterectomised individuals. The doses used are much lower than those used for contraception. Examples of the oestrogens used are **conjugated oestrogens** or **estradiol** (given orally), oestriol (given intravaginally) and **estradiol** (implanted subcutaneously). Examples of the progestogens used are **norethisterone** and **medroxyprogesterone**. Tibolone has both oestrogenic and progestogenic action and is used on its own.

The main *beneficial* effects of HRT are:

- relief from menopausal symptoms (hot flushes, inappropriate sweating, paraesthesias, palpitations, atrophic vaginitis, etc.)
- a reduction in osteoporosis (controversial); see also raloxifene (Ch. 30)
- a possible decrease in the risk of coronary artery disease (this has recently been questioned).

The *unwanted* effects of HRT are:

- a slightly increased risk of venous thromboembolism
- moderate increase in the risk of breast cancer
- an oestrogen-induced risk of endometrial cancer if a progestogen is not also used.

Gonadotrophins and gonadotrophin release

Endogenous gonadotrophin-releasing hormone (GnRH) stimulates secretion of both follicle-stimulating hormone (FSH) and luteinising hormone (LH) from the anterior pituitary (Fig. 31.1) and its action is inhibited by the sex steroids, mainly progesterone.

Long-acting *GnRH analogues* (e.g. **goserelin**) cause continuous stimulation and thus desensitisation of the GNRH receptors; this results in suppression of gonadotrophin release and the suppression of the LH surge, promoting follicle maturation. They can be used in the treatment of infertility and for endometriosis and tumours of the breast or prostate.

GnRH antagonists (e.g. **ganirelix**) also decrease gonadotrophin release and are adjuncts in infertility treatments

Clomiphene, an antiestrogen, acts on the anterior pituitary to inhibit the negative feedback action of oestrogen, thus *increasing* gonadotrophin release; it is used to treat infertility and can result in multiple pregnancies. **Danazol** inhibits gonadal function by suppressing the mid-cycle surge of the gonadotrophins (Fig. 31.1); it is used for endometriosis.

Menotrophin, a preparation of the gonadotrophins FSH and LH is used to treat infertility.

Drugs acting on the uterus

Uterine stimulants: examples are **oxytocin** (a synthetic preparation of the neurohypophyseal peptide), **ergometrine** (an ergot derivative), **dinoprostone** (prostaglandin E_2), **gemeprost** (a prostaglandin E_1 analogue), carboprost (an analogue of prostaglandidn $F_{2\alpha}$). The prostaglandins contract the uterus but relax the cervix.

Uterine stimulants are used by obstetricians as follows:

- to augment or induce labour: dinoprostone (intravaginally); oxytocin (by infusion)
- for the management of the third stage of labour (ergometrine plus oxytocin)
- to treat postpartum haemorrhage: ergometrine plus oxytocin; carboprost if necessary
- to terminate pregnancy: gemeprost (by vaginal pessary)

Uterine relaxants: the main drugs used are β-adrenoceptor agonists, e.g. **ritodrine.** These are given to delay preterm labour.

THE MALE REPRODUCTIVE SYSTEM

The hormonal control of the male reproductive system is outlined in Figure 31.2. FSH acts on Sertoli cells to nurture gametogenesis. Interstitial cell-stimulating hormone (ICSH, the equivalent of LH) stimulates the interstitial cells to secrete *androgens* such as **testosterone**, which controls gametogenesis and the secondary sexual characteristics. Testosterone is converted by 5α-reductase to dihydrotestosterone, which is the main active male sex hormone. As with the female sex steroids, the androgens act on nuclear receptors to modify transcription. Testosterone preparations are used for replacement therapy in testicular failure.

Anti-androgens These (e.g. flutamide) are used in the chemotherapy of prostate cancer.

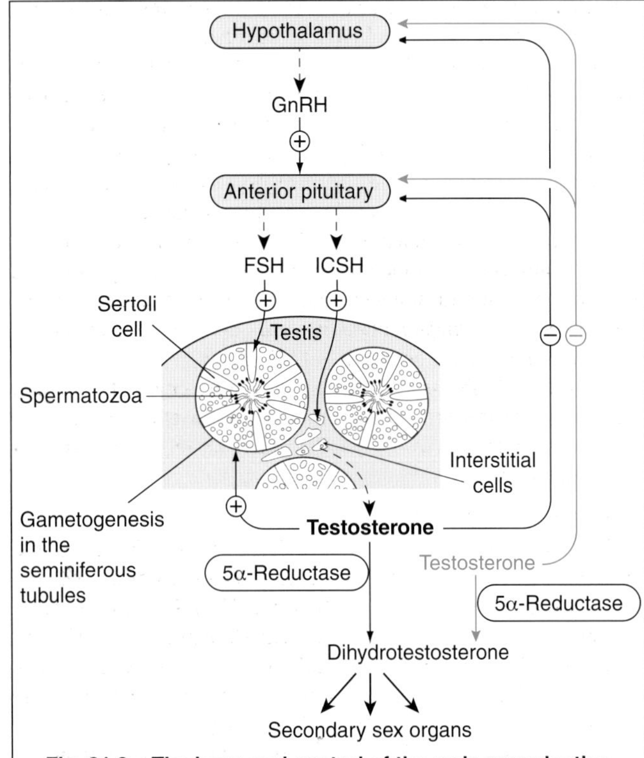

Fig. 31.2 The hormonal control of the male reproductive system and action of some drugs. ICSH, interstitial cell-stimulating hormone; FSH, follicle-stimulating hormone.

Drugs used in erectile dysfunction

Penile erection occurs when sexual stimulation causes relaxation of the arteriolar and non-vascular smooth muscle of the corpora cavernosa. This allows inflow of blood into the tissue which, in turn, compressess the venules and occludes venous outflow. The resulting pressure of the blood causes an erection. Nitrergic nerves have a key role in the process (Fig. 31.3).

Sildenafil

Sildenafil enhances penile erection in response to sexual stimulation but is also able to cause penile erection on its own. Its action in essence is the inhibition of phosphodiesterase type V, which normally reduces cGMP concentration by converting it to 5′-GMP. The concentration of cGMP is increased, causing reduction of the contractile properties of smooth muscle and the promotion of its relaxatory properties (Fig. 31.3). There is thus dilatation of the arterioles and relaxation of the trabecular smooth muscle, with the results described above.

Pharmacokinetic aspects

Sildenafil is taken orally, giving a peak plasma concentration after 30–120 min unless absorption is delayed by food. It has the same mode of action as the organic nitrates (Ch. 19) and so should not be used during therapy with these agents lest it exacerbates their effects.

Unwanted actions

Unwanted actions are due to the action of the drug on other vascular beds and include a fall in blood pressure, headache and flushing.

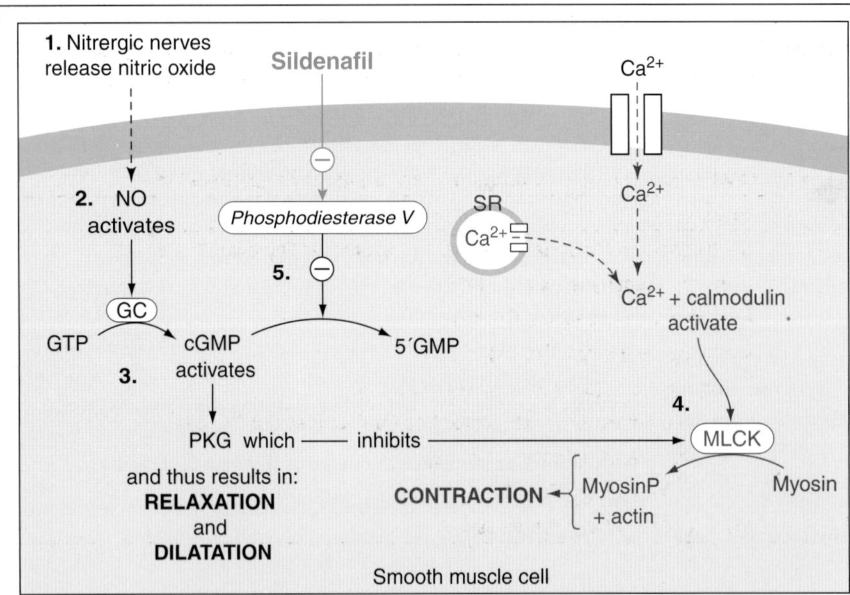

Fig. 31.3 The mechanism of smooth muscle relaxation of the corpora cavernosa that is involved in penile erection, and the action of sildenafil in promoting this. In the figure the contractile elements that are inhibited by cGMP are shown muted.

1. Nitrergic nerves release NO (see Ch. 14)
2. The released NO activates guanylate cyclase (GC) which increases cGMP
3. cGMP activates protein kinase G, which inhibits myosin light chain kinase (MLCK) which with actin, would otherwise cause contraction (4). This action of PKG, along with actions that decreases intracellular calcium and increases K^+ conductance (not shown here, see Fig 19.2) promotes relaxation of the smooth muscle
5. Normally cGMP is inactivated by phosphodiesterase V thus reducing cGMP concentration and promoting the contractile wing of the smooth muscle response

Sildenafil inhibits phosphodiesterase V increasing cGMP and thus its relaxatory properties

32 Outline of transmission and drug action in the CNS

In this chapter we summarise the transmitters in the CNS and how transmission can be modified by drugs.

Drug action

Drugs have important therapeutic effects in a variety of CNS disorders, and normal CNS function can also be modified by general anaesthetics and by drugs taken for non-medical use (alcohol, nicotine, caffeine, etc.). A full understanding of how drugs affect CNS function is currently hampered by our poor understanding of the ways in which the activity of particular neurons influences complex processes such as memory, mood and consciousness. Therefore, although the molecular targets and cellular actions of many centrally acting drugs are well established, the exact way in which the events at neuronal level are converted into therapeutically useful actions, as with antidepressants and anxiolytics, is usually much less clear. The action of drugs in Parkinson's disease (Ch. 35) provides perhaps the best example of how a knowledge of the neuronal pathways and neurotransmitters involved and the pathological deficit provides a rational basis for drug use.

An important consideration in the design of drugs for effects within the CNS is the requirement that they are able to traverse the blood–brain barrier. This barrier serves a valuable role in protecting the brain from many potentially neurotoxic agents which have gained entry into the systemic circulation but it impedes the uptake of most lipophobic drugs into the cerebrospinal fluid. Certain lipophobic drugs are, however, able to make use of active transport systems to enter the brain, e.g. **levodopa** in Parkinson's disease.

Chemical signalling in the CNS

The description of transmitter synthesis, storage and release provided for the peripheral nervous system (Chs 9–11) is largely applicable to CNS neurotransmission. However, chemical transmitters in the CNS operate over quite different time scales.

Neurotransmitters By convention, these are the agents responsible for fast excitatory and inhibitory postsynaptic potentials. Typically they are released by terminal boutons and act on postsynaptic receptors concentrated in postsynaptic densities on a single neuron. Their action is normally rapidly terminated by reuptake or enzymatic degradation. Neurotransmitters commonly act on ionotropic receptors (e.g. NMDA, $GABA_A$) though mediators acting on some G-protein-coupled receptors (GPCRs) may produce quite rapid action and thus also be considered neurotransmitters (e.g. noradrenaline acting on α_1-adrenoceptors can qualify).

Neuromodulators These are more slowly acting and their effects, both pre- and postsynaptically, may be more diffuse, spreading from the site of release to influence many surrounding neurons. Neuropeptides acting on GPCRs (e.g. somatostatin, substance P) are included in this category. Neuromodulators also include arachidonic acid metabolites (e.g. prostaglandins) and nitric oxide, which are not released in the same way as conventional neurotransmitters. Neuromodulators may be released by the same terminals as neurotransmitters—cotransmission. Neuromodulators are involved in synaptic plasticity and modulate the effects of neurotransmitters on action potential firing rate.

Neurotrophic factors These act over the longest time scale, regulating neuronal growth and morphology. Most act on receptor tyrosine kinases to control gene expression (e.g. brain-derived neurotrophic factor).

Drug action in the CNS

As in the autonomic nervous system, drugs can modify each of the processes of transmitter/neuromodulator synthesis, storage, release, action and inactivation in the CNS (Table 32.1). Receptor agonists (e.g. **opioids**; Ch. 41) and antagonists (e.g. **chlorpromazine**; Ch. 38) are employed as well as enzyme inhibitors (e.g. *monoamine oxidase inhibitors*; Ch. 39). Direct modulation of ion channels is an additional mechanism (e.g. **phenytoin**; Ch. 40).

A complication in understanding drug action is that, although a drug's action on its target receptor or enzyme may be manifest within minutes, the clinical effect may be delayed for some days (e.g. antidepressant activity or development of dependence on opioids). These delays are attributed to adaptive changes to drug-induced perturbations and may involve receptor up- or downregulation, modification of transmitter synthesis, etc.

Table 32.1 Summary of the targets of drug action in the CNS, with examples of drugs that act on the targets specified

Target	Example
Transmitter synthesis	Methyldopa (antihypertensive; Ch. 18), aspirin (antipyretic; Ch. 15)
Transmitter storage	Reserpine (antihypertensive; Ch. 18)
Transmitter release	Amphetamine (stimulant; Ch. 42)
Receptor action: agonist	Morphine (analgesic; Ch. 41)
Receptor action: antagonist	Chlorpromazine (antischizophrenic; Ch. 38)
Transmitter reuptake	Cocaine (stimulant; Ch. 42), fluoxetine (antidepressant; Ch. 39)
Transmitter degradation	Phenelzine (antidepressant; Ch. 39)
Ion channel block	Phenytoin (epilepsy; Ch. 40)
Nerve growth	Myotrophin (motoneuron disease)

33 CNS: amino acid transmitters

Within the CNS, *glutamate* is the main fast excitatory transmitter and α-aminobutyric acid (*GABA*) and *glycine* are the fast inhibitory transmitters. Aspartate may have some importance as an excitatory transmitter at glutamate receptors.

Glutamate

Glutamate is synthesised in neural tissues either by transamination of α-ketoglutarate (from the Krebs cycle) or from glutamine by the action of glutaminase. Like most transmitters it is stored in vesicles and released by exocytosis. Its action in the synaptic cleft is terminated mainly by active recapture into the nerve ending.

Glutamate receptors

There are four types of glutamate receptor: three ionotropic and one metabotropic receptor (Fig. 33.1).

The combination of subunits in ionotropic receptors varies widely so that the properties of the channels in different brain regions can also vary. NMDA receptors mediate a slow epsp and have a greater Ca^{2+} permeability. NMDA receptors will only open in response to released glutamate if glycine (or D-serine) occupies its binding sites on the NR1 subunits. (The concentration of glycine in cerebrospinal fluid is normally sufficient to allow this.) An important property of the NMDA receptor is that it is blocked by Mg^{2+} at the resting potential of neurons and the channel will only conduct ions (Na^+, Ca^{2+}) when the block is relieved by depolarisation (produced by AMPA or kainate receptors). Entry of Ca^{2+} through NMDA receptors is involved in synaptic plasticity (e.g. long-term potentiation (LTP) and also in cell damage (excitotoxicity) (Fig. 33.2).

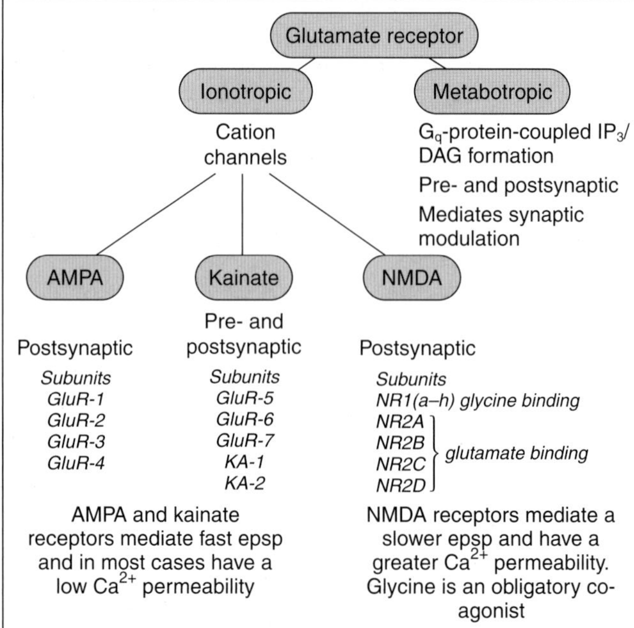

Fig. 33.1 Glutamate receptors. The ionotropic receptors are named after their selective agonists: NMDA, *N*-methyl-D-aspartate; AMPA, α-amino-3-hydroxy-5-methyl-4-isoxazole propionic acid; and kainate. IP_3, inositol trisphosphate; DAG, diacylglycerol; epsp, excitatory postsynaptic potential.

Drugs acting on glutamate receptors

Only a few useful drugs act by affecting glutamate receptors: **ketamine** (which produces dissociative anaesthesia and works partly by blocking the NMDA receptor channel) and possibly **dextromethorphan**, which is a cough supressant. Several other compounds with potent and selective actions on glutamate receptor subtypes have been identified; they are useful tools in the study of these receptors but do not have a recognised clinical value. One example is phencyclidine (angel-dust) a 'street' drug that, like ketamine, may act partially by blocking the NMDA receptor channel.

However, in view of the multiple subtypes of glutamate receptors and their wide distribution, drugs acting on them might eventually provide a variety of useful therapeutic effects. Thus drug-induced changes in LTP and plasticity might affect memory loss, and excitotoxicity might be reduced by NMDA receptor antagonism. Glutamate antagonists might be of value in treating brain damage.

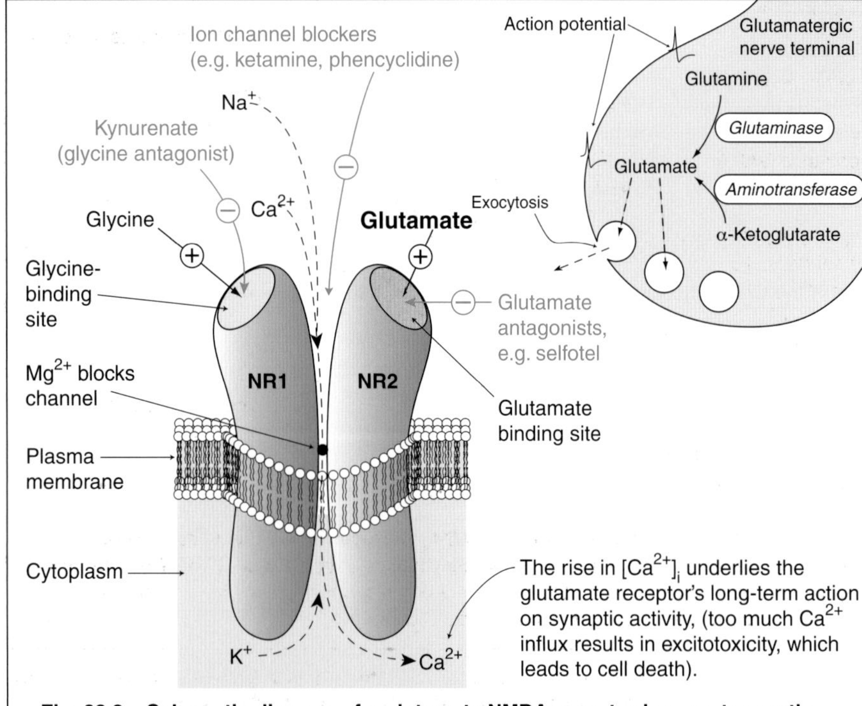

Fig. 33.2 Schematic diagram of a glutamate NMDA receptor in a postsynaptic cell membrane and the action potential-induced exocytosis of glutamate from a glutamatergic neuron. Only 2 of the 4 or 5 subunits are shown. The positions of the receptor sites for glycine and glutamate are purely speculative.)

GABA

GABA is produced from glutamate by glutamic acid decarboxylase (GAD). The activity of released GABA is terminated mainly by reuptake into GABAergic neurons.

GABA receptors

There are two main kinds of GABA receptor: $GABA_A$ and $GABA_B$ (Fig. 33.3).*

$GABA_A$ is a ligand-gated Cl^- channel that occurs postsynaptically (Fig. 33.4). **

Activation of $GABA_A$ receptors tends to clamp the membrane potential close to the Cl^- equilibrium potential (which is usually near to, or more negative than, the membrane potential) and so decreases electrical excitability. Transmitter action at $GABA_A$ receptors typically produces fast inhibitory postsynaptic potentials.

$GABA_B$ is a G-protein-coupled receptor that acts via G_i to:

- inhibit voltage-gated Ca^{2+} channels in nerve endings to reduce transmitter release
- open K^+ channels in nerves to reduce excitability.

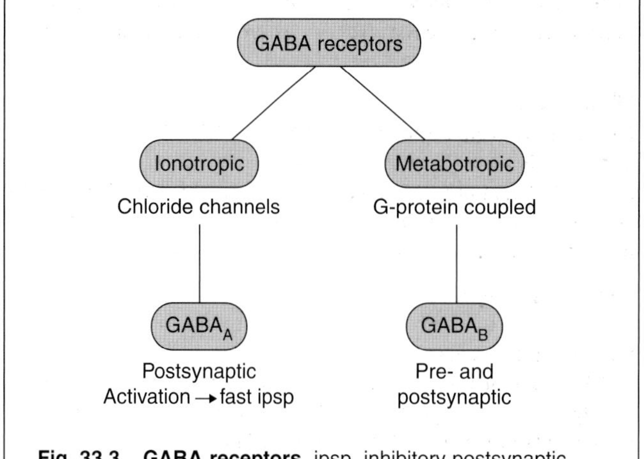

Fig. 33.3 GABA receptors. ipsp, inhibitory postsynaptic potentials.

Drugs acting on GABA receptors

$GABA_A$ receptors are important targets for the therapeutic actions of **benzodiazepines** and **barbiturates**. Useful experimental tools for $GABA_A$ receptors are muscimol, an agonist, and **bicuculline**, a competitive antagonist. The convulsant picrotoxin blocks the ion channel directly. **Benzodiazepines** modulate the binding and activity of GABA by binding to a modulatory site associated with the γ-subunit. Drugs may act as agonists (e.g. **diazepam**), antagonists (e.g. flumazenil) and inverse agonists (e.g. β-carbolines) at the benzodiazepine 'receptor'. Agonists enhance the activity of GABA whereas inverse agonists reduce the activity (see Ch. 37 for further discussion of inverse agonists). Diazepam has anticonvulsant activity whereas flumazenil is proconvulsant. **Barbiturates** and **neurosteroids** such as **alphaxolone** bind to other modulatory sites on the $GABA_A$ receptor to enhance GABA action.

Baclofen is an agonist at $GABA_B$ receptors and has a useful antispastic activity. Phaclofen, an antagonist, is a useful experimental agent.

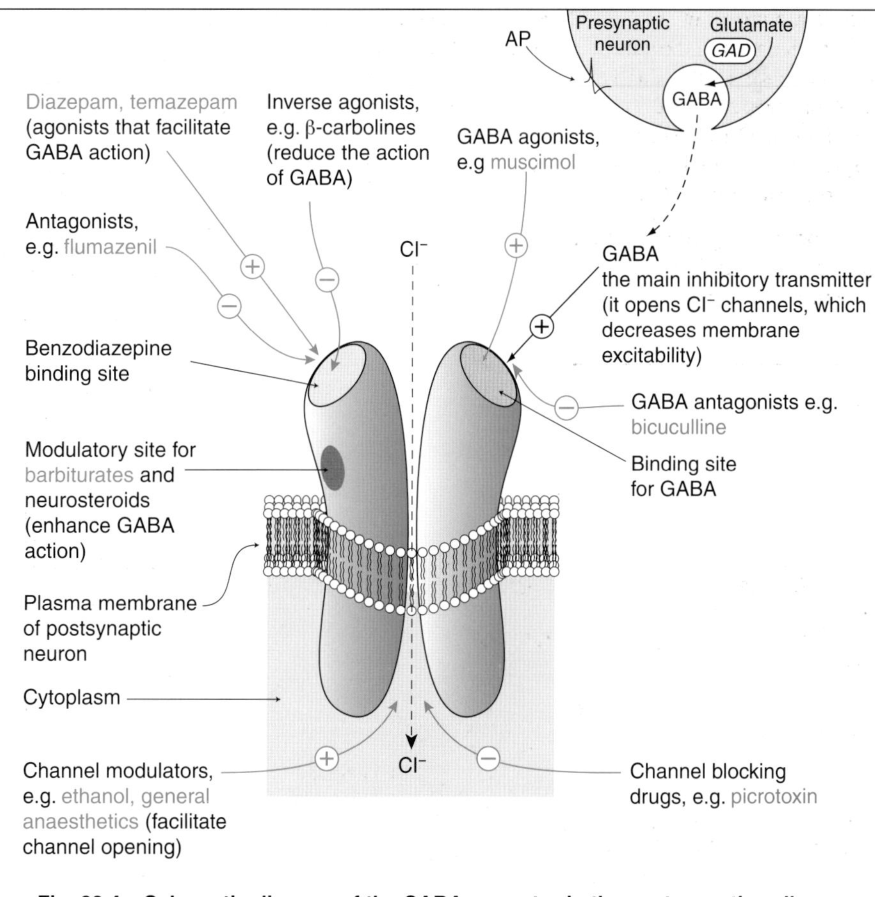

Fig. 33.4 Schematic diagram of the $GABA_A$ receptor in the postsynaptic cell membrane and the action potential (AP)-induced exocytosis of GABA from a nerve ending. The positions of the receptor sites are purely speculative. Only 2 of the 5 subunits are shown. GAD, glutamic acid decarboxylase.

Glycine

Glycine has two important actions; one direct on the inhibitory glycine receptors the other as a coagonist with glutamate on NMDA receptors. It is released particularly from inhibitory interneurons in the brainstem and spinal cord.

Glycine receptors

The glycine receptor is a pentameric ligand-gated Cl^- channel made up of glycine-binding α-subunits (α_1–α_4) and β-subunits. The convulsant action of strychnine results from antagonism at the glycine receptor. No clinically useful drugs are thought to act on these receptors.

*Ionotropic $GABA_C$ receptors (insensitive to bicuculline and benzodiazepines) have recently been identified in the retina.

**These receptors are heteropentamers made up of α (1–6), β (1–4), γ (1–4), δ, ε and π subunits to give receptor subtypes with different properties. The most common $GABA_A$ receptor stoichiometry is α_1 (2) β_2, (2) γ_2.

34 Other CNS transmitters

This chapter deals with non-amino acid transmitters and modulators in the CNS.

Noradrenaline in the CNS

Noradrenaline has both pre- and post-synaptic actions in the CNS. The bodies of noradrenergic neurons are found mainly in the pons (especially in the locus ceruleus), the medulla and brainstem (reticular formation) and project diffusely to the cortex, limbic system, hypothalamus, cerebellum and spinal cord. Synthesis, storage, release, reuptake of NA are essentially as described for peripheral sympathetic neurons in Ch. 11.

The CNS effects of NA are mediated by both α- and β-adrenoceptors acting either pre- or post-synaptically.

As in the periphery α_2-adrenoceptors can cause inhibtion of Ca^{2+} channels to inhibit transmitter release or activate K^+ channels to inhibit excitability. β-receptors may increase cell firing rate by inhibiting the hyper-polarisations which follow action potential discharge.

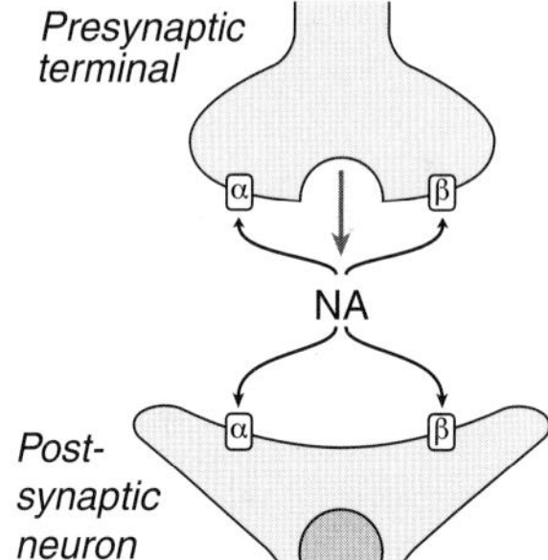

Activation of noradrenergic pathways is thought to increase wakefulness and alertness, whereas reduced activity may contribute to depression (Ch. 39). Noradrenergic mechanisms are also involved in the central regulation of blood pressure.

(Some compounds previously thought to act on α_2-receptors, e.g. clonidine, are now thought to work at least partly through distinct G-protein-coupled imidazoline receptors).

5-HT (serotonin) in the CNS

Serotonergic neurons are found in the Raphe nuclei in the pons and medulla and project to many areas of the brain including the cortex, hippocampus, basal ganglia, limbic system and hypothalamus. Activity in 5HT pathways is known to modulate mood, emotion, sleep, appetite and vomiting and to have some role in pain perception. Synthesis, storage, release and peripheral actions of 5-HT are given in Ch. 12. The synthesis of 5-HT is dependent on the plasma concentration of its precursor tryptophan (itself dependent on dietary intake) and on the activity of tryptophan hydroxylase.

The seven classes of 5-HT receptor, all G-protein coupled except for the ionotropic 5-HT_3 receptor, have been described in Ch 12. The main receptors affecting CNS function are shown here.

The different G-protein-coupled receptors may link to $G_{q/11}$, $G_{i/o}$ or to G_s.

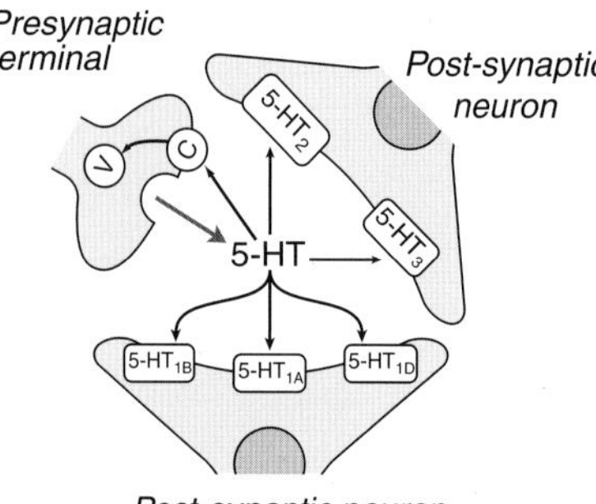

5-HT released from dense core vesicles (V) in serotonergic neurons is mainly inactivated by reuptake by specific carriers (C) different to those for noradrenaline but subject to inhibition by some of the same inhibitors (e.g. tricyclic antidepessants) as well as by selective serotonin reuptake inhibitors (SSRIs, Ch 39).

5-HT_1 receptors in the cortex and amygdala are targets for anxiolytic and antidepressant drugs. 5-HT_2 receptors in the hippocampus and cortex may underlie the hallucinogenic effects of some drugs. 5-HT_3 receptors are found mainly in the brainstem, especially the area postrema, which is concerned with vomiting.

Histamine in the CNS

Histamine is synthesised from histidine by histidine decarboxylase. All three histamine receptor subtypes (Ch. 16) are found in the CNS though histamine amounts are relatively small and few histaminergic pathways have been identified. Nevertheless H_1 antagonists have useful sedative and antiemetic actions. The importance of H_3 receptors is currently unknown though activation of these receptors is shown to inhibit the release of a number of transmitters.

Purines in the CNS

ATP is now well established as a neurotransmitter both in the CNS and periphery and has both ionotropic (P_{2X}) and G-protein-coupled (P_{2Y}) receptors. Adenosine receptors (A_1, A_{2A}, A_{2B}, A_3) are G-protein coupled. Caffeine and some other methylxanthines are A_2 receptor antagonists. Adenosine receptor agonists have potential value as sedatives, anticonvulsants and neuroprotective agents.

Neuropeptides in the CNS

Many peptides (e.g. somatostatin, enkephalins, substance P, neuropeptide Y, see Ch. 13) act as neuromodulators, influencing a wide range of CNS activity. In some cases they are released as co-transmitters with monoamines. Peptide receptors are most usually G-protein coupled; no examples of peptides gating ionotropic receptors are documented.

Dopamine in the CNS

There are three dopaminergic pathways in the CNS. The *nigrostriatal tract*, which contains most of the dopamine in the CNS, runs from the substantia nigra — where the cell bodies of the neurons lie — to the corpus striatum. Another dopaminergic pathway, the *mesolimbic system*, runs from the midbrain to the limbic system and the cortex. A third pathway, the *tuberohypophyseal system*, runs from the hypothalamus to the anterior pituitary. Dopamine is synthesised by the same pathway that produces noradrenaline (and is in fact a precursor of noradrenaline). Like noradrenaline, it is metabolised by monoamine oxidase and catechol-*O*-methyltransferase (yielding dihydroxyphenylacetic acid (DOPAC) and homovanillic acid (HVA).

After release, dopamine can be recaptured by nerve endings using a selective dopamine transporter (T).

Dopamine receptors belong to the GPCR family and comprise five subtypes separated into D_1-like (D_1 and D_5) and D_2 like (D_2, D_3, D_4).

D_1-like receptors couple to G_s-protein to stimulate adenylate cyclase.

D_2-like receptors, acting via G_i /G_o, inhibit adenylate cyclase, reduce calcium currents and increase outward potassium currents. The latter effect reduces electrical excitability and one action is to cause autoinhibition of dopamine release.

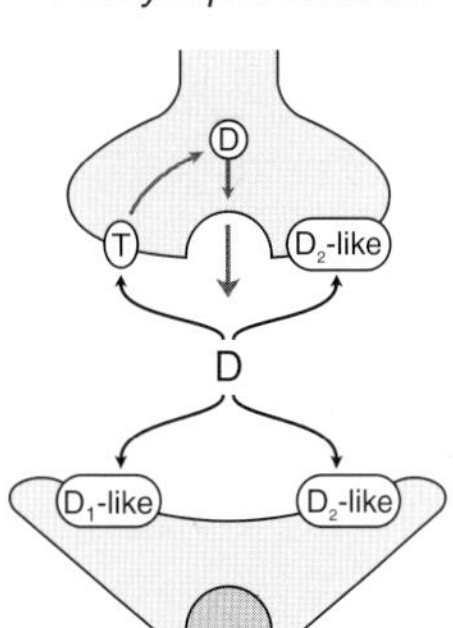

Functions of dopaminergic pathways: The *nigrostriatal pathway* is concerned with motor control and damage to these dopaminergic neurones leads to conditions manifesting motor incoordination notably Parkinson's disease (Ch. 35).
An increase in dopaminergic activity in the *mesolimbic/mesocortical* system induces stereotypic behaviour. An important role of dopaminergic neurones in schizophrenia is suggested by the valuable antischizophrenic action of D_2 receptor antagonists (Ch. 38). The *tuberohypophyseal pathway* regulates hormonal release from the pituitary especially prolactin (reduced) and growth hormone (increased).

Acetylcholine in the CNS

Cholinergic nerves are widely distributed in the CNS, the main pathways being from the magnocellular forebrain nucleus to the cortex, from the pons to the thalamus and cortex and the septohippocampal pathway. Cholinergic neurons also have an important role in the control of motion by the striatum (Ch. 35). Synthesis, storage, release, and inactivation are the same as in the periphery (Ch. 10).

Brain acetylcholine (ACh) has mainly excitatory actions. Both nicotinic and muscarinic receptors are found, both occurring mainly presynaptically. The former are ionotropic, the latter G-protein-coupled (see Ch. 10). Activation of the muscarinic receptors (which are mainly M_1 class) inhibits ACh release. Activation of the presynaptic nicotinic receptors (which are fewer) facilitates glutamate and dopamine release. Some postsynaptic nicotinic receptors mediate fast excitatory transmission. Inhibition of postsynaptic K^+ channels by muscarinic receptors can increase neuronal excitability.

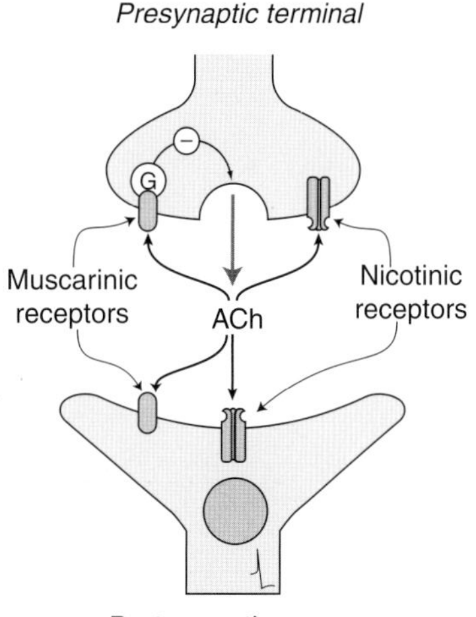

Cholinergic pathways are important mainly in arousal, learning and memory, and motor control; so that hyoscine for example has amnesic effects when used for premedication and anti-cholinesterases are advocated for use in Alzheimer's disease (Ch. 35).
The cholinergic activity in the striatum provides a target for drug action in Parkinson's and Huntington's diseases (see Ch. 35). Cholinergic projections to the cortex influence EEG activity; muscrarinic antagonists increasing slow wave activity which, paradoxically, causes excitement.

Arachidonic acid and its metabolites, including cannabinoids

Eicosanoids (leukotrienes, prostaglandins and HETES, Ch. 15) as well as endogenous cannabinoids are synthesised from arachidonic acid within the brain. Arachidonic acid and the eicosanoids may act as intracellular messengers (for example, modifying ion channel activity) or interact with cell surface receptors. The neuromodulatory roles of eicosanoids are not well established but prostaglandins appear to be involved in temperature regulation (antipyretic action of aspirin) and perhaps in sleep.

G-protein-linked (G_i/G_0) cannabinoid (CB_1) receptors are found in the hippocampus (related perhaps to the memory-impairing action of cannabis) and in the cerebellum, substantia nigra, mesolimbic system and cortex. Metabolism of arachidonic acid yields the endogenous transmitters 2-arachidonyl glycerol and anandamide. CB_1 receptors act via inhibition of adenylate cyclase, inhibition of N- and P/Q-type calcium channels, stimulation of potassium channels and activation of mitogen-activated protein kinase. Synthetic cannabinoids (e.g. nabilone) have potential for use as antiemetics (Ch. 26) and analgesics.

35 Neurodegenerative disorders

The very limited capacity of neurons to divide and re-establish synaptic contacts means that neuronal death produces largely irreversible changes in brain function. The main neurodegenerative disorders are Alzheimer's disease and Parkinson's disease (PD); less-common conditions are Huntington's chorea and motor neuron diseases; the recently described prion diseases such as variant Creutzfeldt–Jakob disease are less common still. A major cause of neuronal death is stroke resulting from brain ischaemia.

Mechanisms of neurodegeneration

Excitotoxicity is neuronal damage produced by disproportionate action of the excitatory neurotransmitter glutamate. High concentrations of glutamate cause an excessive elevation of $[Ca^{2+}]_i$ which leads to membrane damage and cell death (Fig. 35.1).

Oxidative stress This results from the generation of reactive oxygen species (ROS: oxygen and hydroxyl free radicals), which can damage proteins, membrane lipids and nucleic acids. Elevations of ROS are normally prevented by anti-oxidants such as glutathione and vitamins C and E and the activities of superoxide dismutase (SOD) and catalase. However, it seems that, in neurodegenerative diseases, these defence mechanisms can be overwhelmed.

Apoptosis Programmed cell death (see Ch. 4 for detail) is frequently associated with excitoxicity.

Potential drug targets in neurodegenerative disorders Elements of the excitotoxic glutamate cascade, Ca^{2+} entry, intracellular protease activation, free radical damage, the inflammatory response and membrane repair.

STROKE

Brain ischaemia leads to rapid cell death in the hypoxic area followed by a slower neurodegeneration in adjacent areas. The ischaemia causes depolarisation of neurons, which leads to release of glutamate and the consequences shown in Figure 35.1. At present, there are no clinically effective drugs available. If given soon after the vascular occlusion, fibrinolytics (tissue plasminogen activators; e.g. **alteplase** (see Ch. 22)) can improve blood flow and reduce further damage; however, they can make matters worse if the stroke is due to haemorrhage not clot formation.

PARKINSON'S DISEASE

Patients with PD have tremor at rest, muscle rigidity and difficulty in performing voluntary movements (hypokinesis).

Pathogenesis

The motor symptoms of PD are due to a specific loss of dopaminergic neurons in the nigrostriatal pathway, which forms an essential link in the extrapyramidal motor system involved in fine motor control. Excessive activity of the intrinsic cholinergic fibres of the striatum (unchecked by dopamine) is likely to be implicated in the tremor. The imbalance between the two systems is thought to be the main cause of PD. The damage to the dopaminergic neurons is caused by excitotoxicity, oxidative stress and apoptosis. Mitochondrial abnormalities have been detected in PD. Mitochondrial effects of MPTP, a contaminant of meperidine is responsible for a PD-like condition induced in a number of abusers of this drug. PD-like symptoms may be produced, as one might

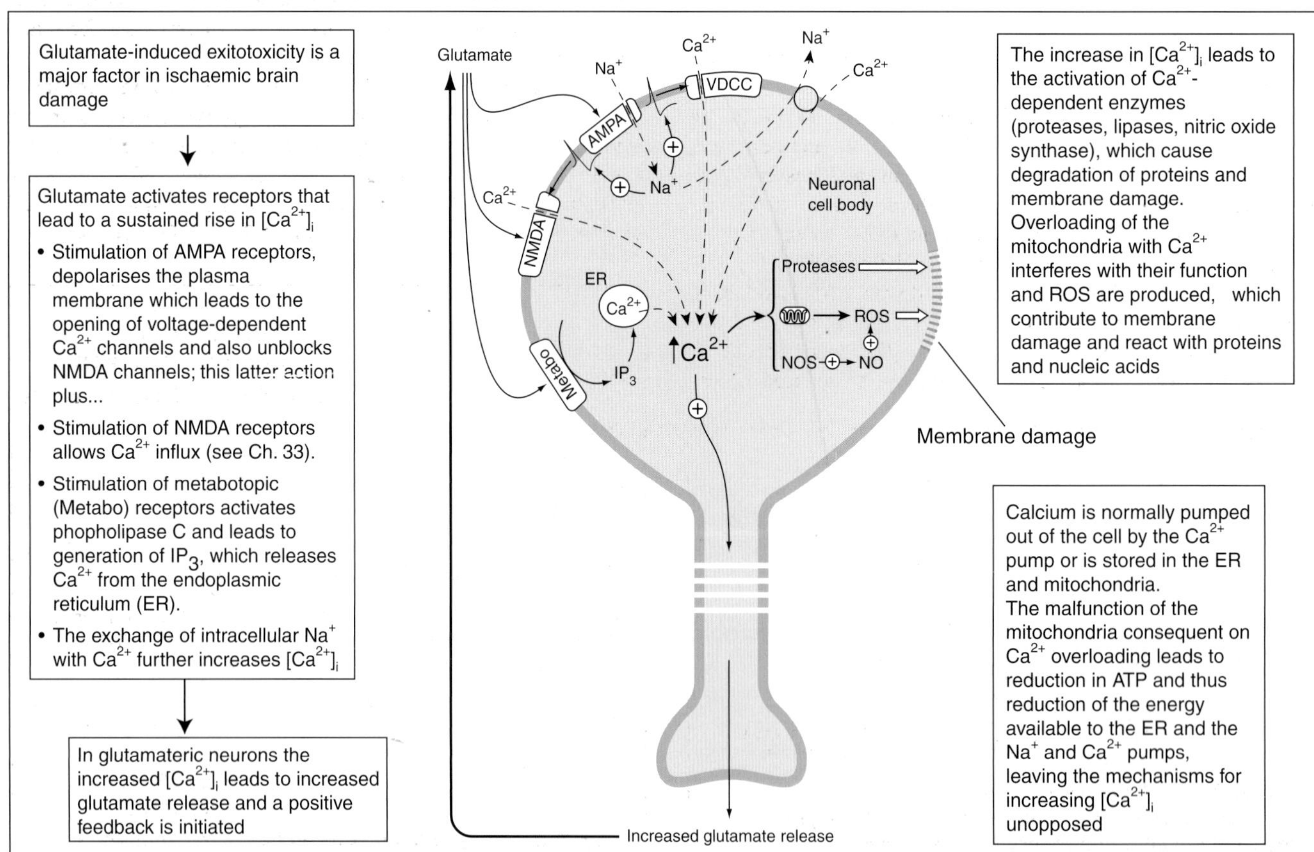

Fig. 35.1 The main mechanisms of excitotoxicity. ROS, reactive oxygen species; NO, nitric oxide; NOS, nitric oxide synthase; VDCC, voltage-dependent Ca^{2+} channel.

expect, by dopamine receptor antagonists. The pathways that are affected in PD are shown in Figure 35.2.

In PD, the destruction of dopaminergic fibres projecting from the substantia nigra to the corpus striatum impairs the fine control of movement exerted by the basal ganglia. This is exacerbated by a resulting enhancement in the action of striatal cholinergic neurons.

Treatment of PD

Drugs used to treat PD act by:

- redressing the loss of dopamine (**levodopa** or dopamine receptor agonists, e.g. **bromocriptine**)
- reducing the unbalanced action of acetylcholine in the striatum (acetylcholine antagonists, e.g. benzatropine)
- inhibiting the breakdown of dopamine in CNS neurons (selegiline)
- releasing dopamine (amantidine).

None of the above drugs halt the progression of the disease. Drugs affecting the dopaminergic system are shown in Figure 35.3.

Levodopa (L-DOPA)

Levodopa is the main treatment for PD.

Actions and mechanism of action Levodopa is decarboxylated to dopamine either within surviving nigrostriatal fibres or in other monoaminergic neurons and provides some restoration of nigrostriatal pathway activity. It is more effective against the akinesia and rigidity than against the tremor. The monoamine oxidase B inhibitor selegiline reduces the breakdown of dopamine in the brain and may enhance the action of levodopa. Combining entacapone (a COMT inhibitor) with levodopa can improve the response.

Pharmacokinetic aspects Levodopa is given orally and is well absorbed. It crosses the blood–brain barrier by active transport and has a half-life of approximatey 2 h.

Unwanted effects These include an acute schizophrenia-like syndrome related to an increase in dopamine concentrations and, more commonly, confusion, disorientation and insomnia or nightmares. More slowly developing effects include dyskinesia (uncontrolled movements, which occur in most patients after 2 years) and 'on–off' effects, which are rapid fluctuations between dyskinesia and hypokinesis/rigidity. Outside the CNS levodopa is converted to dopamine, which causes the unwanted peripheral side effects: postural hypotension and nausea. The latter is due to stimulation of the chemotrigger zone and can be reduced by co-administration of the dopamine antagonist domperidone, whose action is confined to the periphery. These peripheral side effects can be reduced by combining levodopa with a peripheral dopa decarboxylase inhibitor such as **carbidopa** or benserazide. These not only decrease the production of dopamine in the periphery but also substantially reduce the required dose of levodopa.

Dopamine receptor agonists

The dopamine receptor agonists **bromocriptine**, lisuride and pergolide have varying agonist activities on D_1, D_2 and D_3 receptors and can be used in place of, or as adjuncts to levodopa. (Both D_1 and D_2 receptors are involved in the regulation of motor activity by the striatum.) They have similar side effects to levodopa.

Amantadine

Amantadine, an antiviral agent, has a useful action in PD, possibly attributable to an increase in neuronal release of dopamine. It is less effective than levodopa or bromocriptine.

Muscarinic antagonists

Muscarinic antagonists decrease the tremor of PD. The drugs used (e.g. **benzatropine** and trihexyphenidyl (benzhexol)) show some CNS selectivity. Apart from the predictable effects due to parasympathetic block, troublesome side effects in the elderly are sedation and confusion.

ALZHEIMER'S DISEASE

This age-related dementia is associated with a loss of neurons and shrinkage of brain tissue, particularly in the hippocampus and basal forebrain. Amyloid plaques and neurofibrillary tangles characterise the condition. The loss of cholinergic fibres (in basal forebrain nuclei) is thought to be a key factor.

Anticholinesterase drugs have a modest efficacy with predictable parasympathomimetic side effects. The drugs used are tacrine (short acting and can be hepatotoxic), **donepezil** (rather more effective and causes less liver damage), rivastigmine (fewer para-sympathomimetic effects and longer lasting), galanthamine (may work partly by allosteric activation of CNS nicotinic receptors).

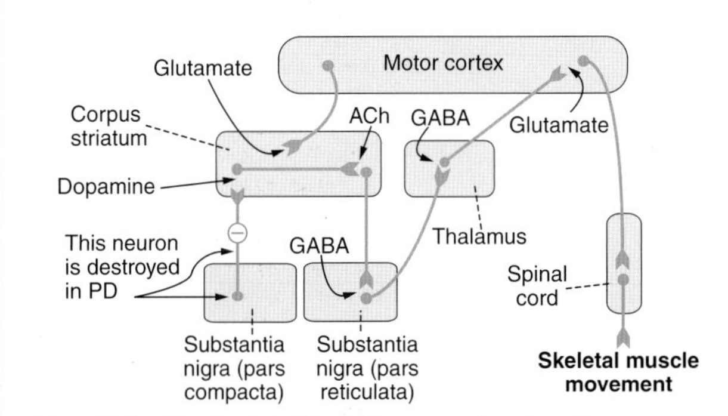

Fig. 35.2 Much simplified diagram showing the pathways between the cortex and the basal ganglia involved in motor control and the specific loss of dopaminergic fibres in Parkinson's disease (PD). ACh, acetylcholine.

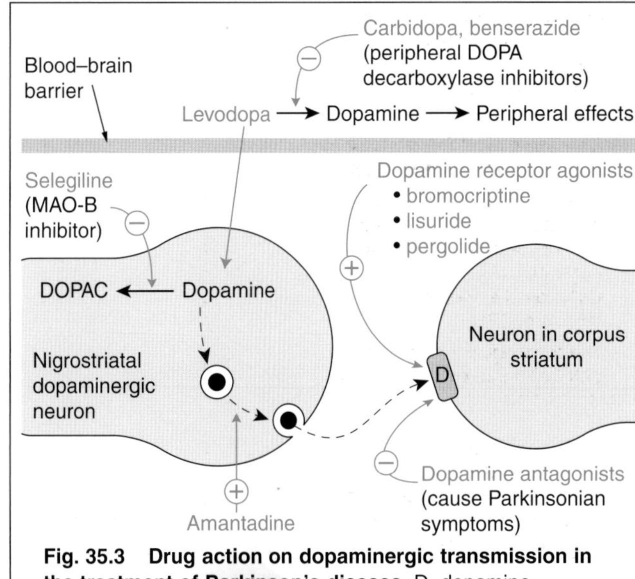

Fig. 35.3 Drug action on dopaminergic transmission in the treatment of Parkinson's disease. D, dopamine receptor; DOPAC, dihydroxyphenylacetic acid.

36 General anaesthetics

General anaesthesia, by producing unconsciousness and loss of sensation and reflexes, facilitates surgery with much reduced distress to the patient. There are two broad categories of general anaesthetics: the inhalation anaesthetics (gases or volatile liquids) and intravenous agents.

Mechanisms of action

Inhalation anaesthetics

Unlike most drugs, the action of the inhalation agents does not seem to involve a well-defined receptor; the agents typically act at high concentration (for example nitrous oxide acts at concentrations of 10 mmol or more, whereas atropine produces more than 50% block of muscarinic receptors at less than 10 nmol (a millionth of the concentration!)). Neither is there a clear structure–activity relationship; most of the agents are small, unreactive molecules and even nitrogen gas produces anaesthesia in sufficiently high concentration. Their potency is well correlated with liposolubility so that cell membranes or, more likely, hydrophobic domains of proteins are likely sites of action (Fig. 36.1).

Electrophysiological studies show that excitatory transmission (glutamatergic and nicotinic) may be inhibited whereas inhibitory transmission at $GABA_A$ receptors is potentiated. In keeping with a particular interaction with receptors, the stereoisomers of some inhalation anaesthetics (e.g. isoflurane) exhibit some differences in potency.

Intravenous anaesthetics

Barbiturates (e.g. thiopental), propofol and etomidate all potentiate the action of GABA on $GABA_A$ receptors, producing a general CNS depression. Ketamine reduces neuronal excitability by blocking NMDA receptors (Ch. 33).

Analgesic action

The analgesic action of these agents may involve the suppression of pain inputs at the spinal level whereas the loss of consciousness probably involves an action on the reticular activating system and thalamocortical tract. The short-term amnesia caused by many anaesthetic agents may result from an effect on the hippocampus.

Stages of anaesthesia

The depression of CNS function commonly proceeds through well-defined stages (Table 36.1). Modern practice allows a rapid transition to surgical anaesthesia so that the unwanted actions in stage II are often avoided.

Table 36.1

Stage	Characteristics
I	*Analgesia.* Still conscious
II	*Excitement.* Loss of consciousness but responsive to painful stimuli; may move, have incoherent speech, vomiting and irregular breathing
III	*Surgical anaesthesia.* Reflexes disappear. Respiration initially more regular but depression develops with increasing depth of anaesthesia; muscle relaxation
IV	*Medullary depression.* Respiratory arrest and cardiovascular collapse. Death

Inhalation agents

Pharmacokinetic aspects

All of these agents are rapidly absorbed across the alveolar membranes of the lungs The rate at which the body equilibrates with the inspired gas, however, varies considerably, as shown in Figure 36.2. The rate of equilibration is determined mainly by the *blood:gas partition coefficient*. Agents with a low coefficient (e.g. nitrous

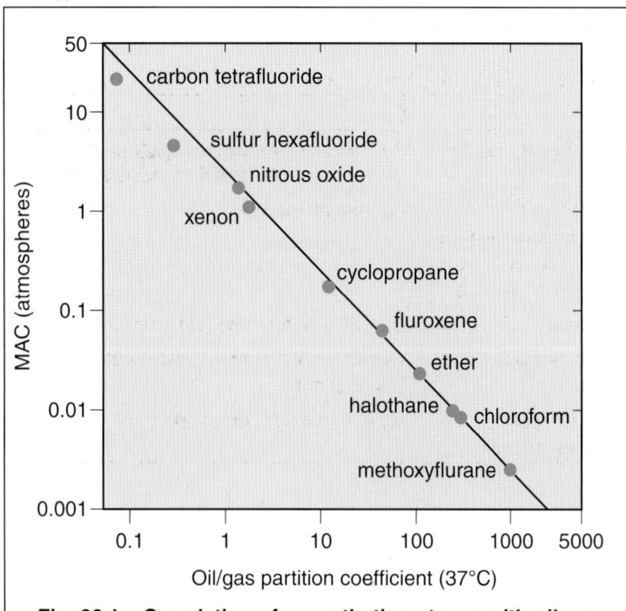

Fig. 36.1 Correlation of anaesthetic potency with oil:gas partition coefficient. Anaesthetic potency in humans is expressed as minimum alveolar partial pressure (MAC) required to produce surgical anaesthesia.

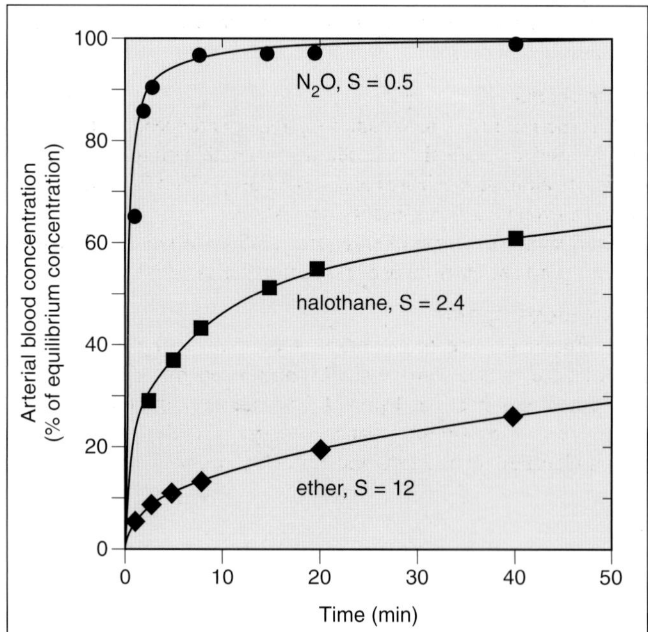

Fig. 36.2 Rate of equilibration on inhalation anaesthetics. S, blood:gas partition coefficient.

oxide) equilibrate quickly and have a rapid effect, whereas agents with a high coefficient (e.g. ether) act more slowly.

Most of these agents are inert and undergo little metabolism; their elimination is then mostly via the lungs. The rate of elimination mirrors the rate of uptake, being quickest for nitrous oxide. In a long surgical operation, there is a slow but potentially large uptake of lipid-soluble agents (e.g. halothane) into adipose tissue. Slow release into the circulation when the anaesthetic is discontinued results in a sustained low level of CNS depression.

Ether

Ether is the archetypal inhalation agent; however, apart from being flammable, it is irritant to the airways and has mostly been replaced by superior agents. Apart from nitrous oxide, all the currently used gaseous anaesthetics are halogenated ethers or hydrocarbons (all contain fluorine). All halogenated anaesthetics are prone to cause *malignant hyperthermia*.

Nitrous oxide

Nitrous oxide has a low potency, and inhalation at maximum possible concentrations will not produce surgical anaesthesia. It is, however, widely used in conjunction with other agents, allowing them to be administered at a lower concentration with a reduction in side effects. It has powerful analgesic actions and is used by itself (50% in oxygen) for pain relief in childbirth and accidents. Prolonged exposure to nitrous oxide may produce bone marrow suppression, resulting in anaemia and leukopenia.

Halothane

Halothane is a potent, non-irritant, volatile anaesthetic with limited analgesic action. It is widely used for maintenance of anaesthesia, but the recognition that it causes severe hepatotoxicity in a small proportion of patients has reduced its popularity and demands caution. It produces some cardiorespiratory depression and may cause cardiac dysrhythmias. Up to 20% of the halothane absorbed is metabolised in the liver. The liver toxicity may be a result of fluoroacetylation of liver cell proteins, which results in an immune response.

Other agents

Enflurane resembles halothane in potency and speed of induction and is used to maintain anaesthesia in combination with nitrous oxide. It can induce seizures and should be avoided in epileptics. It is also a strong cardiorespiratory depressant.

Isoflurane, an isomer of enflurane, desflurane and sevoflurane (a newer agent) are other halogenated anaesthetics in use.

Intravenous agents

The intravenous agents are most often short acting and used to induce anaesthesia, which will be maintained by inhaled agents. Thiopental, etomidate and propofol are all very lipid soluble and cross the blood–brain barrier very quickly to produce unconsciousness in one arm–brain circulation time.

Thiopental

Thiopental, like other barbiturates, has no analgesic action and a low safety margin (cardiorespiratory depression). It is metabolised rather slowly (half-life 8–10 h) producing some CNS depression postoperatively. However, the effect of a single anaesthesia-inducing dose lasts for only 5–10 min because the drug rapidly redistributes from the well-perfused tissues (including brain) to less well-perfused, but higher capacity tissues (muscle initially, then fat).

Etomidate

Etomidate has some advantages over thiopental, causing less cardiorespiratory depression and less hangover. It has little analgesic action. It causes some involuntary movement and postoperative sickness, both of which may be controlled by other drugs. Adrenocortical suppression is possible.

Propofol

The widely used propofol is rapidly metabolised and so avoids the hangover of thiopental. Rapid recovery from its action also allows it to be used on its own, by i.v. infusion, to maintain anaesthesia; this is particularly useful for day-case surgery.

Ketamine

Ketamine, given i.m. or i.v., can produce surgical anaesthesia, suitable for brief procedures, on its own. The anaesthesia is, however, commonly referred to as 'dissociative', since it is possible for the patient to remain conscious but with insensitivity to pain and with short-term amnesia. A high incidence of hallucinations and dysphoria restricts its use in adults but a lower incidence in children makes it suitable for minor paediatric surgery.

Perioperative drugs

Anaesthetic agents alone do not usually provide optimal conditions for operations so drugs may be given prior to inducing anaesthesia (premedication), after induction (e.g. neuromuscular blockers) or during recovery (Table 36.2).

Table 36.2 Perioperative drugs

Use	Drugs
Reduction of anxiety	Benzodiazepine, e.g. diazepam, lorazepam, midazolam (+ useful amnesic action)
Reduction of parasympathomimetic effects: bradycardia, bronchial secretions	Atropine, hyoscine
Analgesia	Morphine or fentanyl (at induction)
Muscle relaxation	Vecuronium, suxamethonium (after induction)
Control of post-operative emesis	Metoclopramide, droperidol

37 Anxiolytics and hypnotics

Anxiolytics are used to treat acute anxiety states. *Hypnotics* are drugs used to treat insomnia.

Anxiety is characterised by psychological symptoms such as nervousness and feelings of forboding, accompanied by a variety of physical symptoms such as agitation, palpitations, sweating, sleeplessness and gastointestinal disturbances. It can be a normal appropriate reaction to disturbing events but can in some circumstances be pathological and disabling, particularly if associated with panic attacks, phobic states or obsessive compulsive disorders.

Insomnia is difficulty in sleeping and may result from anxiety.

Both anxiety states and insomnia can be treated with CNS depressant drugs, which have effects that range from anxiolytic at low concentrations, through sedation and sleep at higher concentrations to anaesthesia and, in toxic doses, coma and respiratory depression. However some sedative and hypnotic drugs are ineffective in anxiety states.

The main drugs used are benzodiazepines, 5-hydroxytryptamine (5-HT, serotonin) 5-HT_{1A} receptor agonists and β-adrenoceptor antagonists. Antihistamines may sometimes be used as hypnotics; barbiturates were once used extensively.

Benzodiazepines

Benzodiazepines are the most important and widely used anxiolytics and hypnotics.

Pharmacological actions

Benzodiazepines cause:

- a decrease in anxiety
- a sedative effect
- the induction of sleep
- a reduction in muscle tone
- an anticonvulsant effect.

The drugs may be used clinically for all the above actions. In general, most benzodiazepines exhibit similar pharmacological actions and choice is made mainly on the basis of duration of action. Shorter-acting agents are preferred as hypnotics to avoid sedative actions throughout the day. Table 37.1 gives a selection from the large number of benzodiazepines available.

Mechanism of action

Benzodiazepines act by binding to distinct 'benzodiazepine regulatory sites' on $GABA_A$ receptors and enhance the action of GABA, effectively increasing its affinity for its site on GABA-activated Cl^- channels (Fig. 37.1; see Ch. 33). The increase in affinity is manifest as a shift of the GABA log dose-response curve to lower concentrations. The overall action of the benzodiazepines on the CNS is to produce a general enhancement of the neuroinhibitory actions of GABA. The action at the $GABA_A$ receptor of benzodiazepines, competitive antagonists such as flumazenil and inverse agonists are shown in Figure 37.2. Flumazenil can be used to treat an overdose of benzodiazepine.

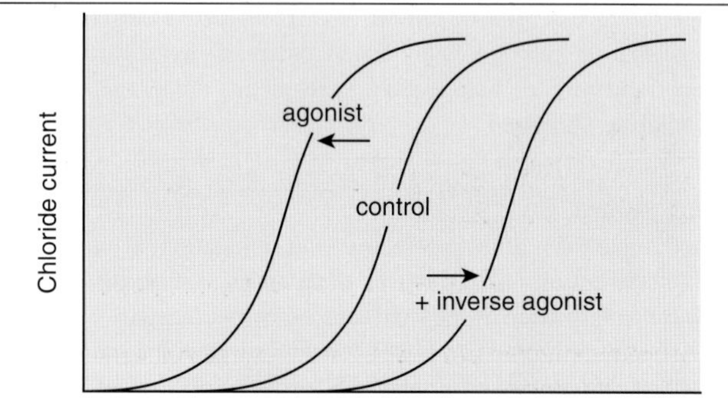

Fig. 37.1 Graph showing that agonists and inverse agonists at the benzodiazepine site have opposite effects on the opening of the $GABA_A$ receptor ion channel.

Table 37.1 Commonly used benzodiazepines and related drugs showing their main clinical uses and half-lives

Drug	Half-life	Main uses
Midazolam	Short (< 10 h)	Premedication, induction
Zolpidem[a]	Short	Hypnotic
Oxazepam	Short	Anxiolytic
Nitrazepam	Medium (10–24 h)	Hypnotic
Temazepam	Medium	Hypnotic
Flunitrazepam	Medium	Hypnotic, jet lag
Lorazepam	Medium	Anxiolytic, premedication
Alprazolam	Medium	Anxiolytic, panic disorder
Clonazepam	Long (>24 h)	Epilepsy
Diazepam	Long[b]	Anxiolytic, premedication, status epilepticus
Chlordiazepoxide	Long[b]	Anxiolytic

[a]Not a benzodiazepine.
[b]Long action due to slowly metabolised active metabolite. The drugs are also used in the treatment of spasticity and withdrawal from alcohol dependence.

Pharmacokinetic aspects

Benzodiazepines are lipid soluble and generally well absorbed from the gut and readily distributed into the brain. Most bind strongly to plasma proteins (up to 90% bound). Some benzodiazepines are metabolised to active agents with longer plasma half-lives. The final excretory product of most benzodiazepines is the glucuronide. Slower metabolism and increased half-lives in the elderly necessitate lower doses.

Unwanted effects

These include drowsiness, confusion, forgetfulness and some loss of motor control. Together these actions impair complex tasks such as driving. In general, benzodiazepines are very safe on their own, although they can produce severe respiratory depression in combination with alcohol. *Tolerance* (not marked for the hypnotic action) and *dependence* can develop. Stopping the drug can, therefore, cause a withdrawal syndrome with both physical and psychological features: rebound anxiety, insomnia, photophobia, feelings of unsteadiness and even seizures. This is more likely to happen with short-acting agents. About a third of long-term users show withdrawal effects when they cease taking the drugs.

$5HT_{1A}$ agonists

5-HT_{1A} receptors occur extensively in the cerebral cortex and the amygdala. They are auto-inhibitory presynaptic receptors and their

1. The $GABA_A$ receptor on CNS neurons has binding sites for GABA and for benzodiazepine (BZD) anxiolytic drugs

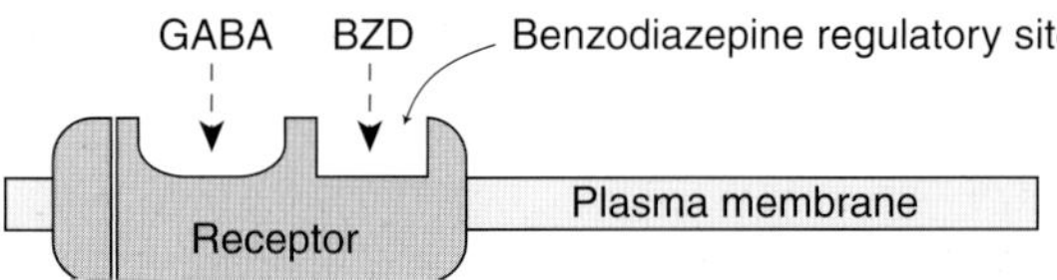

2. The receptor isomerises between a form that can bind the endogenous agonist GABA, which causes the Cl^- channel to open...

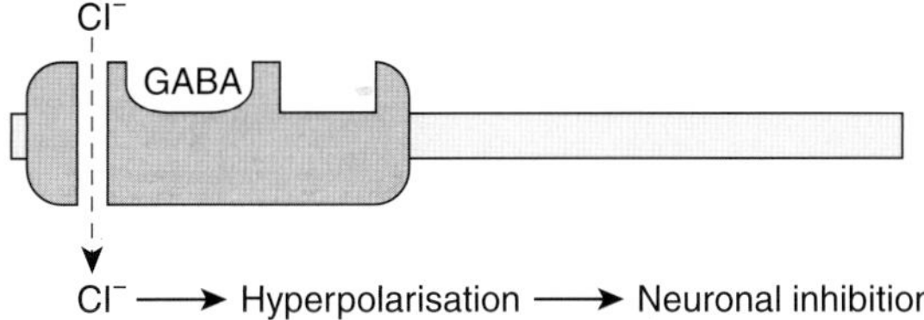

3. ...and an 'inactive' form, i.e. one that has much lower affinity for GABA

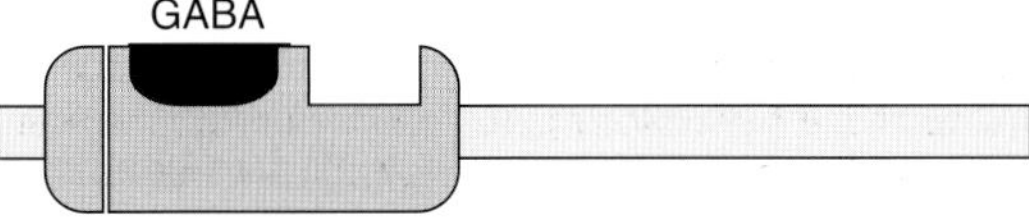

Normally there is equilibrium between the two conformations, with submaximal sensitivity to GABA

4. BZD agonists, such as diazepam, bind preferentially to the active form of the receptor and increase affinity for GABA

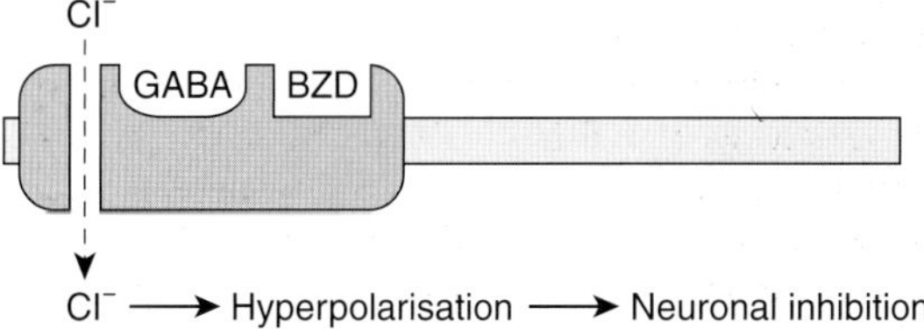

5. Inverse agonists such as the β-carbolines (βcar) bind preferentially to the 'inactive' form of the receptor, thus decreasing the proportion of receptors that bind GABA and reducing its effects

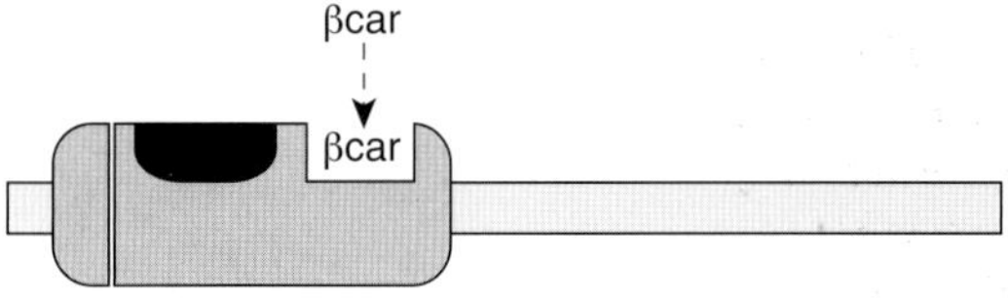

6. Competitive antagonists such as flumazenil (Flu) have equal affinity for the active and inactive configuration and, therefore, on their own, do not disturb the normal equilibrium. But their binding prevents the binding both of conventional agonists and of inverse agonists

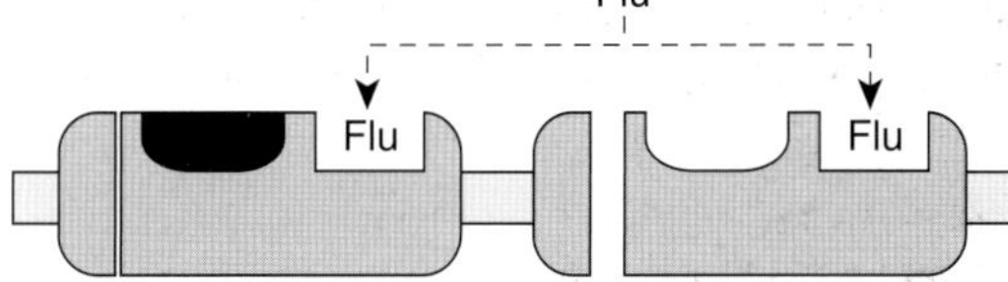

Fig. 37.2 Schematic diagram of the interaction of benzodiazepine agonists, antagonists and inverse agonists with the GABA receptor.

activation results in decreased firing of the serotonergic neurons on which they occur. $5\text{-}HT_{1A}$ receptor agonists will thus have mainly inhibitory effects.

The main drugs are **buspirone**, gepirone and ipsapirone.

Pharmacological actions

The $5HT_{1A}$ agonists reduce anxiety but do not cause the sedation and motor incoordination seen with benzodiazepines.

Mechanism of action

The drugs are believed to work by activating the presynaptic $5HT_{1A}$ autoreceptors, particularly in the dorsal raphe nucleus of the midbrain. The drugs also reduce the activity of some noradrenergic neurons (Ch. 34) and thus decrease arousal reactions (but do not induce sleep). However, there is a delay of several days before clinical effects are seen, which suggests a more complex mechanism of action.

Unwanted effects

These are less of a problem than with the benzodiazepines. They include nausea, nervousness, giddiness, restlessness, headache and light-headedness. The possibility of developing dependence and withdrawal is low.

Beta-adrenoceptor antagonists

Beta-adrenoceptor antagonists (e.g. **propranolol**) can reduce some of the peripheral manifestations of anxiety, notably tremor, sweating, tachycardia and diarrhoea. They have no effect on the central CNS affective component. Accordingly they find use (abuse) in some sports and the performing arts.

Antihistamines

Antihistamines (histamine H_1 receptor antagonists) with sedative action (see Ch. 16) have a useful hypnotic action that is made use of in some cold remedies and for wakeful children. However, many authorities feel that the use of drugs to help children sleep is rarely justified.

Barbiturates

Barbiturates, once used widely as both anxiolytics and hypnotics prior to the introduction of benzodiazepines, are no longer recommended for these clinical uses in view of their low therapeutic index and dependence-producing properties. Barbiturates resemble benzodiazepines in increasing the activity of $GABA_A$ receptors but bind to a different site on the receptor and increase channel opening beyond that seen with GABA itself (Ch. 33). This is responsible for their severe depressant effect on the CNS. They retain useful roles in anaesthesia (Ch. 36) and epilepsy (Ch. 40).

38 Antipsychotic drugs

Antipsychotic drugs, also known as *neuroleptics*, are used mainly in the treatment of schizophrenia, an important disabling mental illness that affects 1% of the population. The *'positive symptoms'* are delusions, hallucinations and thought disorders. The *'negative symptoms'* include social withdrawal, emotional flattening, reduced drive, inability to feel pleasure and poverty of speech. Schizophrenia often becomes overt in adolescence or early adulthood (though signs may be present earlier). Antipsychotic drugs may also be used for agitated depression and severe anxiety (see Ch. 39).

Pathophysiology of schizophrenia

The cause of schizophrenia is not clear. Environmental factors play a part and there is a significant genetic component in that 10–15% of first-degree relatives share the condition. Much evidence now indicates that it is associated with abnormalities of the cerebral cortex—often detectable before birth—and alterations in various neurotransmitter systems (e.g. the dopaminergic pathways).

The dopamine theory of schizophrenia

Clear evidence for a malfunction of dopaminergic transmission comes from the well-established correlation between the potency of dopamine D_2 receptor antagonism and antipsychotic effect (Fig. 38.1). Abnormalities in the mesolimbic and mesocortical dopaminergic pathways are most likely since psychotic symptoms develop after injury or lesions in these areas. The involvement of dopamine is supported by the antipsychotic action of reserpine, which depletes monoamines, and by the action of the amine releaser amphetamine, which can generate psychotic symptoms (e.g. hallucinations). Positron emission tomography also shows increased D_2 receptors in the nucleus accumbens of schizophrenics (but in general the neurochemical evidence for an increase in dopamine receptors is not strong). The positive symptoms seem to be better correlated with changes in dopaminergic pathways than the negative symptoms.

The role of other transmitters

The production of schizophrenic-like symptoms by lysergic acid diethylamide (LSD) and NMDA antagonists (phencyclidine) suggests some malfunction of 5-HT and glutamate transmitter systems. Both 5-HT_2 and 5-HT_{1A} receptors may be involved, the latter showing some increase in the prefrontal cortex of schizophrenics. Recently a greater emphasis has been placed on alterations of glutamatergic pathways.

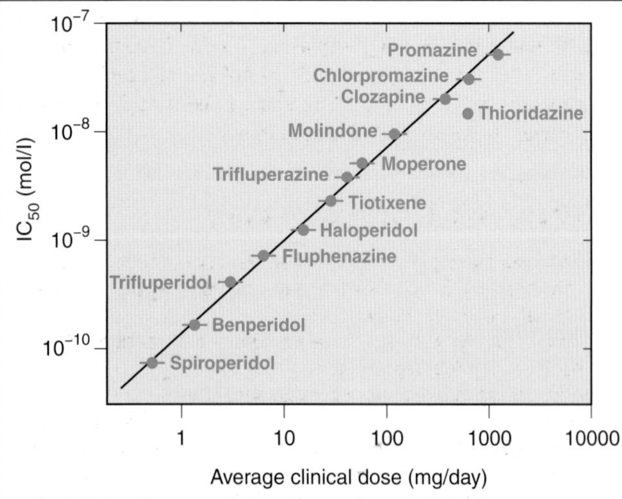

Fig. 38.1 The correlation between the clinical potency of antipsychotic drugs and their affinity for dopamine D_2 receptors. Binding is expressed as the concentration needed to give 50% inhibition of haloperidol binding.

Antipsychotic drugs

Antipsychotic drugs can alleviate the positive symptoms of schizophrenia but have little effect on the negative symptoms; in fact they can produce apathy and decreased initiative. The overall action of the drugs on the CNS is shown schematically in Figure 38.2.

Mechanism of action

All currently used antipsychotics are dopamine D_2-receptor antagonists and have varying activity on the other dopamine receptor subtypes; antagonism of D_2 or D_3 receptors seems to be most relevant. The drugs have a range of actions on other receptors (α_1-adrenoceptors, histamine H_1 receptors, muscarinic receptors, 5-HT receptors) that modifies their effectiveness or side effects (Table 38.1). Effects take some days to develop, suggesting that the antipsychotic effect is not simply due to receptor block, which will closely follow the rise in the concentration of the drug in cerebrospinal fluid.

The early antipsychotic drugs (examples in Table 38.1) are now referred to as 'typical' (or classical) and share a strong tendency to produce extrapyramidal motor symptoms (see below). The typical neuroleptics are often referred to by their chemical structure: **chlorpromazine**, fluphenazine and thioridazine are *phenothiazines*; **haloperidol** is a *butyrophenone* and thiotixene is a *thioxanthene*.

Newer agents (e.g. **clozapine**) are deemed 'atypical' in the sense that they produce fewer extrapyramidal actions and may be effective in cases where the typical agents are not. They are also more effective against the negative symptoms. The improved profile of the atypical agents may reflect reduced activity on D_2 receptors and increased antagonism of $5HT_2$ receptors (implying an alternative mechanism for the antipsychotic action). A role for agonist activity on 5-HT_{1A} receptors, which increase dopamine release in the prefrontal cortex, has been suggested.

Dopamine receptor antagonists have some other useful actions: a central antiemetic action (Ch. 26), a prominent sedative effect (in some cases aided by antihistamine action) and potentiation of analgesics and general anaesthetics.

Unwanted neurological effects

Adverse neurological effects comprise extrapyramidal motor symptoms (parkinsonian effects) caused by D_2 receptor antagonism in the striatum:

- rigidity, a mask-like face and bradykinesia (slowness in movement and in initiating movement)
- dystonias (spasms of the face and neck muscles, which can be relieved with antimuscarinics)
- akathisia (motor restlessness: an uncontrolled drive to move about, countered by β-blockers or benzodiazepines)
- tardive dyskinesias (stereotyped repetitive 'tic'-like movements or worm-like twisting movements; these appear very late in therapy).

Atypical agents (e.g. clozapine and risperidone), have much reduced extrapyramidal effects. Agents with intrinsic anticholinergic action are also less likely to produce the extrapyramidal effects.

Neuroleptic malignant syndrome is a rare but potentially fatal effect of haloperidol, flupentixol or chlorpromazine.

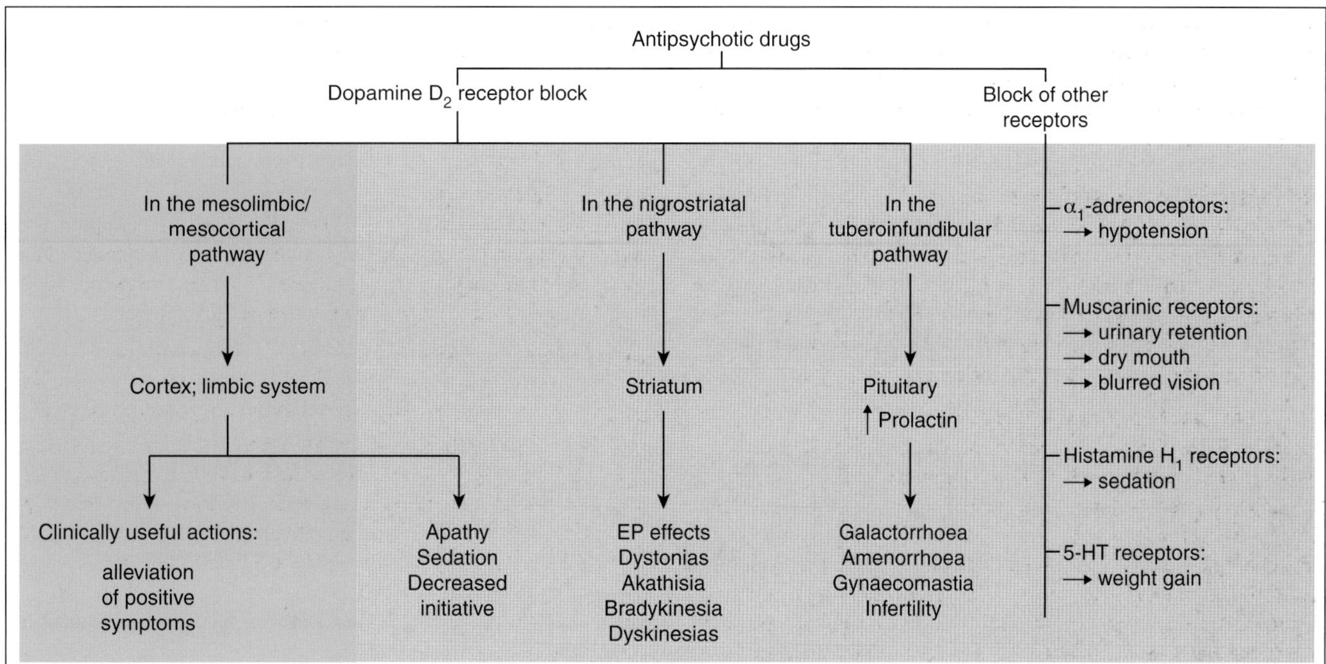

Fig. 38.2 Schematic diagram showing the main effects of antipsychotic drugs. The blue area shows the wanted actions of the drugs; the grey area shows the unwanted actions. The unwanted actions of some individual drugs are shown in Table 38.1. EP, extrapyramidal

Unwanted non-neurological effects

Blockade of the dopaminergic tuberoinfundibular pathway results in increased prolactin secretion (usually insignificant with atypical agents such as clozapine but does occur with resperidone), with consequent breast swelling, galactorrhoea and amenorrhoea.

A range of other effects follow from the actions on other receptor systems (see Fig. 38.2 and Table 38.1).

Chlorpromazine potentiates the respiratory depression of opiates. Clozapine causes serious agranulocytosis in 1% of those treated (risperidone and olanzapine may be as effective as clozapine without causing agranulocytosis). Obstructive jaundice may occur with chlorpromazine and related phenothiazines. Several agents produce weight gain.

Table 38.1 Unwanted effects of some antipsychotic drugs.

Drug	EPS	Sedation	Antimusc	BP↓
Typical				
Chlorpromazine	++	++	+++	++
Fluphenazine	+++	+	++	+
Thioridazine	+	++	+++	++
Haloperidol	+++	+	+	++
Tiotixene	+++	++	++	+
Atypical				
Molindone	++	+	+	+
Clozapine	+	++	+++	++
Olanzapine	+	++	+	++
Risperidone	+	++	+	++

EPS, extrapyramidal symptoms; Antimusc, anti-muscarinic; BP, blood pressure. Number of pluses indicates intensity of effect.

Pharmacokinetic aspects

Most antipsychotic drugs have half-lives of 15–30 h and are given orally or by i.m. injection. There is, however, considerable individual variation, both in the plasma concentration achieved for a given dose and the response to a given plasma concentration. This means that doses need to be determined on an individual basis. The elderly require reduction in dosage. Several neuroleptics have been esterified with long-chain fatty acids to yield depot formulations that are only slowly absorbed from the i.m. injection site (e.g. **fluphenazine decanoate**). These are effective for up to 28 days. Depot formulations can help to ensure effective treatment in the high percentage of schizophrenics who do not take the drugs reliably. There is an increased risk of extrapyramidal motor symptoms with depot formulations. Binding to plasma proteins is commonly high (e.g. >90% for chlorpromazine, haloperidol and olanzapine).

Droperidol is very short acting and can be used in psychiatric emergencies. It is also used in anaesthesia.

Therapy with antipsychotic drugs

- Antipsychotic agents provide effective long-term treatment of schizophrenia in up to 70% of patients, allowing many to lead normal lives in the community.
- The older 'typical' agents are more effective against the positive than the negative symptoms.
- Atypical agents, especially clozapine, may be effective in some patients resistant to the typical agents (e.g. a proportion of patients with chronic schizophrenia) and are better able to control the negative symptoms.
- The extrapyramidal effects and the effects due to increased prolactin are less marked with the atypical agents.
- Intramuscular depot preparations may be used for long-term therapy.

39 Drugs used in affective disorders

Affective disorders are characterised by disturbances in mood and the main types are *depression* and *mania*.

Depression is the most common mental illness. It may be *unipolar* (the mood is always low) or *bipolar* (low mood alternates with mania). It may be *reactive* (i.e. a response to traumatic life events), or *endogenous* (i.e. with no obvious cause). Severe endogenous depression may border on the psychotic and can carry a high risk of suicide.

Pathophysiology

The neurological basis of depression is poorly understood. The monoamine theory, which currently provides the best explanation, states that in depression there is a functional deficit of the transmitters noradrenaline (NA) and 5-HT in the forebrain and in mania there is a functional excess. Evidence for this theory comes from the antidepressant action of drugs acting at NA/5-HT nerve endings:

In support of this theory are the following observations:

- inhibition of NA or 5-HT reuptake improves mood
- inhibition of monoamine oxidase (MAO: which metabolises NA and 5-HT; see below) has an antidepressant effect
- reserpine, which depletes monoamine stores in the nerve endings, causes depression.

Against this theory are the following observations:

- the sympathomimetic drugs cocaine and amfetamine lack an antidepressant action
- some drugs (e.g. iprindole) have an antidepressant effect in the absence of clear effects on NA/5-HT transmission
- there is a 2–4 week delay in the onset of the clinical action of antidepressant drugs despite immediate effects on neurotransmission
- there are inconsistent changes in NA and 5-HT receptor densities and in the turnover of amine transmitters in depressed patients.

Drugs used in affective disorders

The main categories of drugs used in affective disorders are:

- those used to treat unipolar depression, namely the antidepressants
- those used to treat bipolar depression.

Antidepressant drugs

The main classes of antidepressant are:

- inhibitors of the reuptake of monoamine transmitters
  - tricyclic antidepressants (TCAs): e.g. **imipramine**, amitriptyline, clomipramine
  - Selective serotonin reuptake inhibitors (SSRIs), e.g. **fluoxetine**, paroxetine, citalopram
  - miscellaneous reuptake inhibitors, e.g. **maprotiline**, venlafaxine
- MAO inhibitors (MAOIs), e.g. **phenelzine**, isocarboxazid
- atypical antidepressants, e.g. trazodone, bupropion.

Mechanisms of action

Monoamine reuptake inhibitors The explanation of how these drugs act is given by their names. Inhibition of reuptake raises the concentration of transmitter in the synaptic cleft and increases stimulation of postsynaptic receptors (Figure 39.1). The selectivity for NA and 5-HT reuptake varies between the three main groups and between compounds in the same group. The relative potencies in inhibiting 5-HT or NA reuptake are indicated in Figure 39. 2.

MAOIs These inhibit MAO within nerve endings. The cytosolic NA/5-HT concentration thus increases and more leaks out into the synaptic cleft. There are two MAO isoenzymes (A and B). Their actions on the monoamines and the effects of MAOIs are shown in Table 39.1. Selective inhibitors of MAO-A are more effective antidepressants with fewer side effects. The older MAOIs

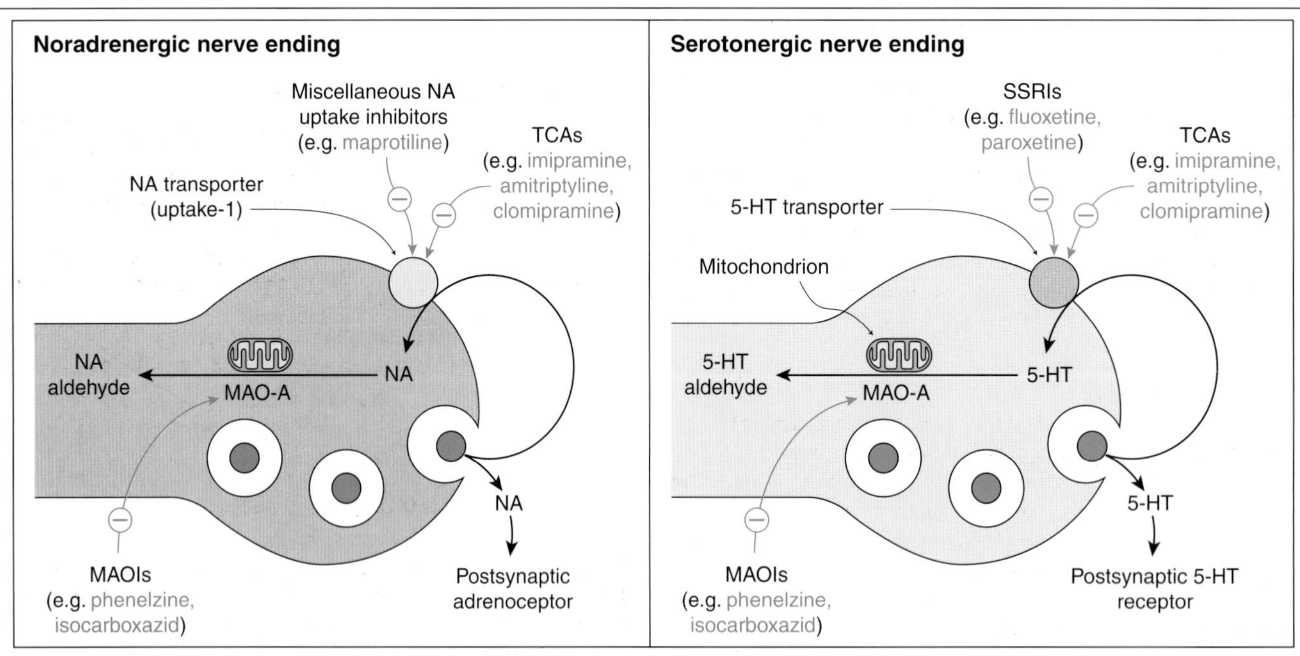

Fig. 39.1 Schematic diagram showing the probable sites of action of antidepressant drugs. TCAs, tricyclic antidepressants; SSRIs, selective serotonin reuptake inhibitors; MAOIs, monoamine oxidase inhibitors.

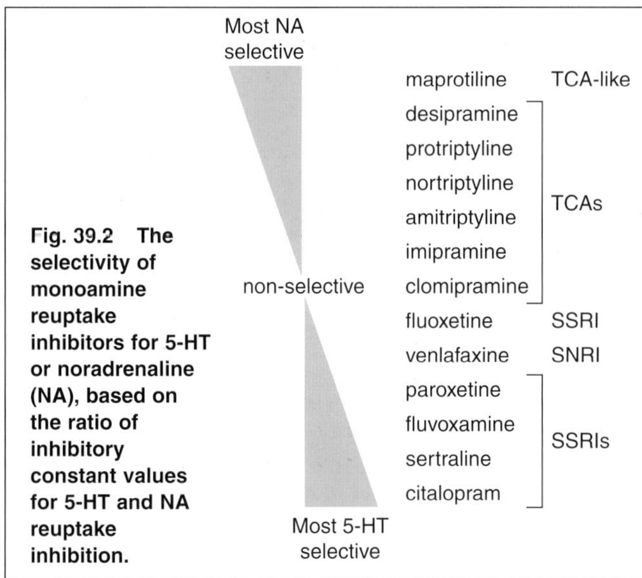

Fig. 39.2 The selectivity of monoamine reuptake inhibitors for 5-HT or noradrenaline (NA), based on the ratio of inhibitory constant values for 5-HT and NA reuptake inhibition.

Table 39.1 The selectivity of drugs for MAOIs

Selectivity	Drugs
Non-selective	Iproniazid, isocarboxazid, tranylcypromine, phenelzine
MAO-A selective	Clorgyline, moclobemide
MAO-B selective	Selegiline

bind covalently to the enzyme and consequently have a long duration of action; some newer drugs bind reversibly (e.g. **moclobemide**) and are safer.

Atypical antidepressants These have less well characterised mechanisms of action; some combine actions on monoamine transporters and on receptors. Trazodone has weak 5-HT uptake inhibition and antagonism of 5-HT receptors; bupropion has dopamine and NA reuptake inhibition; mianserin and mirtazepine have α_2-adrenoceptor antagonism (the latter also has NA reuptake inhibition) and iprindole has dopamine reuptake inhibition.

Time course of action It is important to note that for both the reuptake inhibitors and MAOIs, effects on neurotransmission can be expected fairly rapidly. However, the antidepressant effect is not apparent for 2–6 weeks and is likely to be a consequence of slower changes in receptor density (β_1, α_2-adrenoceptors, 5-HT_{1A} and 5-HT_2-receptors) or perhaps of desensitisation of either pre- or post-synaptic monoamine receptors.

Pharmacokinetics aspects

SSRIs These are given orally and are well absorbed. The half-lives are fluoxetine 24–96 h; citalopram 24–36 h and paroxetine 18–24 h.

TCAs These are very lipid soluble and are well absorbed by mouth. They bind strongly to plasma and tissue components, which results in a large volume of distribution. Many TCAs are tertiary amines with two methyl groups attached to the side-chain nitrogen. Removal of one of these methyl groups (e.g. imipramine to desmethylimipramine or amitriptyline to nortriptyline) yields active drugs. The desmethyl metabolites show a greater ratio of NA/5-HT reuptake inhibition. Many TCAs are subsequently conjugated with glucuronic acid. TCAs have long half-lives and dosage can often be once daily.

Unwanted effects

TCAs Dangerous in overdose. They are chemically related to the antipsychotic phenothiazines and many have a similar spectrum of side effects due to receptor block:

- antimuscarinic actions: dry mouth, constipation, blurred vision, urinary retention
- antihistamine effect: sedation
- α-adrenoceptor block: hypotension.

SSRIs Generally safer and have fewer side effects than TCAs; those that occur include:

- nausea and vomiting
- sexual dysfunction.

Serious adverse effects can occur if SSRIs are given concurrently with MAOIs.

Miscellaneous monoamine reuptake inhibitors These have fewer adverse actions than the TCAs.

Atypical antidepressants Fewer adverse effects than the TCAs. Trazodone causes marked sedation, which leads to low compliance. Mirtazepine can cause weight gain. All antidepressants can cause hyponatraemia, especially in the elderly.

MAOIs These drugs potentiate amine transmitters and indirectly acting amines, e.g. those used as decongestants. They can cause serious unwanted effects if given with tyramine-containing foods (e.g. cheese, red wine). This is referred to as the 'cheese reaction'. Because tyramine is normally rapidly metabolised by MAO in the gut and liver, therapy with MAOIs will lead to high concentrations of this amine in the plasma. The tyramine will then release NA from sympathetic nerve endings which can result in dangerous hypertension. Selective MAO-A inhibitors do not produce such a strong 'cheese-reaction'. MAOIs cause hypotension.

Atypical antidepressants In general, these have fewer adverse actions than the TCAs.

Clinical use of antidepressants

- **SSRIs** and **TCAs** are used primarily to treat depression but are also used effectively in some anxiety disorders: panic disorder (citalopram), obsessive compulsive disorder, bulimia.
- The combination of an atypical agent with an SSRI may be beneficial in antidepressant-resistant patients.
- TCAs produce varying degrees of sedation: sedative agents being used for anxious patients; less-sedative agents for withdrawn patients.
- **MAOIs** are less effective and subject to more drug interactions than the reuptake inhibitors and are considered second line.

Drugs used for bipolar depression

Lithium

Lithium is an important drug for the prophylaxis of bipolar disorder. Its actions may be attributable to inhibition of the formation of inositol trisphosphate (as a result of protein kinase C activation) and/or by mimicking Na^+, thus modifying cell membrane potential and ionic balance. It causes CNS toxicity and in large concentrations, renal damage. Its low therapeutic index makes it essential to monitor its plasma concentration.

40 Antiepileptic drugs

Epilepsy is a condition in which intermittent abnormal high-frequency firing of a localised group of cerebral neurons results in seizures. The discharge may remain localised or may spread to other regions of the brain. The seizures may be *partial* or *general*.

Types of seizure

Partial seizures involve repeated jerking of a limb or complex behavioural changes (pychomotor epilepsy) but no loss of consciousness. In these cases, the abnormal discharge is localised to the relevant area of the cortex.

Generalised seizures can take several forms:

- an initial generalised tonic convulsion followed by jerking of the whole body (clonic convulsion) accompanied by sudden loss of consciousness; this is tonic-clonic epilepsy or *grand mal*
- episodic transient loss of consciousness ('absence seizures'); this is termed *petit mal* and is seen mostly in children.

In generalised seizures, the abnormal electrical activity involves the whole brain.

A state in which generalised convulsions follow each other without consciousness being regained is termed *status epilepticus* and is a medical emergency.

About 75% of those with epilepsy respond well to treatment.

Antiepileptic drugs

Antiepileptic drugs may need to be taken life-long so the fewer adverse effects the better.

The main commonly used antiepileptic drugs are **carbamazepine**, **phenytoin**, **valproate**, **ethosuximide** and benzodiazepines such as **diazepam** and **clonazepam**. Other newer drugs are vigabatrin, gabapentin, lamotrigine, felbamate, tiagabine and topiramate.

Mechanisms of action of antiepileptic drugs

Drugs can inhibit seizures by three main mechanisms (Fig. 40.1).

Table 40.1 gives examples of drugs that act by one or more of these means.

Carbamazepine and phenytoin

These agents inhibit the high-frequency discharge by binding preferentially to inactivated Na^+ channels, thus stabilising them. This prevents the return to the resting state which is necessary for the generation of action potentials (Chs 3 and 43).

Pharmacokinetic aspects They are both given orally. Carbamazepine's half-life is 30 h, but is shorter with repeated administration. Phenytoin is subject to zero-order metabolism (see Ch. 8), which can lead to disproportionate increases in plasma concentration as the dose is increased. There is significant variation between individuals and a given dose can result in considerable differences in the plasma concentrations. Consequently monitoring of the plasma concentration is necessary.

Unwanted effects Both interact with other drugs because they induce the P450 liver enzymes. With phenytoin, the effective plasma concentration and the concentration causing adverse effects are uncomfortably close. It can cause dose-related vertigo, confusion, insomnia and ataxia. Non-dose-related effects include rashes, megaloblastic anaemia, teratogenesis, thickening of the gums and an increase in body hair. Carbamazepine can cause unsteadiness, sedation, mental disorientation and water retention. Both drugs are effective in most types of epilepsy except absence seizures, carbamazepine being preferred because it has fewer adverse effects.

Ethosuximide

Ethosuximide is given orally and has a half-life of about 48 hours. It acts by inhibiting T-type Ca^{2+} channels (see Fig. 40.1) and is used only for absence seizures, for which it is the drug of choice. It can *precipitate* tonic-clonic epilepsy. *Unwanted effects* include gastrointestinal disturbance, sedation and skin rashes.

Valproate

Valproate is given orally and has a half-life of about 15 h. It increases the GABA concentration in the brain and affects several processes involved in seizure generation (Fig. 40.1) but its exact mechanism of action is not clear.

Unwanted effects, which are fewer than with other antiepileptics, include alteration in hair thickness, gastrointestinal disturbance and, rarely, liver failure. It is teratogenic. It is effective in both tonic-clonic and absence seizures.

Benzodiazepines

Benzodiazepines (see Ch. 37) also have a role in the treatment of epilepsy. **Clonazepam** is effective in both tonic-clonic and absence seizures. **Diazepam** is given i.v. for status epilepticus. The main unwanted effect is sedation.

Table 40.1 Sites and mechanisms of action of antiepileptic drugs

Mechanism of action	Drugs
Inhibition of action potential generation/conduction	
Use-dependent Na^+ channel block	**Carbamazepine**, **phenytoin**, **valproate**, lamotrigine
T-type Ca^{2+} channel block	**Ethosuximide**, ?valproate
Enhancement of GABAergic ($GABA_A$) transmission	
Agonist at the BZD site on the $GABA_A$ receptor	**Diazepam**, **clonazepam**
Ligand at the barbiturate site on the $GABA_A$ receptor	Phenobarbital
Inhibiting GABA reuptake or metabolism	**Valproate**, vigabatrin, tiagabine
Reduction of glutamatergic transmission	
NMDA receptor antagonist: glutamate site	?Topiramate
NMDA receptor antagonist: glycine site	Felbamate
AMPA receptor antagonist	?Topiramate
Inhibition of glutamate release	Lamotrigine

The commonly used agents are shown in bold. A question mark indicates uncertainty about the mechanism of action. BZD, benzodiazepine.

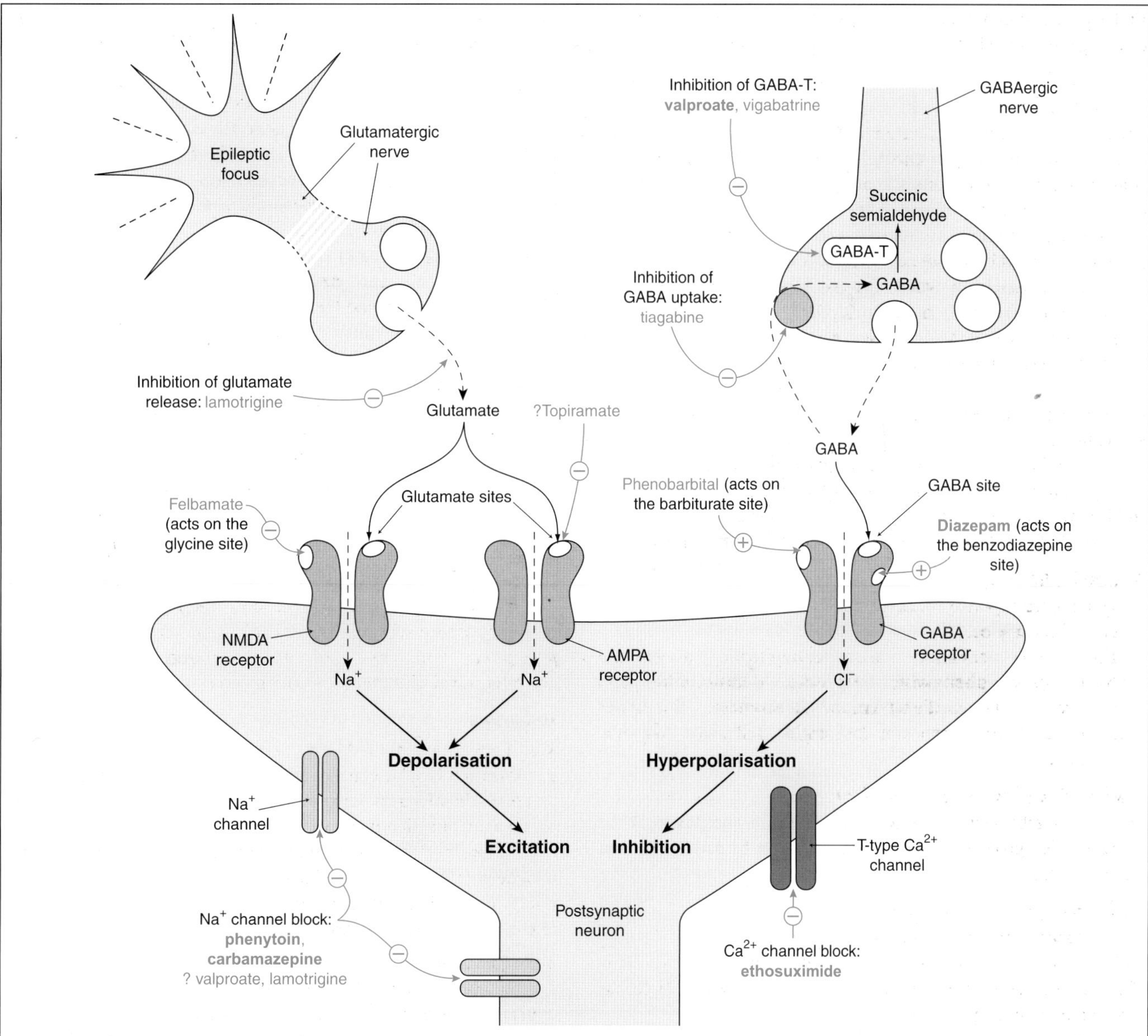

Fig. 40.1 Sites of action of antiepileptic drugs. The neurons undergoing abnormal high-frequency discharge release the excitatory transmitter glutamate; the postsynaptic neuron is depolarised and the discharge propagates. The main drugs used are shown in bold, less frequently used drugs or drugs still being assessed in smaller type. Vigabatrine and tiagabine also block uptake of GABA into, and metabolism in, glial cells. GABA-T, GABA transaminase.

Phenobarbital

Phenobarbital is a second-line antiepileptic drug; see Figure 40.1 for site of action.

Newer antiepileptics

The mechanisms of action of **vigabatrin** and **lamotrigine** are shown in Figure 40.1. Both are given orally. Both affect all types of epilepsy; vigabatrin can, in addition, be effective in epilepsy resistant to other agents.

Antiepileptics still being assessed include gabapentin, felbamate, topiramate and tiagabine.

Unwanted effects Vigabatrin can cause giddiness, sedation, depression and hallucinations. Lamotrigine can cause giddiness, ataxia, skin rashes and gastrointestinal disturbances.

Clinical use of antiepileptic drugs

Commonly used drugs are shown in bold.

- Partial seizures: **carbamazepine**, **valproate**, **phenytoin**, clonazepam, gabapentin, lamotrigine.
- Generalised tonic-clonic seizures: **carbamazepine**, **valproate**, phenytoin, gabapentin, lamotrigine, topiramate. Treatment with a single drug is recommended.
- Generalised absence seizures: **ethosuximide**, valproate, clonazepam, lamotrigine.
- Status epilepticus: **diazepam** i.v., phenytoin

41 Analgesic drugs and the control of pain

Pain is a subjective experience with both sensory and emotional components arising from actual or potential tissue damage. It is frequently a traumatic accompaniment of many diseases and the relief of pain is an important clinical priority. The main pain pathways are shown in Figure 41.1. This chapter concentrates on *opioid* analgesics although other types of drug can have a role.

Analgesia (the relief of pain)

The main pain-relieving drugs are the *opioids*, which modify both the transmission of pain signals to the brain and the subjective perception of the painful stimulus, but other drugs can be helpful in alleviating some types of pain. Mild/moderate musculoskeletal pain can be alleviated by reducing the nociceptive stimulus through decreasing the formation of chemical mediators in areas of tissue damage (Fig. 41.1). *Non-steroidal anti-inflammatory drugs (NSAIDs)*, by reducing the formation of prostanoids, act by this mechanism (Ch. 15). Certain types of pain can be controlled by *local anaesthetics* (Ch. 43) or **nitrous oxide** inhalation (Ch. 36). The pain of trigeminal neuralgia is susceptible to **carbamazepine** (an antiepileptic drug) and the pain of migraine to 5-HT_1-agonists (e.g. **sumatriptan**) or **ergotamine** (Ch. 12). Pain associated with damage to nerves (neuropathic pain) is often resistant to opioids and better treated with antidepressants (Ch. 39).

Opioid analgesics

There are two categories of opioid drugs:

- morphine and related compounds such as diamorphine (heroin) and **codeine**
- synthetic analogues of morphine such as **pethidine**, fentanyl, methadone, **pentazocine**, and buprenorphine.

Mechanism of action

Opioids act on opioid receptors, of which there are four types: μ, δ, κ and ORL (opioid-receptor-like).

Opioid analgesics are agonists on these receptors. Some compounds structurally related to morphine act as partial agonists (nalorphine, levallorphan and buprenorphine) and can have antagonist activity. Some are full antagonists (**naloxone**); these can inhibit/reverse the action of the agonists.

There are a number of endogenous peptide agonists that are essential components of an endogenous analgesia system which underlies the reduced pain sensations that occurs under conditions of stress. These include *β-endorphin, met-enkephalin, leu-enkephalin, dynorphin, nociceptin* and the *endomorphins*. They are derived from the gene products *preproopiomelanocortin, preproenkephalin* and *preprodynorphin* (Ch. 13). Recent work suggests that endomorphins are the normal ligands for the μ-receptor. Table 41.1 gives details of the actions of these various substances on the opioid receptors.

The opioid receptors are coupled to G-proteins, which

- inhibit the action of adenylate cyclase, thus decreasing intracellular cAMP
- couple directly to K^+ and Ca^{2+} channels increasing or decreasing their opening, respectively; this can inhibit presynaptic transmitter release and reduce postsynaptic excitability.

More than 75% of opioid receptors in the dorsal horn are found presynaptically and most of those are μ-receptors.

Pharmacological actions

Morphine will be taken as the reference drug. **Codeine** and dextropropoxyphene are relatively weak analgesics. Tramadol is a codeine analogue with less-marked unwanted action (i.e less respiratory depressant and addictive effect; see below). Its action is due in part to inhibition of 5-HT and noradrenaline reuptake. The actions of the opoids are:

Analgesia Morphine relieves most types of pain, reducing both the sensory and the emotional components. It produces analgesia mainly by (i) inhibition of pain transmission in the dorsal horn, (ii) activation of the descending pathways that inhibit pain transmission in the dorsal horn and (iii) inhibition of activation of the nociceptive afferents in the tissues. The sites of analgesic action are shown in Figure 41.1. Analgesia is mainly due to an action on μ-receptors.

Euphoria A feeling of well-being mediated by μ-receptors is helpful in severe/terminal pain (κ-receptors can cause dysphoria).

Sedation

Cough suppression Opioids inhibit the cough reflex pathways in the brainstem. This can be therapeutically useful; codeine and pholcodine are able to exert this action selectively (Ch. 24).

Antidiarrhoeal action Opioids have inhibitory actions on enteric nerves, which leads to reduced motility and constipation. This is usually an unwanted effect but is useful in the treatment of diarrhoea.

Unwanted actions

Respiratory depression Activation of μ-receptors reduces the sensitivity of the respiratory centre to CO_2. This occurs even with therapeutic doses of morphine and is the main cause of death in overdose. The reversible competitive antagonists **naloxone** and **naltrexone** can reverse opioid-induced respiratory depression but may induce withdrawal reactions in addicts.

Nausea and vomiting Stimulation of the chemoreceptor trigger zone in the medulla by opioids causes troublesome effects in 40% of patients.

Table 41.1 Agents acting at the various opioid receptors

Receptor	μ	δ	κ	ORL
Endogenous agonists	β-Endorphin, endomorphins, leu-enkephalin, met-enkephalin, dynorphin	Enkephalins, β-endorphin	Dynorphin	Nociceptin
Exogenous agonists	**Morphine**, heroin, codeine, fentanyl, pethidine, methadone, dextropropoxyphene, remifentanil	Experimental compounds	Pentazocine	–
Antagonists	Naloxone, naltrexone	Naloxone, naltrexone	Naloxone, naltrexone	

The sensation of pain arises from the activation of the peripheral terminals of nociceptive C and Aδ afferent fibres by thermal, mechanical and chemical stimuli. C fibres are non-myelinated and polymodal and give rise to slow burning pain; Aδ fibres are myelinated, activated by mechanical stimuli and give rise to acute localised pain.

When tissue is damaged, chemical mediators such as bradykinin (see Ch. 15), 5-HT (Ch. 12) and protons depolarise the C fibres (see below) and locally released prostaglandins sensitise the neurons to the action of these mediators (see below). At their central terminals in the DH of the spinal cord, the nociceptive fibres release peptides such as substance P (slow transmitters) and glutamate (a fast transmitter) that activate spinothalamic tract neurons; these carry the pain signals to the contralateral thalamus. From the thalamus, pain signals pass to the cortex and other CNS centres to elicit the conscious sensation of pain and the emotional response

Pain transmission by the DHN is regulated by a 'gating' mechanism, which consists of (i) inhibitory input from GABAergic and enkephalinergic (enkeph) INs in the spinal cord (which are inhibited by the incoming C/Aδ fibres), see projection box, and (ii) descending inhibitory pathways from the midbrain and brainstem, the input of which is coordinated through the PAG

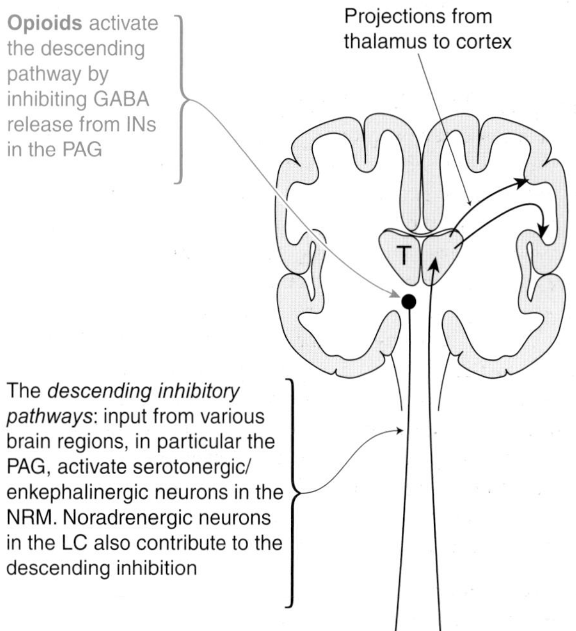

Opioids activate the descending pathway by inhibiting GABA release from INs in the PAG

Projections from thalamus to cortex

T

The *descending inhibitory pathways*: input from various brain regions, in particular the PAG, activate serotonergic/ enkephalinergic neurons in the NRM. Noradrenergic neurons in the LC also contribute to the descending inhibition

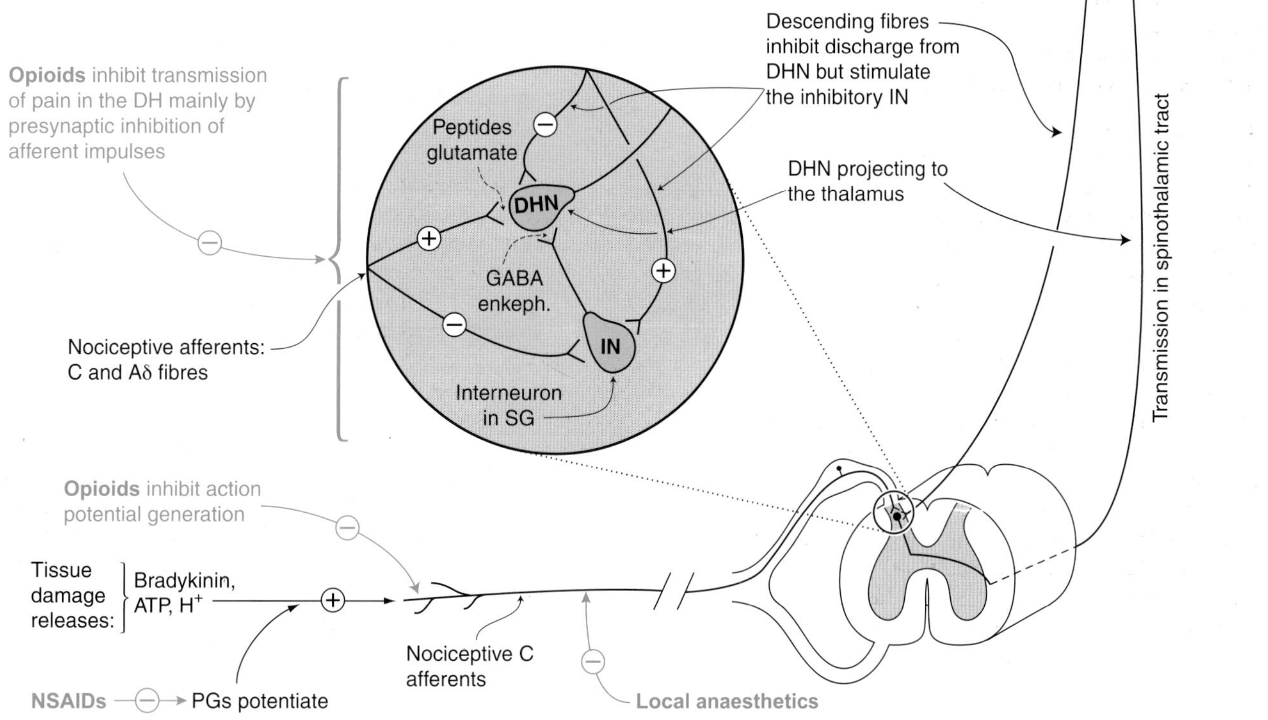

Descending fibres inhibit discharge from DHN but stimulate the inhibitory IN

Opioids inhibit transmission of pain in the DH mainly by presynaptic inhibition of afferent impulses

Peptides glutamate

DHN

GABA enkeph.

IN

Interneuron in SG

DHN projecting to the thalamus

Transmission in spinothalamic tract

Nociceptive afferents: C and Aδ fibres

Opioids inhibit action potential generation

Tissue damage releases: Bradykinin, ATP, H^+

Nociceptive C afferents

NSAIDs ⊖ PGs potentiate

Local anaesthetics

Fig. 41.1 Pain pathways and the action of opioids. Transmission and gating of pain input in the dorsal horn is shown in the projection circle. DH, dorsal horn; DHN, dorsal horn neuron; IN, interneuron;. enkeph, enkephalin; LC, locus ceruleus; NRM, nucleus raphe magnus; PAG, periaqueductal grey matter; SG, substantia gelatinosa; T, thalamus; PGs, prostaglandins.

Pupillary constriction Stimulation of the oculomotor nucleus mediates parasympathetic constriction of the pupil; this is diagnostic of opioid abuse.

Psychological and physical dependence This is very marked with the street use of morphine and other strong agonists but is less troublesome with their use as analgesics (Ch. 44). Withdrawal symptoms may be severe and can be reduced by methadone.

Histamine release Morphine causes release of histamine from mast cells, other opioids having a lesser effect. The released histamine can cause bronchospasm and hypotension; therefore, an alternative should be used for pain relief in asthmatics.

Pharmacokinetic aspects

Morphine and heroin can be given orally (sustained release preparations are available) but are commonly given by injection (i.v., i.m., s.c). Codeine, dextropropoxyphene and phenazocine are given orally. Fentanyl can be given by injection or as a transdermal patch that provides analgesia for up to 3 days. A selective spinal action, with reduced central effects, can be achieved with intrathecal or epidural injection. Buprenorphine is longer acting than morphine and can be given sublingually. Heroin is faster acting than morphine because it is more lipid soluble and penetrates the blood–brain barrier more rapidly. Most opioids are metabolised in the liver, commonly by oxidation or, as with morphine, by production of the glucuronide. A newer opioid, **remifentanil** is very short acting (half-life 3–4min) due to rapid metabolism by plasma and tissue esterases and is less dependent on hepatic and renal function. Some metabolites (e.g. morphine 6-glucuronide) retain analgesic activity. The analgesic action of codeine and heroin is due in large part to their conversion to morphine (by demethylation and deacetylation, respectively).

42 CNS stimulants and psychotomimetics

In this chapter we consider drugs that have mainly stimulant effects of one sort or another on the CNS. A few categories have clinical use; most are drugs misused/abused in society.

Psychomotor stimulants

These include amphetamine (dexamphetamine is its D-isomer), methylamphetamine, methylphenidate, fenfluramine, MDMA (methylenedioxymethamphetamine; ecstasy), cocaine and methylxanthines. (Nicotine (Ch. 44) has some similar effects.) The amphetamines, cocaine and the methylxanthines are used clinically. Table 42.1 has details of psychotomimetics (hallucinogens).

Amphetamines and cocaine

Mechanisms of action These raise the synaptic concentrations of noradrenaline (NA), dopamine (DA) and 5-hydroxytryptamine (5-HT). Four processes contribute to this action:

- stimulation of release into the synaptic cleft
- inhibition of neuronal reuptake
- inhibition of monoamine oxidase (MAO)
- inhibition of vesicular uptake.

Stimulants affect NA, DA and 5-HT transmission to different extents, resulting in different patterns of action. Amphetamines are substrates for the reuptake transporters and, by an exchange process, cause transmitter release. Cocaine potently inhibits the transporters but is not transported and does not stimulate release. The rise in synaptic NA concentration at sympathetic nerve endings confers sympathomimetic activity (e.g. pupil dilation) on cocaine and amphetamines. Cocaine also blocks neuronal Na^+ channels to produce local anaesthesia.

Actions These include euphoria,* elation, improved concentration, appetite suppression, stereotyped behaviour, inhibition of REM sleep, sympathomimetic actions.

Pharmacokinetic aspects Amphetamines are generally well absorbed from the gut and cross the blood–brain barrier easily. (Crack cocaine, the free base form of the drug, is volatile and is usually smoked.) Amphetamine is mostly excreted unchanged in urine; as a base, its excretion is enhanced in acidic urine. Cocaine, an ester, is readily hydrolysed and has a short half-life (circa 1h).

Addiction Amphetamines and cocaine are very addictive though physical withdrawal symptoms are not pronounced. Actions on DA pathways seem to be particularly involved (Ch. 44).

Unwanted actions Psychosis, hallucinations, addiction, insomnia, anorexia, anxiety, aggressiveness, hypertension, dysrhythmias, hyperpyrexia, neurotoxicity, muscle damage (MDMA), teratogenicity (cocaine).

*The euphoria is likely to involve enhanced activity in the DA pathway projecting from the midbrain ventral tegmental area to parts of the frontal cortex and limbic system, in particular to the nucleus accumbens. Increased activity of the NA projections from the locus ceruleus to parts of the cerebral cortex and limbic system is involved in the increased arousal and vigilance induced by these drugs.

Clinical uses of amphetamines

- Attention deficit and hyperactivity disorder (ADHD). The use of stimulants in treating ADHD, a condition characterised by excessive motor activity, may seem paradoxical. However, the increase in mental alertness and concentration subdues the hyperactivity. **Methylphenidate** is recommended for ADHD.

(Note that amphetamines and other uptake inhibitors are appetite suppressants but are not recommended for treatment of obesity.)

Methylxanthines

More detail on xanthines is given in Table 42.1 and in Ch. 24.

Mechanisms of action By inhibiting phosphodiesterase, caffeine and theophylline increase cellular concentrations of cAMP and potentiate responses mediated by β-adrenoceptors and D_1 receptors. This effect occurs only at high doses. The behavioural effects probably involve antagonism of adenosine receptors. Postsynaptic adenosine receptors reduce the firing rate of neurons and presynaptic receptors inhibit transmitter release. Caffeine, by blocking presynaptic receptors, can enhance transmitter release. Caffeine will reverse the sleep-inducing and behavioural depressant actions of adenosine, improving wakefulness and mental alertness.

Pharmacokinetics Caffeine is well absorbed from the gut and is metabolised (mainly by demethylation) in the liver (plasma half-life approx. 6 h).

Table 42.1 CNS stimulants and psychotomimetic drugs

Type	Examples	Mechanisms	Actions	Clinical uses	Unwanted actions
Methylxanthines	Caffeine, **theophylline**	Phosphodiesterase inhibition	Bronchodilatation, diuresis, cardiac stimulation	Asthma (theophylline ethylene diamine (aminophylline); see Ch. 24)	Cardiac arrhythmia, tremors
		Antagonism of adenosine receptors	Improved motor tasks, wakefulness		Agitation, anxiety, rapid breathing, insomnia
Analeptics	Doxapram, nikethamide	Stimulation of neurons in respiratory centre		Apnoea in premature babies, respiratory depression (not often used nowadays.	Convulsions
Hallucinogens (psychotomimetics)	Phencyclidine, **ketamine**	NMDA receptor block, activation of σ-receptors	Stereotyped behaviour	Dissociative anaesthesia (ketamine)	
	LSD, mescaline, psilocybin, DMT, mescaline, MDMA	Elevation of synaptic 5-HT, activation of 5-HT receptors	Altered perception, delusions	None	Nausea and vomiting (mescaline) Long-lasting psychopathological effects (LSD)

LSD, lysergic acid diethylamide; DMT, dimethyltyramine; MDMA, methylenedioxymethamphetamine.

43 Local anaesthetics

Local anaesthetics are drugs used primarily to inhibit pain by preventing impulse conduction along sensory nerves. They achieve this by blocking voltage-sensitive Na^+ channels in the cell membrane. Local anaesthetics are also used as antidysrhythmics (Ch. 17) and in epilepsy (Ch. 40).

The basic electrophysiology of neurons

Sodium channels (Figs 43.1 and 43.2) can exist in three states: *resting* (i.e. closed), *activated* (i.e. open) and *inactivated* (i.e. blocked; explained below).

The resting cell The action of the Na^+ pump in cell membranes normally maintains a high level of K^+ and a low level of Na^+ within the cell (Ch. 3). In the resting cell, the membrane is more permeable to K^+ than to Na^+. The efflux of K^+ makes the cell interior negative with respect to the outside, giving a membrane potential between –60 and –90 mV. In the resting cell, the Na^+ channels are *closed.*

Activation! The action potential When a nerve cell is stimulated locally (e.g. by noxious stimuli acting on a pain fibre or by neurotransmitter action on a receptor linked to a cation channel) the Na^+ channel opens, leading to a local increase in the membrane permeability to Na^+. The resultant increased influx of positive Na^+ causes membrane depolarisation and an action potential is generated. This is a regenerative process, as the action potential itself causes more Na^+ channels to open, allowing its propagation along the nerve.

Inactivation Within 5 ms the Na^+ channels are inactivated (i.e. they close and are transiently refractory to being opened) allowing the cell to repolarise. (The delayed opening of K^+ channels in response to the membrane depolarisation also contributes to repolarisation.) The rapidity of the sequence of events means that repetitive firing can proceed at high frequency.

Local anaesthetics

Important examples are **procaine**, **lidocaine** (lignocaine), **tetracaine** (amethocaine), bupivacaine and prilocaine. Cocaine was the first local anaesthetic to be used but has few clinical applications now.

Mechanism of action

Local anaesthetics are nearly all weak bases (pK_a 8–9) and have similar chemical structures (Fig. 43.3). They act by blocking Na^+

Sodium channels consist of one α subunit, which forms the aqueous channel, and one or two modulatory β subunits. The α subunit contains 4 linked domains each comprising 6 transmembrane helices (segments S1-S6); shown in A.

The S4 segments contain several positively charged amino acids and it is proposed that the outward movement of the S4 segments in response to membrane depolarisation causes a structural change which opens the channel.

Loops between S5 and S6 in each domain (labelled 'P loop' and shown as black lines in B) penetrate the membrane and line the outer part of the channel.

Inactivation of the channels is caused by the loop connecting domains III and IV — shown in black in A — folding up into the channel and blocking it like a trap door.

The local anaesthetic binding site is on S6 in domain 4 (which is shown in blue).

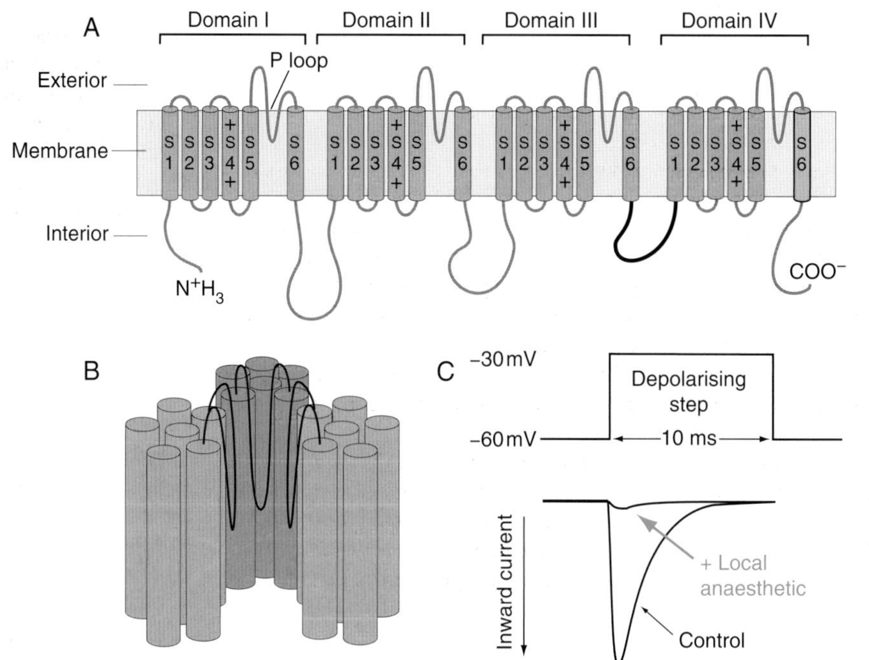

Fig. 43.1 Schematic diagram of sodium channel. A. The four linked domains. B. Suggested arrangement of the domains to form the channel (the front domain is omitted to show the pore). C. Activation and inactivation of Na^+ current during a depolarising voltage step.

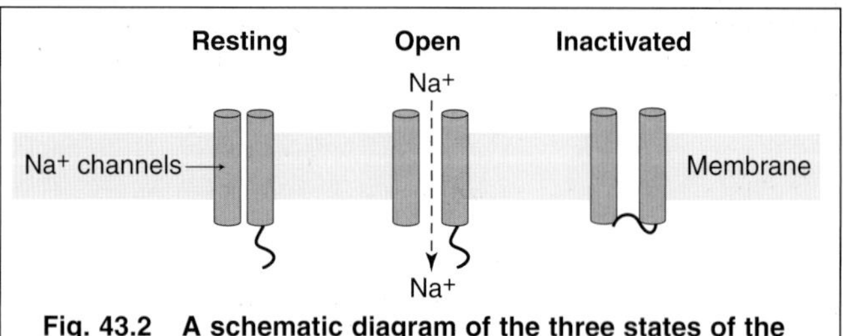

Fig. 43.2 A schematic diagram of the three states of the sodium channel.

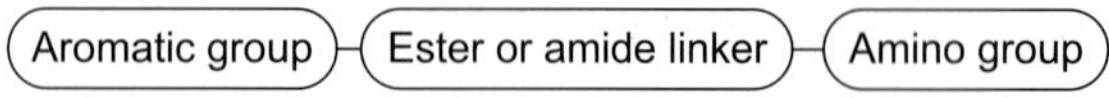

Fig. 43.3 Simplified outline of the structure of local anaesthetics.

channels and stopping the propagation of action potentials in nerve. (Figs 43.1 and 43.4). Local anaesthetics gain access to their binding site either from the cell interior or by lateral diffusion in the cell membrane. In both cases, it is essential for the drug to adopt its lipid-soluble, uncharged form to gain access (Fig. 43.4). This, of course depends on pH and can explain the reduced activity of local anaesthetics in inflamed tissue, where the lower pH increases ionisation. Many local anaesthetics show *use-dependence*, that is they are more effective in blocking channels once these have been activated. This may be because the drug's binding site is within the channel and accessible only when the channel opens or it may result from greater affinity for the inactivated state of the channel.

Local anaesthetics usually block small diameter fibres at lower concentrations than large fibres. Accordingly, pain sensation is blocked before other sensory inputs but it is not usually possible to achieve local anaesthesia without loss of other sensory modalities or local paralysis.

Pharmacokinetics

The plasma half-life of most local anaesthetics is 1–2 h, but their action persists for longer due to retention at the site of administration. The duration of action can be increased by the use of a vasoconstrictor (epinephrine (adrenaline) or felypressin). The esters (tetracaine, benzocaine, procaine, cocaine) are hydrolysed rapidly by plasma esterases once they reach the bloodstream; whereas most amides (prilocaine, bupivacaine) are relatively resistant to plasma esterases and are subject to N-dealkylation and hydrolysis in the liver at a slower rate.

The variable lipid solubility of local anaesthetics determines the rate at which they penetrate tissues to cause nerve block and also their suitability for action on mucous membranes.

Table 43.1 summarises the properties of three local anaesthetics. Cocaine and lidocaine penetrate membranes readily: procaine poorly. Benzocaine differs from other local anaesthetics in lacking the amine group; this results in increased lipophilicity and allows rapid entry into tissues, a fast onset and long duration of action.

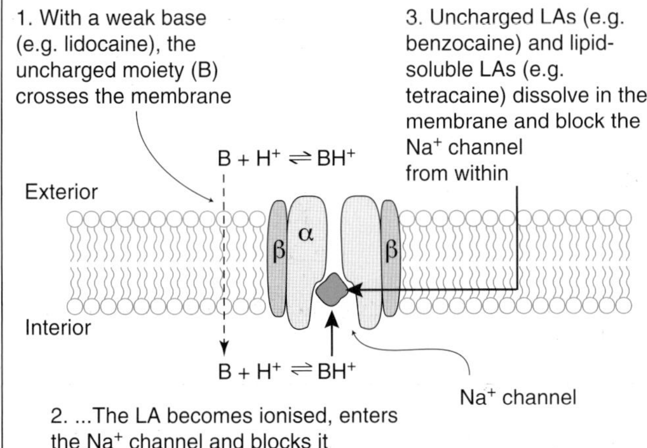

Fig. 43.4 Access of local anaesthetics (LAs) to channel-blocking site as uncharged species via the membrane or as charged species from the cell interior.

Table 43.1 Summary of the pharmacokinetic aspects of some local anaesthetics (LAs)

LA	Onset of action	Duration of action	Metabolism
Lidocaine	Rapid	Moderate	Amide-linked LAs are degraded in the liver
Bupivacaine	Slow	Long	
Tetracaine	Slow	Long	Ester-linked LA, hydrolysed by plasma esterases

Unwanted effects

The unwanted effects of local anaesthetics are due to their entry into the systemic circulation. CNS effects, prominent with procaine, less with lidocaine and prilocaine, are paradoxically stimulatory and include restlessness and tremor; though larger doses are depressant. Respiratory depression may be a cause of death. Local anaesthetics also cause myocardial depression and vasodilatation, which may result in a serious lowering of blood pressure. (Cocaine has additional effects related to its ability to inhibit monoamine uptake into nerve-endings (not shared by other local anaesthetics). Sympathomimetic effects arising in this way include a rise in blood pressure.) Hypersensitivity reactions, manifest as allergic dermatitis, may occur.

Clinical use and administration of local anaesthetics

- Surface anaesthesia. Lidocaine and tetracaine are used for local anaesthesia of skin, cornea, etc.
- Infiltration anaesthesia. Most LAs are suitable. Given by injection for minor surgery. Epinephrine (adrenaline) or felypressin may be coadministered to cause local vasoconstriction and reduce loss to circulation, thus prolonging action.
- Intravenous regional anaesthesia. A pressure cuff maintains local concentration and prevents entry into the general circulation. Lidocaine and prilocaine are suitable.
- Nerve-block anaesthesia. Most LAs are suitable. Injection close to the nerve trunk produces regional anaesthesia for surgery or dentistry. Vasoconstrictors may be used to enhance duration.
- Spinal anaesthesia. Lidocaine or tetracaine can be injected into the subarachnoid space to act on spinal roots and spinal cord. This is used for lower body surgery when general anaesthesia is undesirable.
- Epidural anaesthesia. Lidocaine or bupivacaine are injected into the epidural space. This is used for spinal anaesthesia and also childbirth.

44 Drug dependence and drug abuse

Many drugs are taken for non-medical purposes, most commonly to generate a sense of well-being or to give pleasure. Drug dependence arises with centrally acting drugs producing a psychological 'reward' and follows repeated administration. It is reinforced by a need to avoid unpleasant withdrawal effects and by the ritual of drug taking itself. Dependence (addiction) is characterised by:

- *psychological dependence*: craving, compulsive drug-seeking behaviour
- *physical dependence*: habituation/tolerance associated with a withdrawal (abstinence) syndrome
- *tolerance*: the need to increase dose to maintain the desired effect.

Drug abuse is important because of the damage done to the individual's health and the cost to society—in healthcare costs, criminal behaviour, etc. Drugs abused for their central effects include: opioids (Ch. 41), stimulants/psychotomimetics (amphetamines, cocaine, LSD, Ch. 42), anxiolytics (benzodiazepines, Ch. 37) and depressants (barbiturates (Ch. 39), solvents). Here we specifically consider, **nicotine**, **ethanol** and **cannabinoids**. Apart from alcohol and tobacco, the important drugs of abuse are controlled under the Misuse of Drugs Act; categories A to C reflecting their addictive power. Their unauthorised possession is a criminal offence. Drugs misused to improve competitive performance (e.g. anabolic steroids) are not considered here.

Pathophysiology

Dependence-producing drugs enhance dopaminergic transmission in the important reward pathway from the midbrain to the limbic system and especially to the nucleus accumbens. Tolerance seems to involve adaptive changes to the effects of the drugs. Thus the inhibitory effect of opioids on adenylate cyclase activity in the brain is countered by a rise in the amount of enzyme synthesised. This increased enzyme activity can at least partially explain a rebound, withdrawal effect when the drug is discontinued. Downregulation of receptors and receptor desensitisation may also be involved. A genetic predisposition towards addictive behaviour has been identified.

NICOTINE

Nicotine is taken mainly by tobacco smoking, or less often chewing, and is strongly addictive.

Mechanism of action

Effects are due to activation and desensitisation of central nicotinic acetylcholine receptors. The behavioural effects depend on dose and may be excitatory or depressant and smokers may indeed seek either a calming effect or a stimulant effect. Nicotine is reported to enhance learning in rats. Long-term use is associated with a large increase in the number of nicotinic receptors in the CNS. (Tolerance might have been expected to correlate with a decrease in receptor density; the paradoxical increase is most likely due to a high proportion of receptors being in the desensitised state.) Slow release from nicotine patches is used with counselling to assist in quitting the habit.

Pharmacokinetic effects and unwanted effects

Nicotine is rapidly absorbed in the lungs and also well absorbed from patches applied to the skin. It is mostly metabolised by oxidation in the liver and has a half-life of 2 h. Peripheral side effects of nicotine are those expected of stimulation of autonomic ganglia and the adrenal medulla, e.g. tachycardia and a rise in blood pressure. Stimulation of the posterior pituitary causes antidiuretic hormone (ADH) release and, consequently, decreases urine flow. *Adverse effects of tobacco smoking* are mainly due to nicotine, tars and carbon monoxide (CO). (In heavy smokers, up to 15% of haemoglobin may be converted to carboxyhaemoglobin.) Lung, throat and bladder cancer and bronchitis are mainly caused by the tars. The increases in coronary heart disease and stroke in smokers are most likely caused by nicotine and CO. Nicotine and CO from smoking in pregnancy may be responsible for low birth weight.

ETHANOL

Alcohol dependence is widespread and heavy drinking is a factor in many hospital admissions.

Pharmacological actions

Ethanol has CNS depressant actions similar to those of gaseous anaesthetics and the molecular mechanism is likely to involve similarly enhancement of $GABA_A$ receptor action, inhibition of NMDA receptors and inhibition of the opening of voltage-gated Ca^{2+} channels. Ethanol has a relatively low potency and large quantities are needed to elicit pharmacological actions. Little effect is seen below a plasma concentration of 10 mmol/l, and 100 mmol/l (500 mg/100 ml) or more is needed to cause death (by respiratory depression). Activation of the reward pathways described above probably occurs by depression of an inhibitory input. Inebriation produces the well-known euphoria and increased self-confidence. Less-desirable effects are motor incoordination and aggressive behaviour. Vasodilatation can cause heat loss and hypothermia. Ethanol inhibits ADH secretion from the pituitary, causing diuresis. Other hormonal effects are feminisation of men due to reduced testosterone levels and a Cushing's syndrome-like action due to enhanced glucocorticoid action. It is suggested that a modest consumption of ethanol has a beneficial effect on coronary heart disease partly due to increasing plasma high density lipoproteins. The abstinence syndrome includes tremors, nausea and sweating and in alcoholics may progress to 'delerium tremens' (the DTs) with confusion, hallucinations and aggression. DTs may be alleviated by benzodiazepines. In heavy drinkers, tolerance raises the plasma concentration at which performance deteriorates.

Pharmacokinetic effects and unwanted actions

Ethanol is well absorbed from the gut and is eliminated mainly (90%) by oxidation to acetaldehyde and acetic acid (Fig. 44.1). Metabolism is saturated at relatively low plasma concentrations due to the limited availability of NAD^+, leading to zero-order elimination with a fixed rate of approximately 10 ml/h. A small proportion (higher after enzyme induction in heavy drinkers) is oxidised by the P450 system. Limited amounts of ethanol are eliminated unchanged in the breath and urine and provide the basis for police tests of alcohol consumption. **Disulfiram** inhibits aldehyde dehydogenase and thus elevates the plasma concentration of acetaldehyde. This produces a range of unpleasant symptoms, which is intended to discourage alcohol consumption. Long-term alcohol abuse can lead to brain damage and dementia and to severe liver damage. The poor

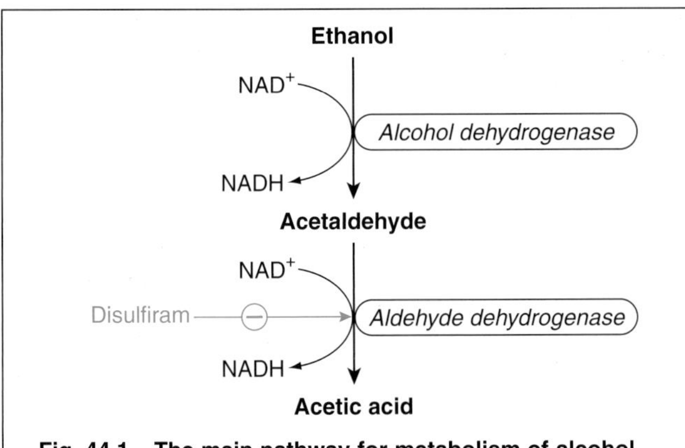

Fig. 44.1 The main pathway for metabolism of alcohol. Disulfiram causes a build up of acetaldehyde.

diet of alcoholics contributes to deteriorating health. The *fetal alcohol syndrome*, characterised by facial deformities and mental retardation in the baby, follows heavy ethanol consumption in pregnancy.

CANNABINOIDS

Cannabinoids are taken for relaxation and enhancement of sensory perception. They are only weakly addictive and produce mild withdrawal symptoms. The most active compound in cannabis (hashish, marijuana) is Δ^9–tetrahydrocannabinol (THC).

Pharmacological actions

These compounds act on G-protein-coupled cannabinoid receptors. CB_1 receptors are responsible for the CNS effects, coupling to G_i, to inhibit adenylate cyclase, activate K^+ channels and inhibit Ca^{2+} channels. (CB_2 receptors are found in the periphery and affect immune responses.) Anandamide, derived from arachidonic acid, is an endogenous agonist.

Clinical use

Cannabinoids (e.g. nabilone) improve appetite and have a useful antiemetic action, which is made use of in cancer chemotherapy. Trials are currently investigating the use of cannabinoids in treating severe pain (particularly neuropathic) and symptoms of multiple sclerosis.

Pharmacokinetic effects and unwanted actions

Cannabinoids are usually taken by smoking, though oral absorption from cannabis cakes occurs readily. Cannabinoids are very lipid soluble and strongly protein bound. Distribution to adipose tissue causes them to be retained in the body for several days. THC is mostly metabolised to inactive products by microsomal oxidation, though a small proportion of a more active metabolite is produced. Biliary excretion is greater than urinary excretion. A single dose of THC acts for 2–3 h. Learning, memory and motor control may be adversely affected. Cannabinoids may also aggravate schizophrenia and depression. Sympathomimetic actions such as tachycardia occur. Unlike alcohol, heroin and amphetamine, they are relatively safe in overdose.

45 Antibacterial agents

Antibacterial agents are drugs used to treat bacterial infections. Many species of bacteria cause disease in humans; these are termed *pathogens*. It was once thought that these pathogenic bacteria had a special ability to cause infections whereas bacteria that lived happily and innocuously within the mammalian organism, termed *commensals*, lacked this ability. It is now known that commensals—and also bacteria in the environment that are normally harmless—are virtually all capable of being pathogenic. In the healthy host, the immune/inflammatory response prevents these 'inoffensive' organisms from giving rise to infections; however, if the immune system is compromised, as in HIV infection or after the use of immunosuppressant drugs, these bacteria can and do cause disease.

The effect of an antibacterial agent can be *bactericidal*, i.e. it kills the bacterium, or it can be *bacteriostatic*, i.e. it stops the bacterium growing. With these latter drugs, the enfeebled organism is eliminated by the host's defence mechanisms. If these mechanisms are impaired, only bactericidal drugs are effective.

The term *antibiotic*, originally developed to describe a chemical agent produced by one microorganism that killed or prevented the growth of another microorganism, is now subsumed in the term *antibacterial agent*. Antibacterial agents, to be effective, need to manifest selective toxicity, i.e. they should be toxic to the bacterium but innocuous in the human host. Humans and bacteria have the same blueprint—DNA—and many biochemical processes are common to both. Nevertheless, there are components and metabolic processes in the bacterial cell that are sufficiently different from those in humans to be potential targets for antibacterial drugs.

TARGETS FOR ANTIBACTERIAL DRUGS

Figure 45.1 describes the potential targets for selective antibacterial attacks.

The terms Gram-positive and Gram-negative

Many organisms are classified as Gram-positive or Gram-negative. These terms refer to whether or not the bacteria stain with Gram's stain but it has more significance than that of an empirical staining reaction. Gram-positive and Gram-negative bacteria differ from each other in several important respects that have implications for the effects of antibiotics.

One important difference is in the structure of the cell wall—which provides support for the plasma membrane and is subject to an internal pressure of approximately 5 atmospheres in Gram-negative organisms and 20 atmospheres in Gram-positive organisms. The wall must, therefore, be able to resist these pressures. Its main constituent is peptidoglycan (Fig. 45.1). Gram-negative bacteria have a single layer of peptidoglycan; that in Gram-positive bacteria can be up to 40 layers thick. Each peptidoglycan

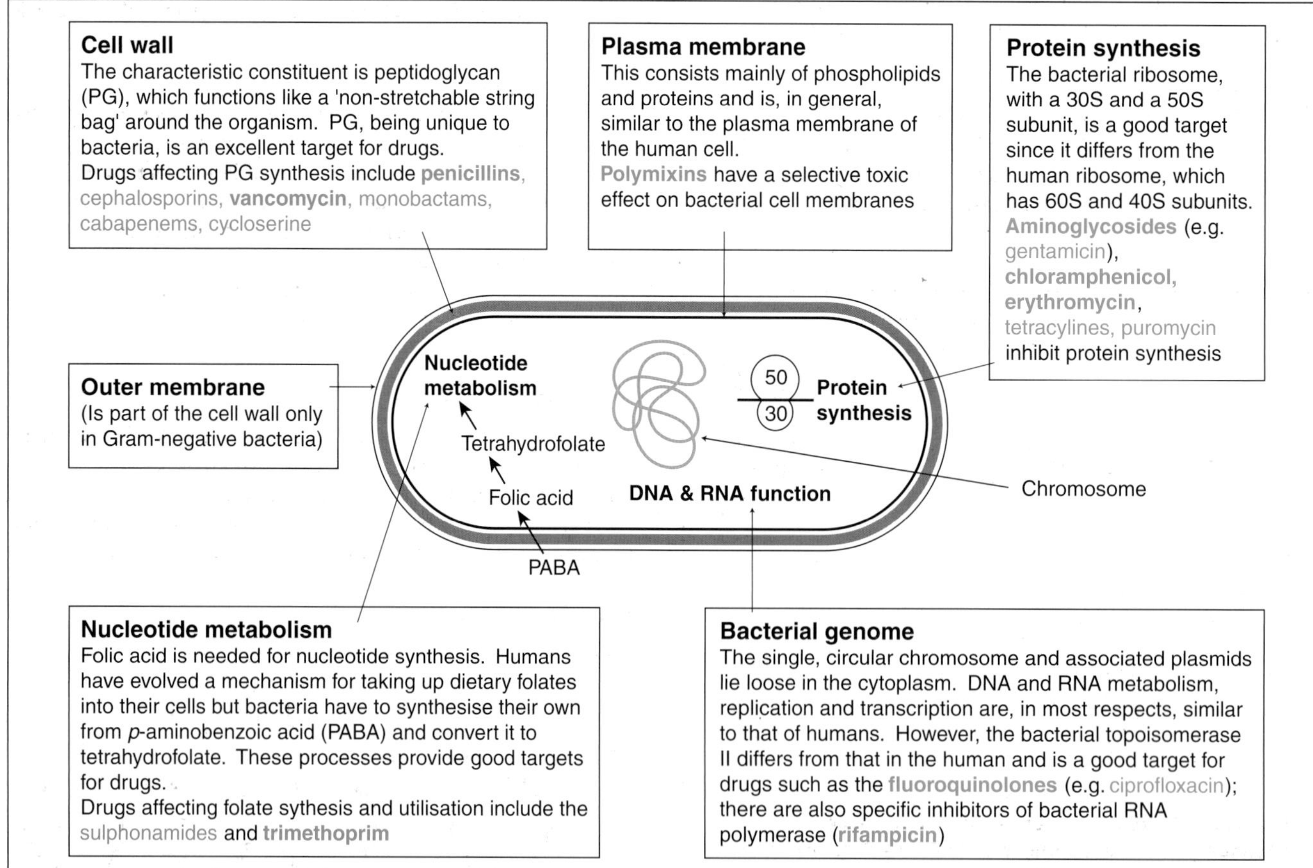

Fig. 45.1 The structural elements and biochemical processes in the bacterial cell that provide potential targets for attack by antibacterial agents.

layer consists of numerous backbones of amino sugars; some having short peptide side-chains that are cross-linked to form a lattice (Fig. 45.2).

There are other differences between the cell wall in Gram-positive and Gram-negative bacteria that are pharmacologically relevant.

The cell wall of *Gram-positive organisms* is a relatively simple structure, 15–50 nm thick of which 50% is peptidoglycan and about 40% consists of acidic polymer. The latter, being highly polar, favours the penetration of positively charged antibacterials, such as streptomycin, into the cell.

In *Gram-negative organisms*, the cell wall is thinner but more complex, and it also has an outer membrane (similar in some respects to the plasma membrane) that connects to the single layer of peptidoglycan. The outer membrane contains transmembrane water-filled channels, termed *porins*, through which hydrophilic antibacterial agents can move freely. In addition, complex polysaccharides on the outer surface comprise the *endotoxins* that determine the antigenicity of the organism. In vivo, these can trigger various aspects of the inflammatory reaction.

The lipopolysaccharide of the cell wall is also a major barrier to penetration by benzylpenicillin, methicillin, the macrolides, rifampicin, fusidic acid and vancomycin.

Difficulty in penetrating this complex outer layer is probably the reason why some antibiotics are less active against Gram-negative than Gram-positive bacteria and is the basis of the extraordinary insusceptibility to most antibiotic drugs of *Pseudomonas aeruginosa*, a pathogen that can cause life-threatening infections in neutropenic patients and patients with burns and wounds.

Resistance to antibacterial agents

The genetic determinants of resistance

Chromosomal determinants Mutations of the chromosomal genes in the bacterium are important in methicillin-resistant staphylococci, and in infections with mycoplasma and organisms causing tuberculosis.

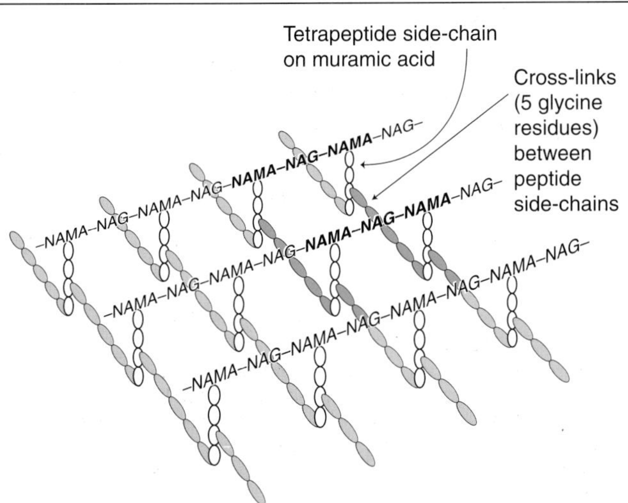

Fig. 45.2 Schematic diagram of a single layer of peptidoglycan such as might be found in *Staphylococcus aureus*. The darkened area at top right is used to explain the action of β-lactam antibiotics in Figs 45.4 and 45.5. NAMA, *N*-acetylmuramic acid; NAG, *N*-acetylglucosamine.

Extrachromosomal determinants Many bacteria have, lying free in the cytoplasm, genetic elements that can replicate on their own. These are closed loops of DNA (termed *plasmids*) that can carry resistance genes—often with resistance to several antibiotics. Some stretches of plasmid DNA can be transposed from one plasmid to another and from a plasmid to the chromosome, replicating the while. These stretches are called *transposons* and they can spread resistance between plasmids (Fig. 45.3).

Transfer of resistance genes between bacteria This occurs mainly by conjugation, in which protein tubules called 'sex pili' connect two bacteria, allowing transfer of plasmids between them. Genes can also be transferred by phages (bacterial viruses).

The biochemical mechanisms of resistance

Production of enzymes that inactivate the drug Examples are β-lactamases, which inactivate many penicillins, acetyltransferases, which inactivate chloramphenicol and kinases and other enzymes that inactivate aminoglycosides.

Modification of the drug-binding sites This occurs with aminoglycosides, erythromycin and penicillin.

Decreased accumulation of the drug in the bacterium Plasmid-mediated efflux of the drug causes tetracycline resistance in both Gram-positive and Gram-negative organisms and fluoroquinolone resistance in *Staphylococcus aureus*. Reduced penetration can cause resistance to aminoglycosides, chloramphenicol and glycopeptides.

Alteration of the target enzymes An example is the plasmid-mediated synthesis of a dihydrofolate reductase that is insensitive to trimethoprim, or of a dihydropteroate synthetase with low affinity for sulphonamides but unchanged affinity for *p*-aminobenzoic acid (PABA).

Resistant pathogens

Many pathogenic bacteria have developed resistance to the commonly used antibiotics; important examples are:

- some strains of staphylococci ('methicillin-resistant staphs'; MRSA) and enterococci are resistant to virtually all current antibiotics; these organisms can cause virtually untreatable nosocomial (acquired in hospital) infections
- some strains of *Mycobacterium tuberculosis* have developed resistance to most antituberculosis agents.

ANTIBACTERIAL AGENTS

Antibacterial agents will be dealt with under the following headings:

1. Drugs that affect bacterial peptidoglycan synthesis
2. Drugs that affect bacterial protein synthesis
3. Drugs that affect bacterial DNA and RNA synthesis and function
4. Drugs that affect bacterial folate synthesis and utilisation
5. Antituberculosis drugs
6. Antileprosy drugs.

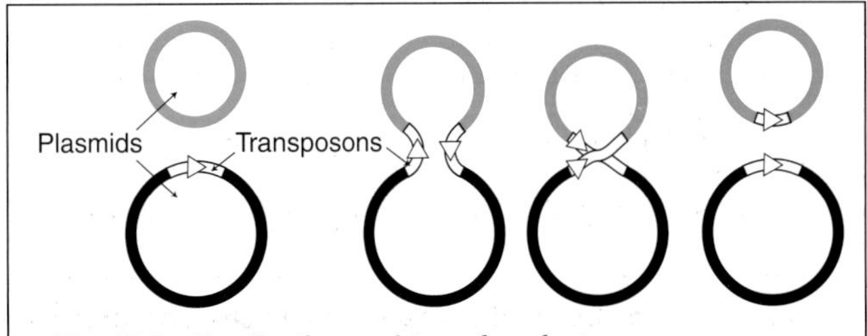

Fig. 45.3 Replication and transfer of a transposon between plasmids.

Drugs that affect peptidoglycan synthesis

These drugs include the penicillins, cephalosporins, monobactams, carbapenems and glycopeptides. The first four are termed β-lactam antibiotics because they all have a β-lactam ring in their structure (see Fig. 45.6, below).

Mechanism of action The **β-lactams** inhibit the synthesis of the peptidoglycan 'corset' by inhibiting the enzyme that inserts the crosslinks to the peptide chains that are attached to the peptidoglycan backbone (Figs 45.4 and 45.5). **Glycopeptides** (e.g. vancomycin) inhibit an earlier reaction. The effect is to weaken the 'corset' enclosing the bacterium. Since the internal osmotic pressure within the organism is high, this leads to rupture of the bacterial cell. These drugs are thus *bactericidal*.

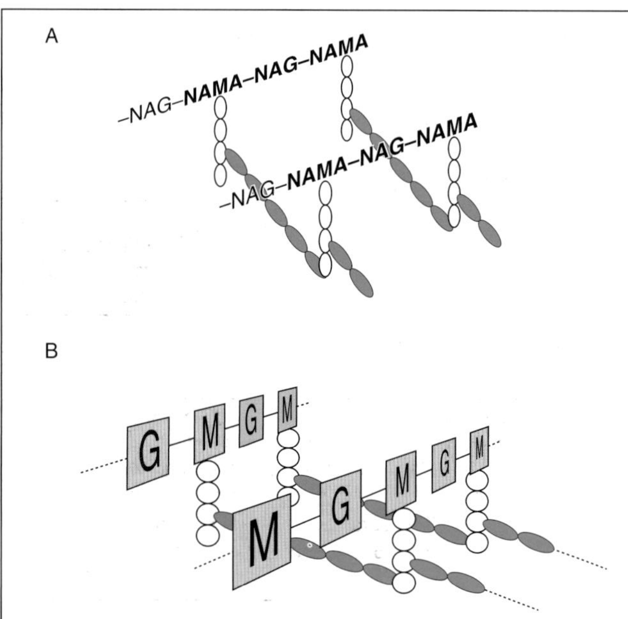

Fig. 45.4 A section of the peptidoglycan 'corset'. This was shown darkened in Figs 45.2 and 45.5. It has been modified in (A) and modified again in (B) to show the segment depicted in Fig. 45.5. G, *N*-acetylglucosamine (NAG); M, *N*-acetylmuramic acid (NAMA).

Penicillins

The main types of penicillin are given in Table 45.1 and their basic structure in Figure 45.6. All act by binding to penicillin-binding proteins before interfering with cell wall synthesis. They then inactivate an inhibitor of autolytic enzymes in the cell wall, leading to rupture as the 'corset' gives way. Many organisms are now resistant.

Resistance to penicillins The main mechanism of resistance is the production of β-lactamases, which disrupt the β-lactam ring. The concomitant use of a β-lactamase inhibitor that binds to the bacterial enzyme may overcome this (e.g. clavulanic acid; Fig. 45.6). Other mechanisms of resistance are modification of the binding sites and reduced permeability of the outer membranes.

Pharmacokinetic aspects The drugs pass into all body fluids: joints, pleural and pericardial cavities, bile, saliva and milk. They cross the placenta but not the blood–brain barrier (unless the meninges are inflamed). Excretion is via the urine and can be blocked by **probenicid**.

Unwanted effects The penicillins are not directly toxic (though they can cause convulsions if injected intrathecally) but are very likely to cause allergic reactions: skin rashes (common), anaphylaxis (rare but life threatening).

Clinical uses of the penicillins

- First choice drugs for many infections, particularly for bacterial meningitis and infections of bone, joints, skin, soft tissues, throat, bronchi (in obstructive airway disease) and urinary tract.
- Gonorrhoea, and syphilis.
- Note that many organisms (particularly staphylococci) may be resistant.

Cephalosporins and cephamycins

These are chemically related to penicillin. Examples are **cefaclor**, **cefadroxil**, and cefotaxime.

The *mechanism of action* is the same as for the penicillins: interference with cell wall synthesis. Many Gram-negative bacteria now produce a β-lactamase that inactivates these drugs.

Unwanted effects Mainly hypersensitivities.

Table 45.1 The main types of penicillin

Type of penicillin	Absorption in GIT	Main properties and similar agents
Beta-lactamase sensitive, e.g. benzylpenicillin (penicillin G)	Poor	The first choice for many infections but destroyed by β-lactamases; many staphylococci now resistant. Given i.m. or i.v., (but *not* intrathecally). Active against most Gram-positive cocci and Gram-negative bacteria. Phenoxymethylpenicillin is well absorbed in the GIT but is less potent
Beta-lactamase resistant, e.g. flucloxacillin, methicillin	Reasonable	Active against the same organisms as benzylpenicillin but less potent. Used mainly for infections with organisms that produce β-lactamase. Many staphylococci now resistant
Broad-spectrum: amoxicillin	Very good	Active against more organisms than benzylpenicillin but less potent; destroyed by β-lactamases but can be given in combination with clavulanic acid. Given orally, i.m, i.v. Many bacteria now resistant. Skin reactions can occur. (Ampicillin is similar but less well absorbed)
Antipseudomonas, e.g. piperacillin	Poor	Susceptible to β-lactamases. Spectrum as for broad-spectrum drugs, plus pseudomonads. Most strains of *S. aureus* are resistant. Given i.v. or by deep i.m. injection. Ticarcillin is similar and is also effective against some Gram-negative organisms (e.g. *Proteus*); it can be combined with clavulanic acid

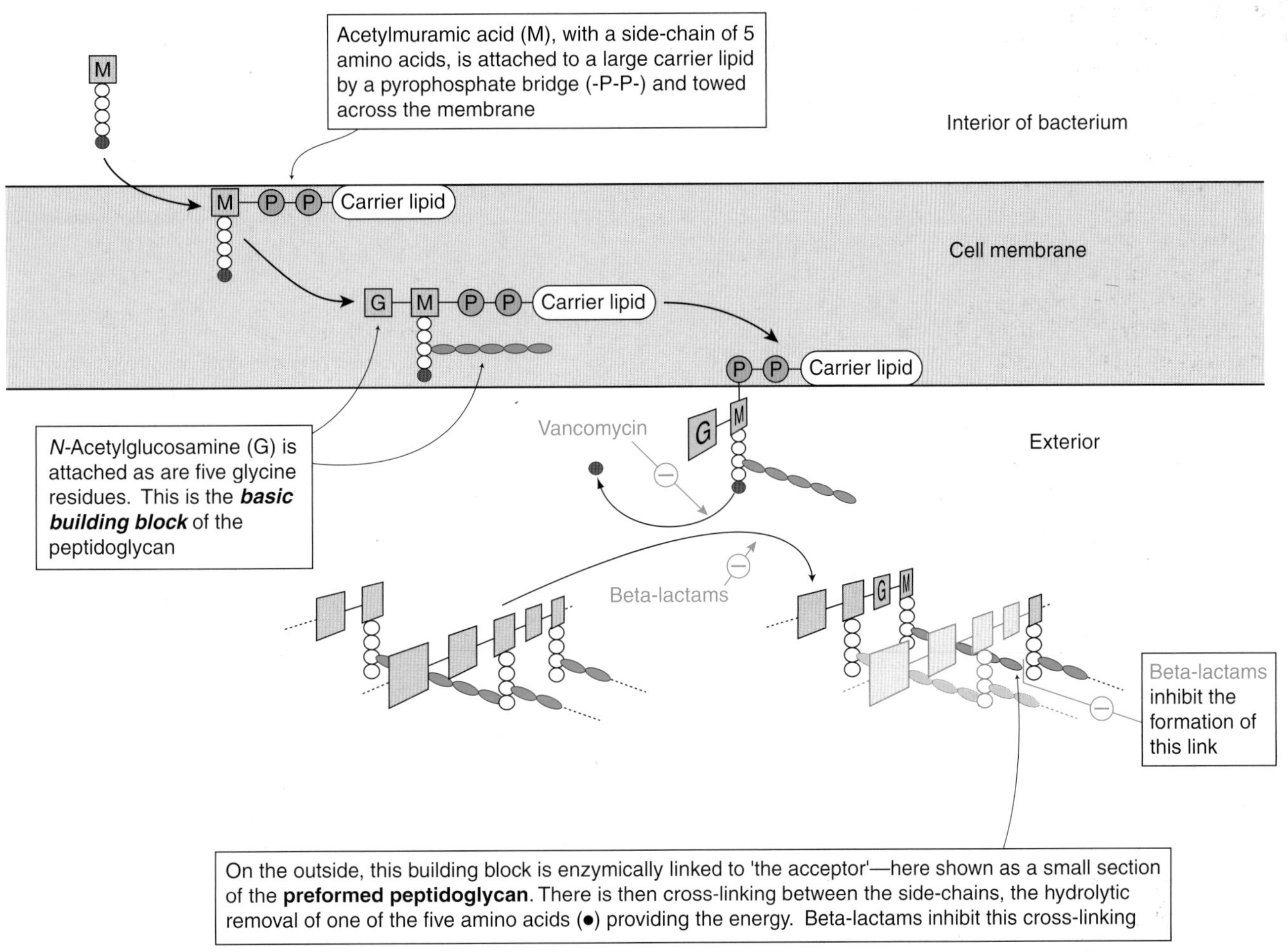

Acetylmuramic acid (M), with a side-chain of 5 amino acids, is attached to a large carrier lipid by a pyrophosphate bridge (-P-P-) and towed across the membrane
Interior of bacterium
Carrier lipid
Cell membrane
Carrier lipid
Carrier lipid
N-Acetylglucosamine (G) is attached as are five glycine residues. This is the basic building block of the peptidoglycan
Vancomycin
Exterior
Beta-lactams
Beta-lactams inhibit the formation of this link
On the outside, this building block is enzymically linked to 'the acceptor'—here shown as a small section of the preformed peptidoglycan. There is then cross-linking between the side-chains, the hydrolytic removal of one of the five amino acids (•) providing the energy. Beta-lactams inhibit this cross-linking

Fig. 45.5 The synthesis of peptidoglycan and the site of action of drugs affecting it. The figure shows the process of biosynthesis and the establishment of a cross-link in a segment such as the one depicted in Fig. 45.2 for a bacterium such as *S. aureus*.

Pharmacokinetic aspects Cefaclor is given orally; others are given i.m. or i.v. They pass into all body fluids: joints, pleural and pericardial cavities, bile, saliva and milk and also cross the placenta. They cross the blood–brain barrier poorly unless the meninges are inflamed. They are excreted mainly in the urine but partly in the bile.

Amidase
β-Lactamase
Penicillin nucleus
Clavulanic acid
(inhibits many β-lactamases)

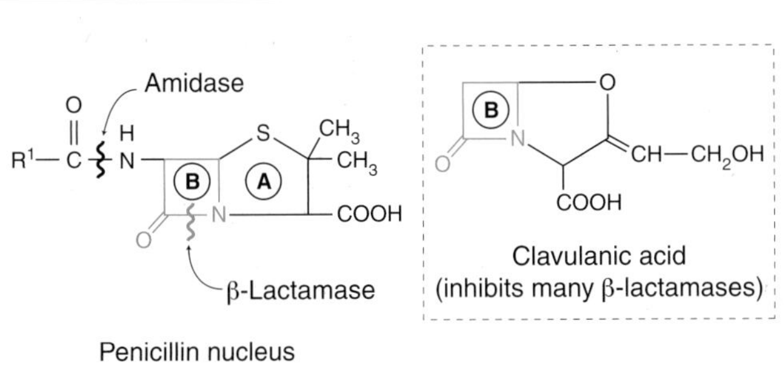

Fig. 45.6 Structures of penicillin and clavulanic acid. Substituents at R^1 determine the pharmacological characteristics of different types of penicillin. A, thiazolidine rings; B, β-lactam ring.

Other β-lactams

Carbapenems These broad-spectrum antibiotics (e.g. **imipenem**; used with **cilastin**, which blocks its breakdown by the kidney) are resistant to many, but not all, β-lactamase-producing organisms. Given i.v. and excreted in urine.

Monobactams Aztreonam is active only against Gram-negative aerobic bacteria and is resistant to most β-lactamases.

Glycopeptides

Examples are **vancomycin** and teicoplanin. The glycopeptides act by interfering with cell wall synthesis (Fig. 45.5). Vancomycin is not absorbed from the gastrointestinal tract (GIT). It is given i.v., is widely distributed and is excreted by the kidney. It is used only for multiple-resistant staphylococcal infections and is given by mouth for local effect within the GIT in pseudomembranous colitis.

Clinical use of cephalosporins and cephamycins

- Second choice for many infections such septicaemia, meningitis, pneumonia, biliary-tract and urinary-tract infections if these are caused by susceptible organisms.

Drugs that inhibit bacterial protein synthesis

The main drugs that inhibit protein synthesis are the aminoglycosides, chloramphenicol, tetracyclines, macrolides, fusidic acid and clindamycin. Figures 45.7 and 45.8 show bacterial protein synthesis and sites of action of drugs.

Aminoglycosides

These are bactericidal, broad-spectrum agents whose action is enhanced by inhibitors of cell wall synthesis. They are given by injection and excreted in the urine. An important example is **gentamicin**. Excretion is renal and poor kidney function will result in accumulation and greater risk of toxicity.

Dose-related ototoxicity and nephrotoxicity, usually irreversible, can occur and blood levels must be monitored. Ototoxicity will be exacerbated if given with furosemide (frusemide) (which can also be ototoxic). Neuromuscular transmission can be impaired and the drugs are contraindicated in myasthenia gravis.

Resistance—due to plasmid-controlled inactivating enzymes—is increasing. The enzymes have less effect on **amikacin**.

Streptomycin is reserved for treatment of tuberculosis.

Macrolides

The main macrolide is **erythromycin**, which has an antibacterial spectrum fairly similar to penicillin and has been used as an alternative drug. It is also active against mycoplasma and chlamydial infections. It is used for respiratory tract infections, campylobacter enteritis and Legionnaires' disease. Its use for penicillin-resistant staphylococcal infections has been compromised by the development of plasmid-controlled resistance due to alteration of its binding site for the ribosome. Clarithromycin and azithromycin are active against *Haemophilus influenzae* and azithromycin kills *Toxoplasma gondii* cysts. Given orally or by i.v. infusion.

Tetracyclines

Examples are **tetracycline** and **doxycycline**. These are orally active, bacteriostatic, broad-spectrum antibiotics and are the drugs of choice for rickettsial, mycoplasma and chlamydial infections, brucellosis, cholera, plague and Lyme disease. Many organisms are now resistant. Absorption is decreased in the presence of food. Doxycycline is excreted in the bile. GIT disorders are commonly seen. These drugs are deposited in growing bone and are contraindicated in children and pregnant women.

Chloramphenicol

Chloramphenicol is a potent broad-spectrum antibiotic given orally or i.v. It can cause serious idiosyncratic depression of the bone marrow: a rare but severe pancytopenia or fatal aplastic anaemia. Poor inactivation and excretion in the newborn can cause 'grey baby' syndrome, which has a 40% mortality.

Its use is reserved for *H. influenzae* infections resistant to other agents and meningitis in patients in whom penicillin cannot be used. It is also useful in bacterial conjunctivitis. It is effective in typhoid fever—but so are less-toxic drugs.

Clindamycin

Clindamycin acts against many penicillin-resistant staphylococci and some anaerobes such as *Bacteroides.* Its use can result in pseudomembranous colitis: a severe inflammation of the colon caused by toxins produced by clindamycin-resistant faecal organisms.

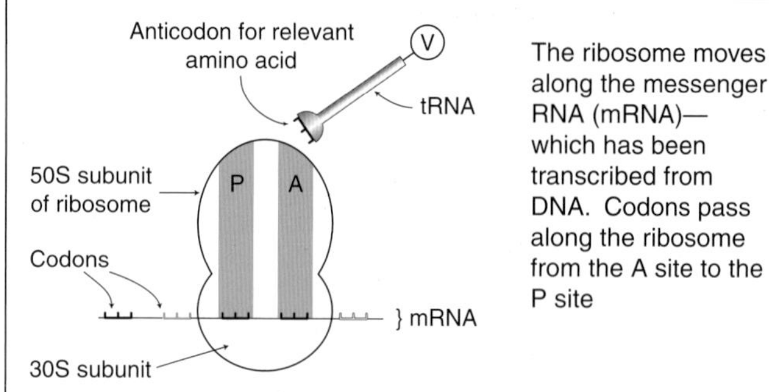

Fig. 45. 7 Outline of the basic structure and function of the bacterial ribosome.

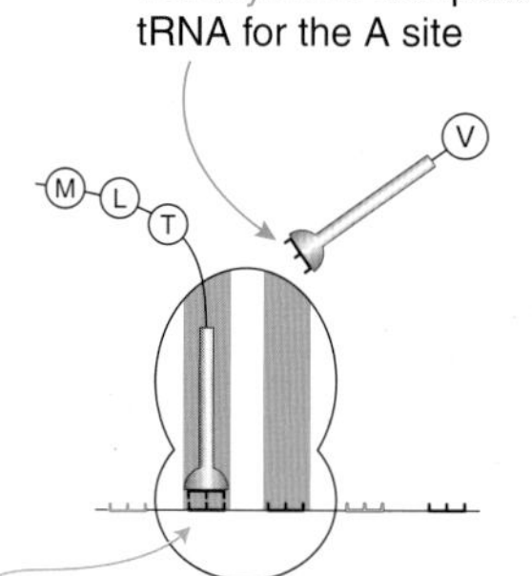

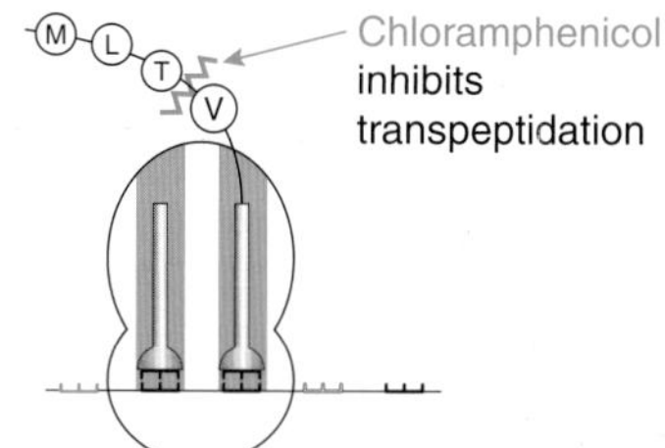

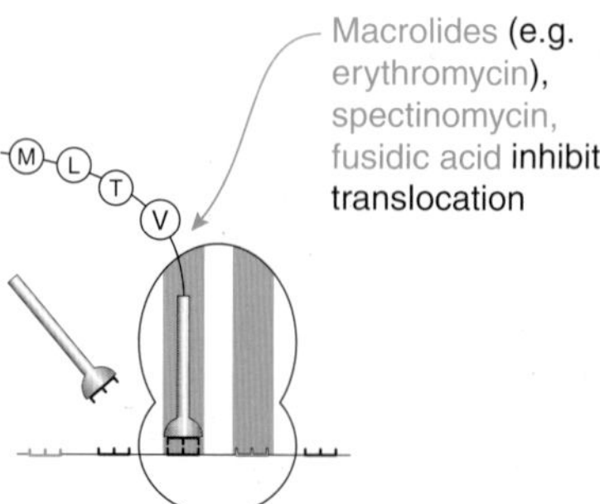

Fig. 45.8 The main steps in protein synthesis and the mechanism of action of drugs. Recent information about the E site has not been included.

Drugs affecting DNA synthesis

The main drugs are the fluoroquinolones.

Flouroquinolones

Examples are **ciprofloxacin**, norfloxacin and cinoxacin. These are broad-spectrum antibacterial agents that are particularly effective against Gram-negative organisms. They are also active against chlamydia and mycobacteria.

Mechanism of action The drugs inhibit topoisomerase II (DNA gyrase): the enzyme that produces the supercoil in the chromosome (Fig. 45.9), which is essential for transcription and replication.

Pharmacokinetic aspects Ciprofloxacin is given orally or by i.v. infusion. It is well absorbed from the GIT—except in the presence of magnesium and aluminium. It accumulates in the kidney, prostate and lung and concentrates in phagocytes. Elimination is partly by metabolism in the liver and partly by excretion in the urine.

Clinical use of the fluoroquinolones

- Complicated urinary tract infections.
- Gonorrhea.
- Cervicitis.
- Prostatitis.
- Typhoid fever.
- Septicaemia caused by sensitive organisms.
- Respiratory tract infections (but not if caused by pneumococci).

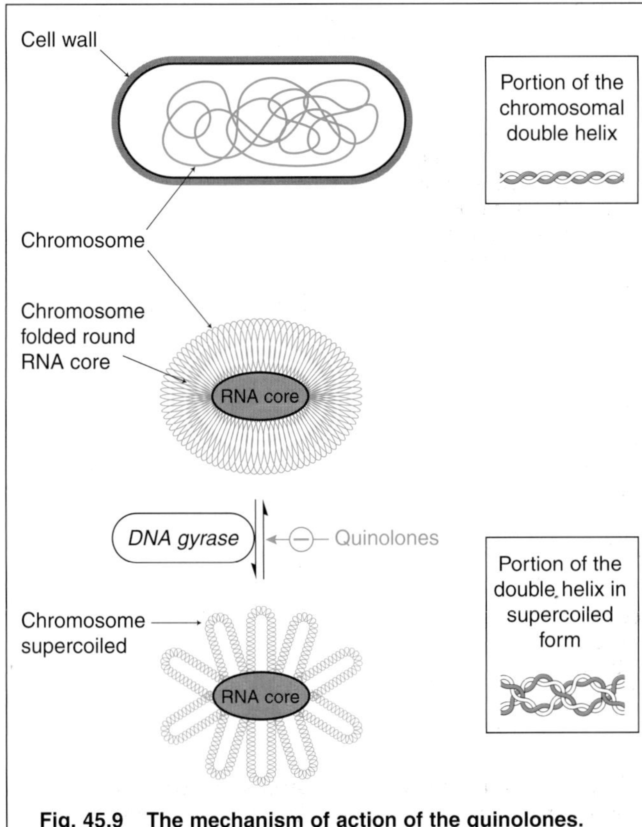

Fig. 45.9 The mechanism of action of the quinolones.

Unwanted effects GIT disorders and skin rashes can occur as can joint pains, allergic reactions and photosensitivity.

As the drugs can inhibit GABA binding to GABA receptors, CNS disorders such as convulsions may occur.

Drugs affecting bacterial folate synthesis and utilisation

The main drugs are sulfonamides, trimethoprim and co-trimoxazole. The mechanism of action is shown in Figure 45.10.

Sulphonamides

Examples are: **sulfamethoxazole** (short acting), **sulfalene** (sulfametopyrazine; long-acting) and sulfadiazine.

Sulphonamides are given orally, pass into inflammatory exudates and cross the placenta. They are inactivated in the presence of pus.

Unwanted effects Allergic reactions (rashes, fever), bone marrow depression and crystalluria can occur. (Alkalinising the urine and giving plenty of fluids prevents the last of these.)

Resistance Common and plasmid mediated.

Trimethoprim

Trimethoprim is active against most common pathogens. It is given orally, is well absorbed and widely distributed; it is excreted in the urine.

Unwanted effects GIT disturbances, blood disorders and skin rashes.

Antituberculosis drugs

Tuberculosis is now the world's main cause of death from a single agent and treatment has become a problem because of the development of multidrug-resistant strains of *Mycobacterium tuberculosis*.

First-line drugs used in treatment are isoniazid, rifampicin, ethambutol and pyrazinamide.

Second-line drugs are capreomycin, cycloserine, ciprofloxacin and streptomycin.

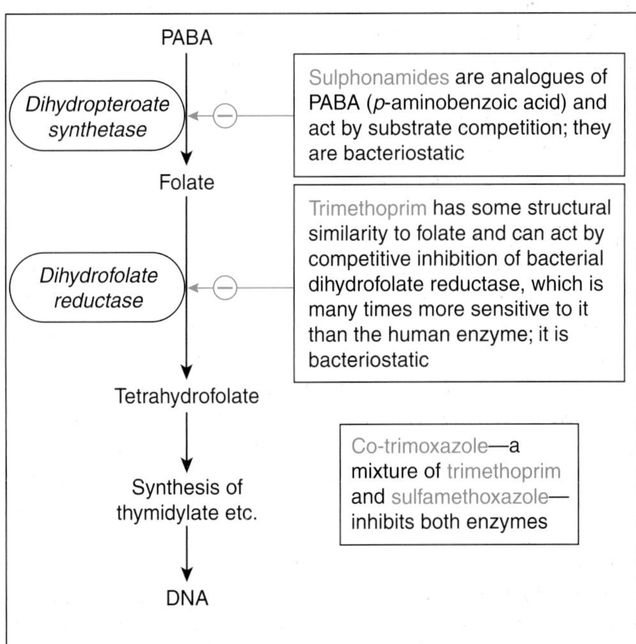

Fig. 45.10 The mechanism of action of drugs affecting folate metabolism or utilisation.

Clinical uses of trimethoprim, co-trimoxazole and the sulphonamides

- Trimethoprim on its own is used for urinary tract and respiratory infections.
- Co-trimoxazole is used only for *Pneumocystis carinii* pneumonia, norcardiasis and toxoplasmosis.
- Sulphonamides are now only used:
  - —with trimethoprim for a few special conditions
  - —for respiratory nocardial infections
  - —for sexually transmitted chlamydial infections and chancroid.

To reduce the emergence of resistant organisms, compound therapy is used: a first 2-month phase of isoniazid, rifampicin and pyrazinamide; then a 4-month phase of isoniazid and rifampicin.

Isoniazid

Isoniazid acts only on mycobacteria, being bacteriostatic on resting organisms and bactericidal on proliferating ones. Its mechanism of action is not understood.

Pharmacokinetic aspects It is given orally and is well absorbed. It is widely distributed, passing into the cerebrospinal fluid (CSF) and into necrotic tuberculous lesions. It enters into mammalian cells and is taken up by tubercle bacilli. It is acetylated in the liver—slowly in some individuals ('slow acetylators') fast in others—the former responding more efficiently to therapy. Elimination is partly by acetylation and partly by excretion unchanged in the urine.

Unwanted effects These are dose related, the most frequent being allergic reactions. Adverse effects in liver, blood, joints and blood vessels can occur. Isoniazid decreases the metabolism of several antiepileptic drugs.

Resistance This does occur but not cross-resistance with other antimycobacterial drugs.

Rifampicin

Mechanism of action Inhibition of the bacterial but not the human RNA polymerase. Rifampicin enters phagocytic cells and kills the intracellular tubercle bacilli. Rifampicin has very potent antimycobacterial action and is also effective against most Gram-positive and many Gram-negative species.

Pharmacokinetic aspects It is given orally, widely distributed and excreted in urine and bile. It imparts an orange tint to saliva, sweat and tears. Induction of hepatic metabolising enzymes results in decreased action of warfarin, narcotic analgesics, glucocorticoids and oral contraceptives.

Unwanted effects They are not common but include skin rashes, fever, GIT disturbances and, rarely, serious liver damage. CNS symptoms, allergic reactions and a 'flu-like syndrome can occur.

Resistance Modification of the bacterial RNA polymerase to give rise to reistance is reported.

Ethambutol

Ethambutol acts only against mycobacteria, being taken up by them and inhibiting their growth.

It is given orally and can cross into the CSF. It is partly metabolised and partly excreted unchanged in the urine.

Unwanted effects These are uncommon but optic neuritis can occur as can GIT disturbances and joint and CNS symptoms.

Resistance This is likely to occur if the drug is used on its own.

Pyrazinamide

Pyrazinamide is active against intracellular organisms in phagolysosomes in macrophages.

It is well absorbed and can cross into CSF; it is excreted by the kidneys.

Unwanted effects Include gout, GIT upsets and fever.

Resistance Develops quite readily but cross-resistance with isoniazid does not occur.

Capreomycin

Capreomycin is a peptide antibiotic given i.m.

Unwanted effects Kidney damage, deafness and ataxia can occur.

Cycloserine

Cycloserine is a broad-spectrum antibacterial agent affecting not only tubercle bacilli but many other organisms. It acts at an early stage of cell wall synthesis. Given orally, it is widely distributed in tissues and body fluids (including the CSF) and is excreted in the urine.

Other drugs

Streptomycin is an aminoglycoside (see above for mechanism of action) now rarely used for treatment of tuberculosis. Ciprofloxacin is dealt with above.

Antileprosy agents

There are two forms of leprosy: 'paucibacillary' leprosy in which few bacilli are present and in which the lesions are 'tuberculoid'; and 'multibacillary' leprosy in which numerous bacilli are present and the lesions are termed 'lepromatous'.

The drugs available are dapsone, clofazamine and rifampicin; the last is covered above.

Dapsone

Dapsone is related chemically to the sulphonamides and probably acts by a similar mechanism. It is given orally and is widely distributed through body water and tissues. It undergoes enterohepatic cycling but some is acetylated and excreted in the urine.

Unwanted effects These are fairly common and include methaemoglobinaemia, GIT disturbances, allergic skin rashes, neuropathy and, occasionally, exacerbation of lepromatous lesions.

Resistance This is increasing and necessitates combined treatment with other drugs.

Clofazimine

Clofazimine is a dye that is given orally and is taken up by macrophages. Its effect only starts after 6–7 weeks and it has an 8-week half-life.

Unwanted effects Include reddening of the skin and urine and GIT disturbances.

46 Antifungal drugs and anthelminthic drugs

ANTIFUNGAL DRUGS

The incidence of fungal infections has been increasing with the spread of AIDs and the increased use of broad-spectrum antibiotics that reduce the non-pathogenic bacteria which normally compete with fungi. Fungal infections can occur on the surfaces of the body or, more seriously, within the body; the latter are seen more frequently in immunocompromised patients.

Amphotericin

Amphotericin has a very wide spectrum of antifungal activity.

It interacts with ergosterol and forms a transmembrane ion channel in the fungal membrane It affects only fungi because cholesterol not ergosterol is the main sterol in human cells. Given orally, it is not well absorbed but acts in the gastrointestinal tract. It can be given by intravenous infusion and intrathecally. It is eliminated very slowly (over weeks) in the urine. *Unwanted effects* with parenteral amphotericin are common and can be serious: renal toxicity, hypokalaemia, anaemia, anaphylactic reactions.

Flucytosine

Flucytosine is converted to 5-fluorouracil, an anti-metabolite, within fungal cells. It has a narrow spectrum of action affecting mainly yeast and cryptococcal infections. It is given orally or by intravenous infusion and is widely distributed in the body. *Unwanted effects* are infrequent.

Azoles

This group includes imidazoles and triazoles; both are effective in a wide range of fungal infections, the triazoles having a broader spectrum than the imidazoles.

Mechanism of action: Azoles inhibit the fungal P450 enzymes that are necessary for the synthesis of ergosterol – an essential component of the fungal membrane. Examples of triazoles are fluconazole and itraconazole. Examples of imidazoles are ketoconazole and clotrimazole.

Fluconazole is given orally or intravenously and is widely distributed, passing into the CSF and other bodily fluids. Itraconazole is given orally and undergoes extensive first-pass metabolism.

Unwanted effects of fluconazole are mild. Itraconazole can cause GIT disturbances. Ketoconazole can be hepatotoxic.

Terbinafine

Terbinafine inhibits the synthesis of ergosterol, a crucial component of fungal cell membranes Given orally, it is selectively taken up by the nails, the skin and fat. Unwanted effects are mild.

ANTHELMINTHIC DRUGS

The main helminths (worms) that infect humans live either within the alimentary tract or in the tissues.

Worms living in the alimentary canal include the nematodes (the common round worms, and the less common hookworms, threadworms and whipworms) and the cestodes (tapeworms).

Worms living in the tissues include the trematodes or flukes which cause schiztosomiasis (aka bilharziasis), the tissue round worms and the hydatid tape worm.

Mebendazole

Mebendazole is a broad-spectrum anthelminthic. It inhibits helminth microtubule synthesis, resulting in impairment of glucose uptake. The worms die slowly and can take several days to be voided. It is given orally but 10% is absorbed. *Unwanted effects* are few but can include gastrointestinal disturbances and allergic reactions.

Levamisole

Levamisole causes a tonic paralysis of the worm by stimulating the nicotinic receptors at the neuromuscular junction. It is given orally. *Unwanted effects* include mild nausea and vomiting in a small percentage of patients.

Piperazine

Piperazine is effective mainly against Ascaris (common round worm) infection. It paralyses the worm by blocking its neuromuscular junction and the worm is then expelled by the peristaltic action of the host's intestine. It is given orally, readily absorbed and excreted unchanged within 24 hours. Unwanted effects are few but can, rarely, include minor CNS disturbances.

Praziquantel

Praziquantel causes an increase in the calcium permeability of the cell membranes resulting in paralysis and death of the worm. Given orally, it is well absorbed and rapidly metabolised in the liver to inactive products. *Unwanted effects* are few.

Ivermectin

Ivermectin acts at the worm's neuromuscular junction causing paralysis either by intensifiying GABA-mediated inhibition or by activating an invertebrate-specific glutamate-gated chloride channel. It is rapidly absorbed and widely distributed. *Unwanted effects* are rare.

Niclosamide

Niclosamide is effective against tapeworms. It either interferes with oxidative phosphorylation or activates ATPases. The adult worm is killed but the ova are unaffected. It is not absorbed. *Unwanted effects* are rare and can include gastrointestinal disturbances.

Clinical uses of antifungal drugs

- Amphotericin + flucytosine, or fluconazole on its own, are used for systemic candidiasis, cryptococcosis, and mucormycosis
- Amphotericin infusion is used for systemic aspergillosis and histoplasmosis
- Clotrimazole or itraconazole are used for ringworm and athlete's foot.
- Terbinafine is used for fungal nail infections.

Clinical uses of anthelminthic drugs

- Thread worms: mebendazole, piperazine
- Tapeworms: niclosamide, praziquantel; for hydatid disease: albendazole
- Round worms : levasmisole, mebendazole, piperazine
- Hookworm: mebendazole
- Schistosomes: praziquantel
- Filariae: ivermectin

47 Antiviral drugs

Viruses consist essentially of DNA or RNA in a protein coat. They have no ribosomes or protein-synthesising apparatus although some contain enzymes. They replicate by taking over the metabolic processes of the host. Because a virus virtually (in some cases, actually) becomes part of its host cell, selective chemotherapy is difficult.

The human immunodeficiency virus (HIV)—an RNA retrovirus—will be taken as an example of viral infection of a host cell (Fig. 47.1). Antiviral drugs will be dealt with under two headings: anti-HIV drugs and other antiviral agents.

Viral infection of a cell

The binding sites on the host cell to which the virus attaches are normal membrane constituents: receptors for cytokines, neurotransmitters or hormones, ion channels, integral membrane glycoproteins, etc. Thus the virus that causes infantile diarrhoea attaches to the β-adrenoceptor; the rabies virus attaches to the acetylcholine receptor on skeletal muscle. With many viruses, the receptor–virus complex enters the cell by receptor-mediated endocytosis during which the virus coat may be removed. Some by-pass this route.

On entering and infecting a host cell, the virus genome itself acts as—or is transcribed into—virus-specific messenger RNA, which then directs the synthesis of new virus particles. DNA viruses enter the host cell nucleus to accomplish this. Most RNA viruses replicate without involving the host cell nuclear material. RNA retroviruses (e.g. HIV, responsible for the acquired immunodeficiency syndrome (AIDS)) have an enzyme, reverse transcriptase, that makes a DNA copy of the viral RNA; this DNA copy is integrated into the host genome and directs the generation of new viral particles (Fig. 47.1).

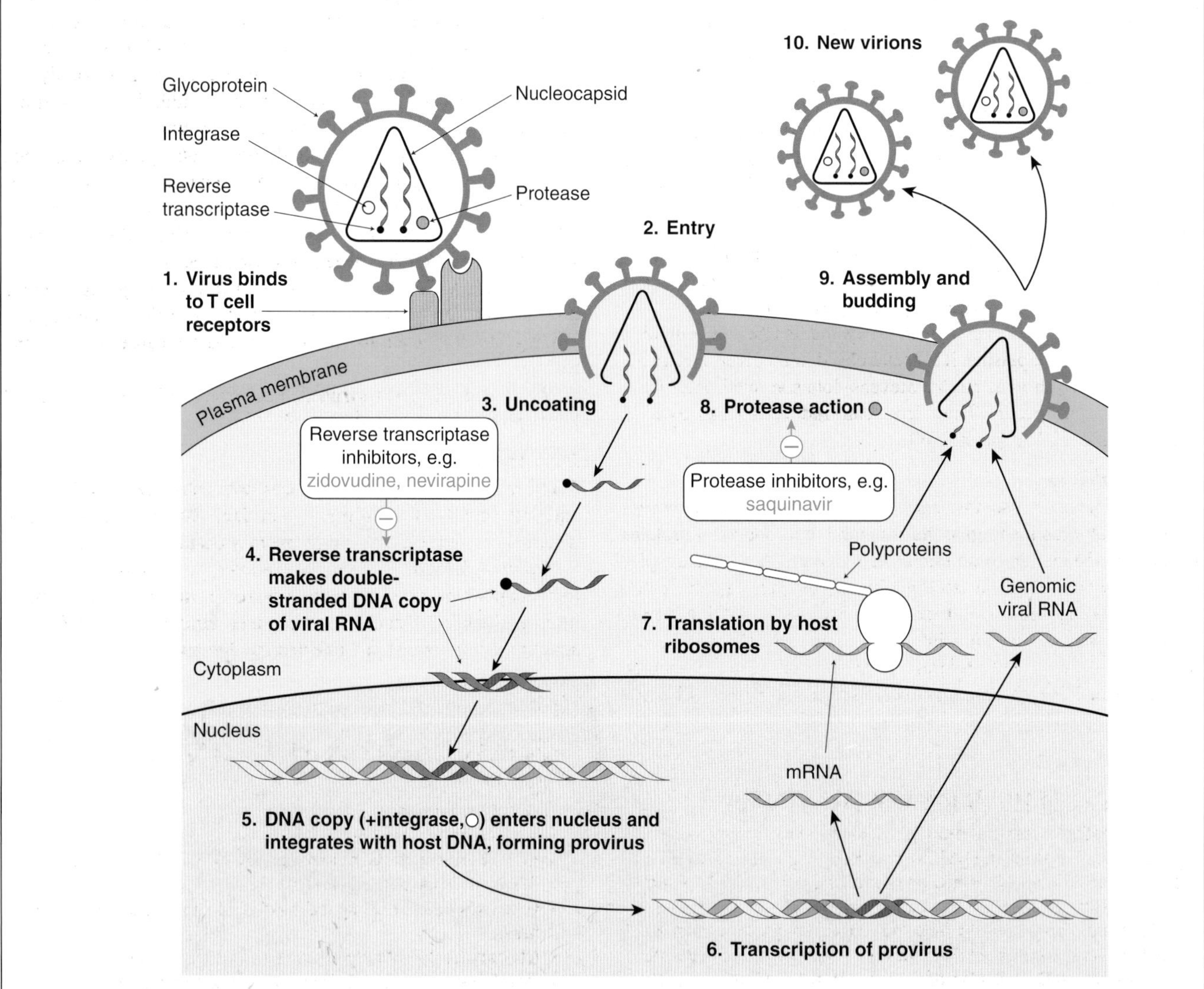

Fig. 47.1 Schematic diagram of the infection of a T cell with the HIV retrovirus, showing the principal viral structures, the main steps in viral replication (1–9) and the sites of action of anti-HIV drugs.

Anti-HIV drugs

The two main groups of anti-HIV drugs are reverse transcriptase inhibitors (RTIs) and protease inhibitors. Combinations of these is essential in treatment to prevent the development of tolerance.

Reverse transcriptase inhibitors

Nucleoside RTIs

Nucleoside RTIs (NRTIs) inhibit the action of the viral reverse transcriptase. The drugs are analogues of endogenous nucleosides and are phosphorylated by host cell enzymes to give a 'false' 5-trisphosphate. This competitively inhibits the equivalent trisphosphates of the host cell needed by the reverse transcriptase for the formation of the viral DNA. Examples are **zidovudine**, abacavir, didanosine, lamuvidine, zalcitabine and stavudine.

Zidovudine (AZT, azidothymidine) This analogue of thymidine is usually given orally but can be given by i.v. infusion. The cerebrospinal fluid (CSF) concentration is 65% of the blood level and the half-life of the 'false' trisphosphate is 3 h. Most is metabolised in the liver but 20% is excreted via the kidney. *Unwanted effects* with long-term use include blood dyscrasias, gastrointestinal (GIT) disorders, CNS disturbances, myopathy, rashes, fever and a 'flu-like syndrome. Short-term use in fit individuals usually causes only minor, reversible adverse effects. *Resistance* is likely to occur in late-stage HIV disease.

Abacavir This guanosine analogue is given orally; it is well absorbed and inactivated in the liver. The CSF concentration is one third that of the plasma. *Unwanted effects* include skin rashes, GIT disturbances and, rarely, a serious general hypersensitivity reaction.

Non-nucleoside RTIs

The non-nucleoside RTIs (NNRTIs) are chemically diverse compounds that denature the catalytic site of the reverse transcriptase. Examples are nevirapine and efavirenz.

Nevirapine This drug is given orally and its CSF concentration is 45% of that in the plasma. It is metabolised in the liver. *Unwanted effects* include rash and, rarely, Stevens–Johnson syndrome. Drug interactions can occur. This drug can reduce mother-to-child transmission of HIV by about 50%.

Protease inhibitors

In the final stage of assembly and budding, a viral protease cleaves precursor polyproteins to give the structural and functional proteins of the new virions. Protease inhibitors prevent this step. Examples are **saquinavir**, indinavir and nelfinavir. All are given orally, saquinavir being subject to first-pass metabolism. All inhibit the P450 liver enzymes so drug interactions are possible. In general, these drugs are well tolerated. *Unwanted effects* include gastrointestinal disturbances, insulin resistance and hyperlipidaemia. With long-term use, redistribution of fat is seen (some fat accumulation, some fat loss).

Other antiviral drugs

The antiviral agents for infections other than HIV can be classified according to their mechanism of action.

Inhibition of penetration of host cell

Amantadine Inhibits both the uncoating stage and the later assembly and release of new virions. It is given orally. Minor CNS and gastrointestinal disturbances occur infrequently. Resistance may be seen.

Zanamivir This is a neuraminidase inhibitor and prevents the release of new virions. It is given as a powder by inhalation and is well tolerated.

Palivizumab This is a humanised monoclonal antibody raised against a specific surface glycoprotein of the respiratory syncytial virus; it neutralises the virus. It is given i.m.

Inhibition of transcription of the viral genome

Aciclovir The drug is inactive until converted to the trisphosphate. The first phosphorylation is only effectively carried out by the viral kinase (so the step can only occur in infected cells); subsequent steps are catalysed by host cell kinases. Aciclovir selectively inhibits viral DNA polymerase. It can be given orally, i.v. or topically and is degraded fairly speedily within host cells. It has minimal unwanted effects. Resistance can occur.

Ganciclovir This also undergoes phosphorylation and suppresses DNA replication in a similar manner to aciclovir. It is given i.v. or orally and persists in the host cell for approximately 20 h. *Unwanted effects* include myelosuppression, which occurs in 40% of patients, and it is potentially carcinogenic.

Foscarnet This non-nucleoside analogue of pyrophosphate inhibits viral DNA polymerase by attaching to the pyrophosphate binding site. It is given by i.v. infusion and can cause serious renal toxicity.

Tribavirin This is a synthetic nucleside that is given by aerosol for respiratory viral infections.

Immunomodulators

Interferon-α This cytokine induces host cells enzymes that have antiviral activity. It is given i.v. or i.m. Blood dyscrasias, GIT disturbances and 'flu-like symptoms may occur.

Immunoglobulins Normal pooled plasma contains immunoglobulins that can neutralise some viruses. Hyperimmune immunoglobulins specific for particular viruses can be effective against the viruses that had infected the donors.

Treatment of HIV/AIDS with anti-HIV drugs

A combination of several drugs is used (known as highly active antiretroviral therapy (HAART)) consisting of two NRTIs with either a NNRTI or one or two protease inhibitors. The drugs do not cure HIV infection but can slow progress of the disease and prolong life. They have to be taken indefinitely and a balance must be struck between the therapeutic and adverse actions. Patients with AIDS will also be taking numerous other drugs for the inevitable intercurrent infections so drug interactions are a hazard.

Clinical uses of non-anti-HIV antiviral agents

- **Amantadine**: influenza A.
- **Aciclovir**: herpesviruses.
- **Ganciclovir**: cytomegalovirus (CMV) infection, especially CMV retinitis in AIDS patients.
- **Ribavirin**: respiratory syncitial virus, influenza, possibly Lassa fever.
- **Foscarnet**: CMV (fairly effective).
- **Interferons**: hepatitis B; may also be useful in AIDS.
- **Hyperimmune immunoglobulin**: hepatitis B, varicella-zoster, CMV, rabies, tetanus.

48 Antiprotozoal drugs

The main protozoans that produce disease in humans are those causing malaria, amoebiasis, pneumocystis infection, trypanosomiasis and leishmaniasis.

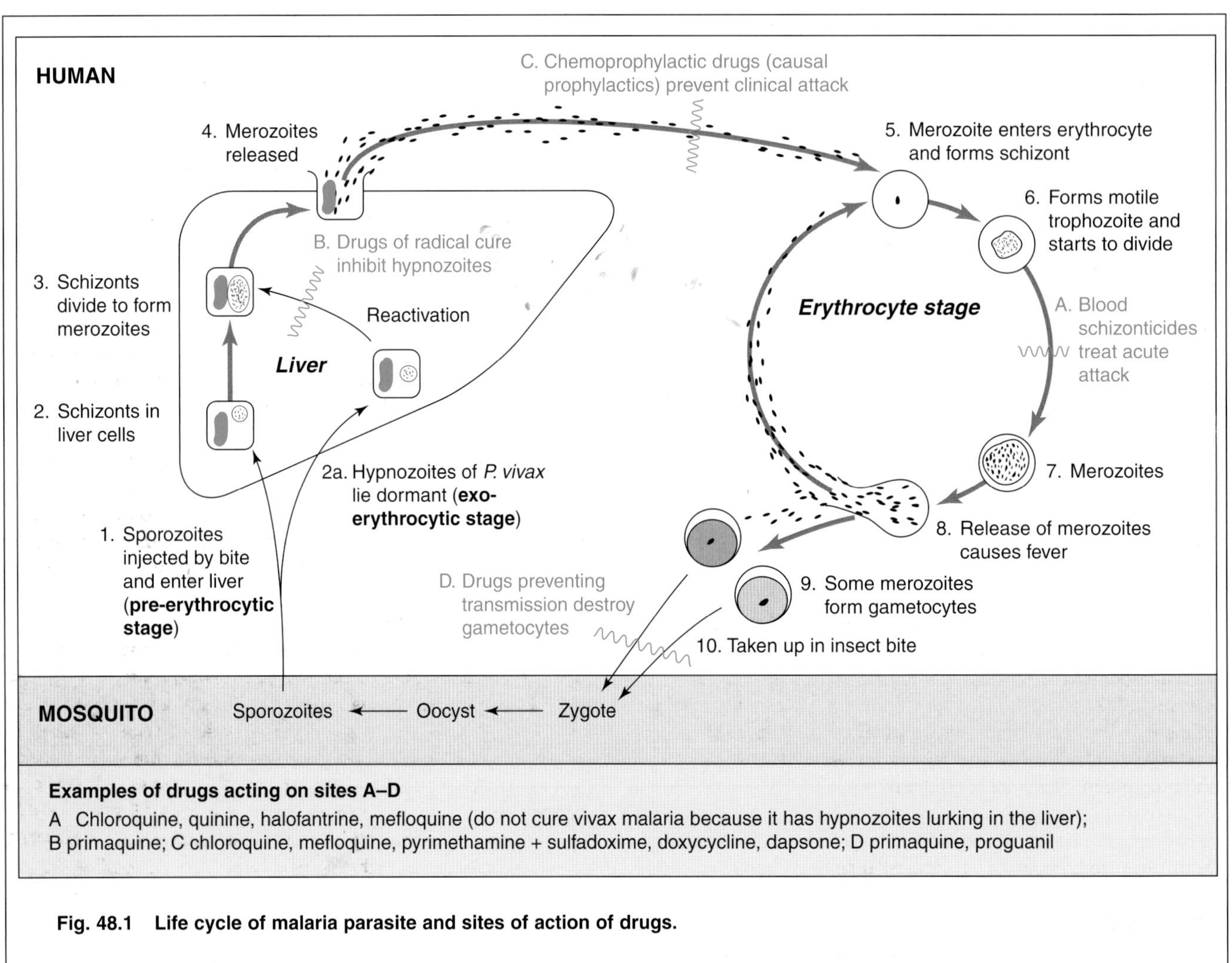

Fig. 48.1 Life cycle of malaria parasite and sites of action of drugs.

MALARIA

Malaria, a mosquito-borne disease caused by various *Plasmodium* species, is a major killer in the developing world and sporadic cases occur elsewhere as a result of air travel. The female anopheline mosquito injects sporozoites during a blood meal. Figure 48.1 shows the subsequent sequence of changes in the parasite and their relation to the bouts of fever.

The main malarial parasites are *P. vivax* and *P. falciparum*, both of which cause fever every third day (tertian malaria), *P. vivax* causing benign and *P. falciparum* malignant tertian ('malignant' because it is a very severe form of the disease and can be fatal). *P. vivax* gives rise to hypnozoites in the liver; these lie dormant and can produce relapses months or years later. *P. falciparum* does not form hypnozoites and thus has no exo-erythrocytic stage. *P. malariae*, which is rare, has a 72 h cycle (quartan malaria) and also has no exo-erythrocytic stage.

Antimalarial agents

Chloroquine reduces the necessary digestion of haemoglobin by the plasmodium and also inhibits the parasite's haem polymerase (the enzyme that inactivates the toxic free haem generated by the organism, which is fatal for it). It is usually given orally (half-life 0.5 h) but can be given by injection. It is widely distributed in the body but much is concentrated in the parasitised red cells. Unwanted effects include nausea, vomiting and dizziness. Large doses cause retinopathy and bolus injections can cause dysrhythmias. *P. falciparum* is resistant in most parts of the world and *P. vivax* is resistant in some places.

Halofantrine is given orally; the parent drug has a half-life of 1–2 days and the active metabolite 3–5 days. Unwanted effects include GI tract disturbances and, occasionally, cardiac dysrhythmias.

Quinine is given orally (half-life 10 h) but can be given by i.v. infusion. It is usually given with pyrimethamine (see below) and

Clinical use of antimalarial drugs

	For the clinical attack	For chemoprophylaxis
All infections except chloroquine-resistant *P. falciparum*	Oral chloroquine or sulfadoxine + pyrimethamine	Oral chloroquine or proguanil
Chloroquine-resistant *P. falciparum*	Oral quinine + doxycycline or Oral halofantrine	Oral chloroquine plus either proguanil or pyrimethamine + dapsone

either dapsone (given orally; half-life 24–48 h) or sulfadoxine, a long-acting sulfonamide (half-life ~ 8 days). It causes GI tract upsets, tinnitus, headache, blurred vision and allergic reactions. Large doses affect the heart (dysrhythmias) and/or the CNS (delirium). 'Blackwater fever' may be associated with the use of this drug.

Mefloquine is given orally (half-life 30 days) and has a slow onset of action. Like chloroquine, it inhibits the plasmodial haem polymerase. It can cause GI tract disturbances and is known to produce neuropsychiatric symptoms.

Pyrimethamine is a folate antagonist inhibiting folate utilisation having greater affinity for the plasmodial than for the mammalian system. It is only used with either dapsone or sulfadoxine. It is given orally and is slow acting (half-life 4 days). It has few unwanted effects.

Proguanil has a similar action to pyrimethamine. It is a slow-acting schizonticide (half-life 16 h) with some action on the pre-erythrocytic stage of *P. vivax*. It is given orally.

Primaquine is given orally (half-life 3–6 h) and usually with chloroquine. It can cause haemolysis in individuals with genetic deficiency of red cell glucose 6-phosphate dehydrogenase.

Doxycline is a broad-spectrum tetracycline antibiotic that acts by inhibiting plasmodial protein synthesis.

OTHER PROTOZOAL INFECTIONS

Amoebiasis

Amoebiasis is caused by the ingestion of the cysts of *Entamoeba histolytica*. The cysts develop into motile trophozoites in the GI tract, which can invade the intestinal wall and, rarely, migrate to the liver. The presence of the organism in the GI tract usually causes dysentery; its presence in the liver causes amoebic abscesses. Some individuals remain symptom-free 'carriers', i.e. they excrete the cysts, which can infect others.

Amoebicidal drugs

Metronidazole kills the motile form of *E. histolytica*. It is given orally (half-life 7 h) but can also be given i.v. and rectally. It has few unwanted effects but has a bitter taste and interferes with alcohol metabolism.

Clinical use of amoebicidal drugs

- Acute severe dysentery: metronidazole (or tindazole) followed by diloxanide
- Chronic amoebiasis: diloxanide
- Hepatic amoebiasis: metronidazole followed by diloxanide
- Treatment of carriers: diloxanide.

Diloxanide is given orally and has a direct action in the GI tract against the non-motile form of the amoebae.

Leishmaniasis

The leishmania parasite has two forms, a flagellated form in the sandfly (the insect vector) and a non-flagellated form that occurs in the bitten human. Infected humans develop cutaneous and/or visceral leishmaniasis. The protozoon is ingested by mononuclear phagocytes and it remains alive intracellularly.

The main drug used in treatment is **sodium stibogluconate**, which is given i.m. or by slow i.v. injection daily in a course lasting 10–20 days. Coughing may occur during injection. *Unwanted effects* are GI tract disturbances, muscle pain, cardiovascular disturbances.

Other drugs used are amphotericin, and pentamidine isethionate.

Pneumocystis infection

Pneumocystis carinii is widely distributed in the mammalian kingdom but only causes disease (pneumocystis pneumonia; PCP) in individuals who are immunosuppressed. It is a common presenting symptom and a leading cause of death in patients with AIDs.

Drug treatment. The drug of choice is **co-trimoxazole**, which is a mixture of trimethoprim (a folate antagonist related to pyrimethamine) and sulfamethoxazole (see Fig. 45.10). Together these interfere with thymidylate synthesis and, therefore, with DNA synthesis. It is given orally in high doses. The second-line drug is pentamidine, given parenterally. Other drugs are trimethoprim–dapsone and atovaquone.

Trypanosomiasis

The trypanosomes *T. gambiensi* and *T. rhodesiense* cause sleeping sickness, which can be treated with **suramin** or **pentamidine**. Suramin is endocytosed by the parasite and damages it; the parasite is then cleared by host responses. The drug is given i.v. very slowly. It is relatively toxic especially to the kidney. Optic atrophy, blood dyscrasias and skin rashes can occur. Pentamidine is taken up by the parasites and rapidly kills them. It is given i.m. daily for 10–15 days.

Trichomoniasis

Trichomonas vaginalis causes vaginal infection in females and, sometimes, urethral infection in males. It is treated with **metronidazole**.

Toxoplasmosis

Toxoplasma gondii is a protozoal infection of cats. Oocysts from cat faeces can cause disease in humans. The treatment of choice is **pyrimethamine–sulfadiazine**.

49 Cancer chemotherapy

The term 'cancer' refers to a malignant tumour. Cancer cells can manifest, in greater or lesser degree: uncontrolled proliferation, invasiveness, the ability to metastasise and/or infiltrate normal tissues and loss of function due to lack of the capacity to differentiate. Benign tumours manifest only uncontrolled proliferation.

Pathology

The two main alterations in DNA underlying cancerous change in a cell are (i) mutation/inactivation of tumour-suppressor genes and (ii) mutation/activation of *proto-oncogenes*. Proto-oncogenes are genes that normally code for the growth factor-induced and apoptotic pathways and thus control the cell cycle and cell proliferation. Oncogenes code for cancerous changes. The development of cancer, however, is a multistage process, involving not only more than one genetic change but also other non-genetic factors (hormonal effects, co-carcinogen actions, etc.) that increase the likelihood that the mutation(s) will result in cancer. The formation of new blood vessels (angiogenesis) is required for the growth of the tumour, the infiltration of cancer cells into nearby tissue and their metastasis to other organs.

Most anticancer agents are cytotoxic, i.e they damage or kill cells; they do not affect the underlying pathogenetic mechanisms, namely the changes in growth factors and/or their receptors, in the cell cycle and apoptototic pathways, in telomerase expression or in tumour-related angiogenesis. Most are mainly antiproliferative, acting primarily on dividing cells (Fig. 49.1) and have no specific inhibitory effect on invasiveness, the loss of differentiation or the tendency to metastasise. Because the drugs inhibit cell proliferation, they will also affect rapidly dividing normal cells. Therefore, they can depress the bone marrow, impair healing, depress growth, cause sterility and hair loss, be teratogenic; most cause nausea and vomiting.

Newer agents and some in the pipeline (Fig. 49.2) more successfully affect the factors involved in the pathogenesis of cancer specified above. Anti-angiogenesis anticancer agents are under investigation.

Anticancer drugs

Most currently used anticancer drugs have the adverse effects specified above; only the adverse effects particular to each drug are given below. Cells damaged by cytotoxic anticancer drugs undergo apoptosis (see Ch. 4).

Alkylating agents and related drugs

These agents directly interfere with DNA synthesis.

Cyclophosphamide This alkylating nitrogen mustard agent can form covalent bonds with bases (usually guanine) in the DNA. It has two alkylating groups and can cross-link the two strands, interfering with cell division and triggering apoptosis. It is given orally or i.m. and is metabolised in the liver and the tissues to give *phosphoramide mustard* (the active moiety) and *acrolein*, which is responsible for bladder toxicity. *Unwanted effects* include nausea and vomiting and acrolein-mediated haemorrhagic cystitis. The last effect can be ameliorated by giving the sulfhydryl donor mesna. Another alkylating nitrogen mustard is chlorambucil.

Cisplatin This platinum coordination compound can cross-link DNA and trigger apoptosis. It is given by infusion. It causes very severe nausea and vomiting (which can be ameliorated by the

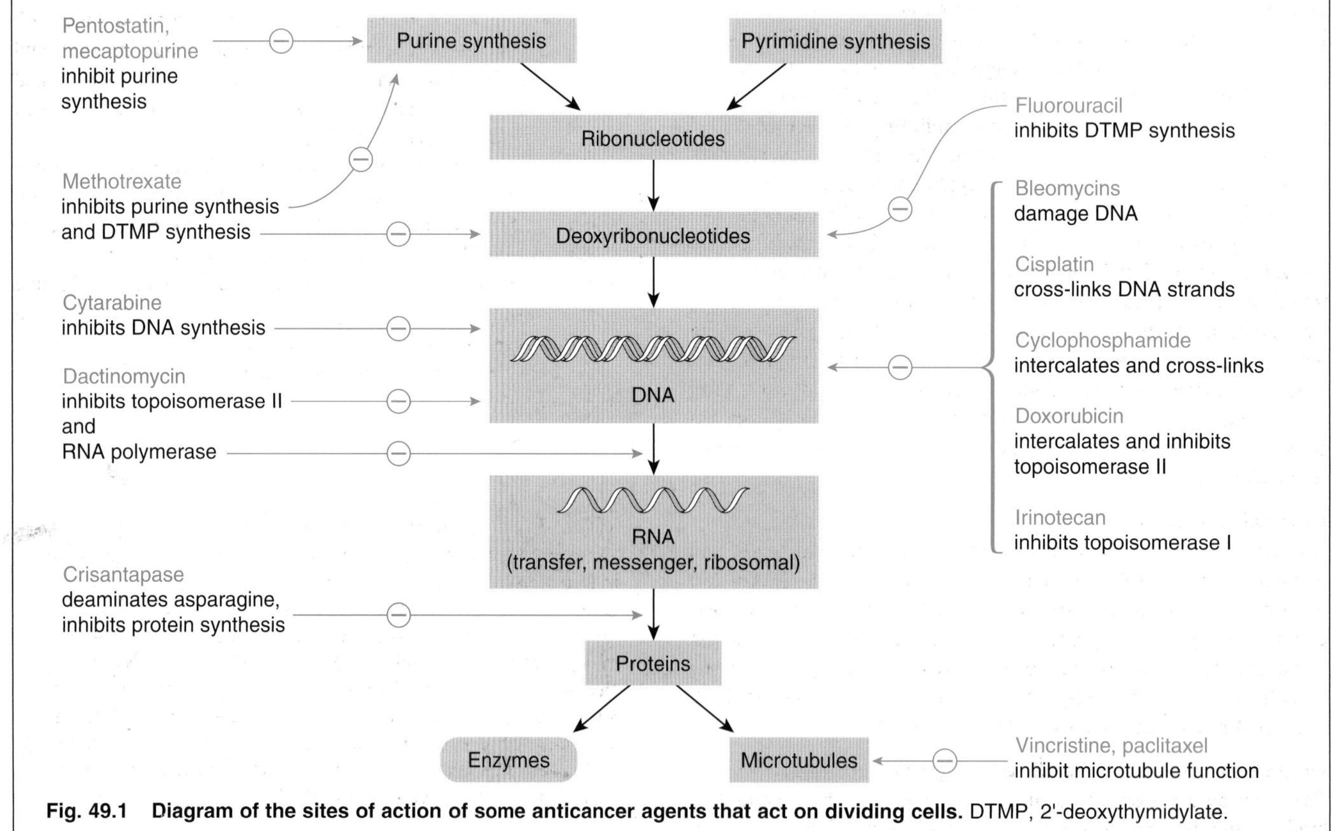

Fig. 49.1 Diagram of the sites of action of some anticancer agents that act on dividing cells. DTMP, 2'-deoxythymidylate.

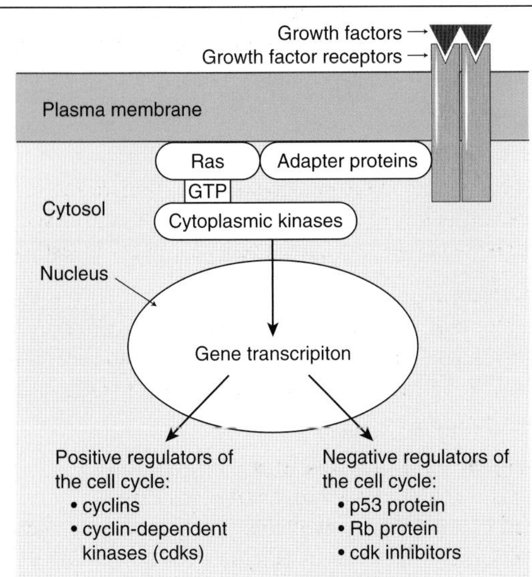

Proto-oncogene	Proto-oncogene products	Cancer	Anticancer drugs
Gene for EGF receptor	EGF receptor (an rtk)	Breast	Trastuzumab inhibits the EGF rtk; used to treat breast cancer
Gene for PDGF	PDGF receptor (an rtk)	CM leukaemia	Imatinib inhibits the PDGF trk; used to treat CM leukaemia
c-ras	Ras proteins	30% of all tumours	Ras inhibitors are in clinical trial
abl	A cytoplasmic tyrosine kinase (ctk)	CM leukaemia	Imatinib inhibitis the ctk coded for by *abl:* used to treat CM leukaemia

Mutation of the nuclear proto-oncogenes can alter expression of the regulators of the cell cycle, e.g. more than 50% of human tumours have mutations of the tumour supressor gene that codes for p53 protein

Fig. 49.2 Schematic diagram indicating some mutations of some proto-oncogenes that can result in cancer (i.e. the proto-oncogenes for growth factor receptors and the cell cycle pathways) and the sites of action of some new drugs. PDGF, platelet-derived growth factor; EGF, epidermal growth factor; Rb, retinoblastoma; CM, chronic myeloid; rtk, receptor tyrosine kinase.

antiemetic $5HT_3$ antagonist ondansetron) and can result in kidney damage unless copious fluids and diuretics are given. It has low myelotoxicity.

Antimetabolites

Antimetabolite agents interfere with DNA synthesis. For most, the *unwanted effects* are bone marrow depression and damage to the intestinal epithelium with resultant gastrointestinal disturbances.

Methotrexate is a folate antagonist; it inhibits the enzyme dihydrofolate reductase, competing with dihydrofolate in the generation of tetrahydrofolate, thus inhibiting the formation of thymidylate (Ch. 23). It is given orally and taken up into cells, where it persists for weeks in the form of polyglutamate derivatives. High-dose regimens must be followed by 'rescue' with folinic acid (a form of tetrahydrofolate). *Fluorouracil*, a pyrimidine analogue, is converted to a fraudulent nucleotide which interferes with thymidylate synthesis. It is given by injection. *Cytarabine*, pyrimidine analogue, is converted in the cell to the trisphosphate which inhibits DNA polymerase. *Fludarabine*, purine analogue, has a similar mechanism of action to cytarabine. It is given i.v. *Pentostatin*, purine analogue, inhibits adenosine deaminase, an enzyme important in the generation of inosine—an early stage of ribonucleotide synthesis.

Cytotoxic antibiotics

Anticancer antibiotics act directly on the nucleic acids. *Doxorubicin* intercalates in the DNA and inhibits the action of topoisomerase II. It is given by infusion and the unwanted effects include dose-related cardiac damage. *Bleomycins* cause DNA fragmentation and the unwanted effects include pulmonary fibrosis and allergic reactions. They have low myelotoxicity. *Dactinomycin* intercalates in the DNA and inhibits RNA polymerase and topoisomerase II.

Plant derivatives and miscellaneous agents

These act by a variety of means. *Vincristine* is a vinca alkaloid; it binds to tubulin and interferes with spindle formation in dividing cells. It is given i.v. often in conjunction with a glucocorticoid. It is relatively non-toxic, having low myelotoxicity, but can cause sensory changes and muscle weakness. *Paclitaxel*, a taxane, stabilises microtubules in the polymerised state and interferes with spindle formation. It is given by i.v. infusion. Unwanted effects may include serious myelosuppression and cumulative neurotoxicity. Hypersensitivity is common and necessitates pretreatment with glucocorticoids. *Etoposide* inhibits mitochondrial function and topoisomerase II action. *Irinotecan* inhibits topoisomerase I and interferes with DNA function. It has fewer unwanted effects than most cytotoxic anticancer drugs.

In hormone-sensitive tumours, inhibition of tumour growth can be brought about by antagonists or synthesis inhibitors of those hormones, or by hormones with opposing action. Some examples are **glucocorticoids** (Ch. 28), which inhibit lymphocyte proliferation and are used for leukaemias, **tamoxifen**, an anti-oestrogen effective in hormone-dependent mammary cancer, and flutamide, an androgen antagonist used in prostate cancer.

Radioactive isotopes can damage tumours directly. **Radioactive iodine** is used for thyroid tumours.

Treatment regimens with anticancer drugs

The detailed clinical uses of anticancer drugs are the province of the oncologist. Anticancer drugs are usually given in combinations that increase anticancer action without increasing toxicity. For example, methotrexate, which depresses the bone marrow, can be given with a drug that has low myelotoxicity (e.g. cisplatin or bleomycin). Drugs are usually given in large doses intermittently, in several courses, with 2–3 weeks between courses, because this permits the bone marrow to regenerate during the intervals. Resistance can occur to most anticancer drugs and will complicate treatment.

A.1 Appendix 1: The Schild plot and pA_2

The Schild plot, named after H O Schild, was devised as a means of identifying reversible, competitive antagonism and to obtain an estimate of the affinity of a competitive antagonist for a receptor.

In reversible, competitive antagonism, the antagonist shifts the log concentration–response curve for the agonist to the right, without changing its shape (Fig. A.1). It is assumed that the agonist, (A) and antagonist (B) bind independently to the receptor (R):

$$A + R \rightleftharpoons AR \qquad B + R \rightleftharpoons BR$$

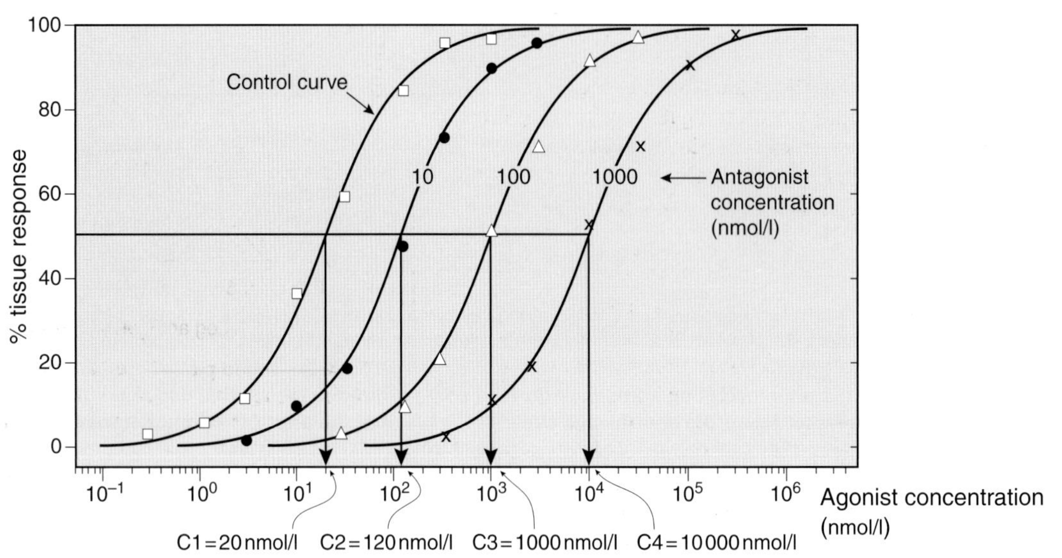

Fig. A.1 Log concentration–response curves to an agonist in absence and presence of three concentrations of competitive antagonist. See text.

Application of the Law of Mass Action shows that the proportion of receptors occupied by the agonist, p_{AR}, is given, in the absence of antagonist, by:

$$p_{AR} = \frac{[A]}{K_A + [A]} \qquad (1)$$

and, in the presence of antagonist, by:

$$p_{AR} = \frac{[A]}{K_A\left(1 + \frac{[B]}{K_B}\right) + [A]} \qquad (2)$$

where K_A and K_B are the equilibrium dissociation constants for binding of agonist and antagonist to the receptor.

Schild made the reasonable assumption that, for simple competitive antagonism, a particular response in the presence of the antagonist required the same proportion of receptors to be occupied by the agonist as in its absence. In the presence of the antagonist, a higher concentration of agonist would be required and for any given response it would be increased by a factor CR, the concentration ratio. This is the ratio of the concentrations of agonist in the presence and absence of antagonist producing the same response. Equating occupancies in the absence and presence of antagonist for a specified response gives:

$$\frac{[A]}{K_A + [A]} = \frac{CR[A]}{K_A\left(1 + \frac{[B]}{K_B}\right) + CR[A]} \qquad (3)$$

Simple algebra allows equation 3 to be simplified to:

$$CR - 1 = \frac{[B]}{K_B} \qquad (4)$$

This is the Schild equation. As expected, equation 4 indicates that the CR will increase as [B] increases and is large for small values of K_B. The Schild plot uses the logarithmic form of this equation:

$$\log(CR - 1) = \log[B] - \log K_B \qquad (5)$$

A plot of log(CR – 1) versus log[B] is of the form $y = mx + c$ and should, therefore, yield a straight line. There is no multiplier for log[B]; in other words, m, which denotes the slope, should have a value of 1.

When log(CR – 1) is zero, log[B] equals $\log K_B$.

The Schild relationship can also be shown to apply to the more realistic del Castillo–Katz model of receptor action. (See Jenkinson D H 2003 In Textbook of receptor pharmacology, 2nd edn, J C Foreman & T Johansen (eds). Boca Raton, FL, CRC Press.)

Figures A.1 and A.2 provide a simple worked example of the Schild analysis of competitive antagonism.

In Figure A.1, we see that increasing concentrations of antagonist produce progressively larger shifts of the concentration–response curve to the right. The concentrations (C1–C4) producing a specified response, here 50%, can be read from the x-axis. The CR values for the three concentrations of antagonist are then: 120/20, 1000/20 and 10000/20. Table A.1 shows the values needed for the Schild plot.

Table A.1 Antagonist concentrations and concentration ratios (CR) for worked example.

Antagonist concentration [B] (nmol/l)	Log[B]	CR	CR – 1	Log(CR – 1)
10	1	6	5	0.699
100	2	50	49	1.69
1000	3	500	499	2.70

The values of log[B] and log(CR-1) are plotted in Figure A.2. The data provided yield points that lie on a straight line with a slope very close to 1. Such findings are in keeping with reversible competitive antagonism. Since the Schild plot has a slope of 1, the x-value at log(CR – 1) = 0 provides an estimate of Log K_B. In this example, K_B has a value of about 2 nmol/l (antilog of 0.3).

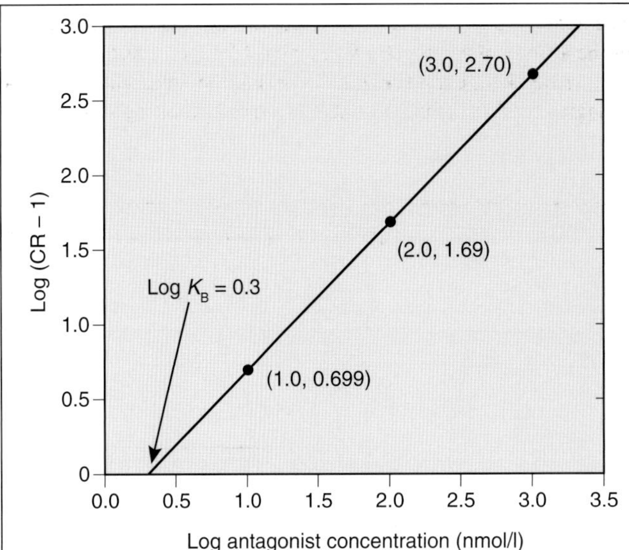

Fig. A.2 Schild plot of the data in Table A.1. The straight line and slope of 1 is indicative of reversible, competitive antagonism. The x-intercept then gives an estimate of log K_B.

pA_2

The term pA_2 is much used to describe the activity of a receptor antagonist. It was introduced by H O Schild, and is simply the negative logarithm of the antagonist concentration which produces a concentration ratio of 2. It is thus given by the intercept of the Schild plot on the x-axis (when log (CR-1) = log1 = 0). It is possible to determine a pA_2 value for a Schild plot which is neither linear nor has a slope of 1. In these circumstances reversible competitive antagonism has not been demonstrated and it is inappropriate to take the x-intercept as a measure of log K_B for the antagonist. (Regrettably many studies do erroneously equate pA_2 (an empirical measure) with –log K_B.)

Index

Note: Page numbers followed by *f* and *t* refer to figures and tables respectively

A

B

C

D

E

M

N

O

P